Dr. Patrick Walsh's
GUIDE TO
SURVIVING
PROSTATE CANCER

Dr. Patrick Walsh's
GUIDE TO
SURVIVING
PROSTATE CANCER

Patrick C. Walsh, M.D.
and Janet Farrar Worthington

WARNER BOOKS

A Time Warner Company

The information herein is not intended to replace the services of trained health professionals. You are advised to consult with your health care professional with regard to matters relating to your health, and in particular regarding matters that may require diagnosis or medical attention.

Warner Books, Inc., 1271 Avenue of the Americas, New York, NY 10020

Visit our Web site at www.twbookmark.com.

 A Time Warner Company

Printed in the United States of America

First Printing: August 2001
10   9   8   7   6   5   4   3   2

Library of Congress Cataloging-in-Publication Data

Walsh, Patrick C.
    Dr. Patrick Walsh's guide to surviving prostate cancer / Patrick C. Walsh and Janet
Farrar Worthington.
        p.   cm.
    Includes index.
    ISBN 0-446-52640-1
    1. Prostate—Cancer—Popular works.   I. Title: Doctor Patrick Walsh's guide to surviving
prostate cancer.   II. Worthington, Janet Farrar.   III. Title.

RC280.P7 W365   2001
616.99'463—dc21

                                                                    2001026260

Text design by Stanley S. Drate/Folio Graphics Co. Inc.

To all the patients, past and present, who inspired us to write this book, with deep gratitude for the lessons they have taught us—which we now share with others.

Acknowledgments

This book would not have been possible without the work and experience of many people, too many to name here. We tried, but the result looked like a telephone book—and had about as much personal meaning. So instead of listing all, and inevitably missing one or two, of the sources upon which we've drawn to produce this guide, we would simply like to thank those colleagues, patients, friends, and family members who have helped us the very most, including:

Donald S. Coffey, Ph.D., H. Ballentine Carter, M.D., Jonathan I. Epstein, M.D., Mario Eisenberger, M.D., Michael A. Carducci, M.D., Theodore L. DeWeese, M.D., Alan W. Partin, M.D., William B. Isaacs, Ph.D., John T. Isaacs, Ph.D., William G. Nelson, M.D., Ph.D., Ronald Rodriguez, Ph.D., M.D., Angelo M. De Marzo, M.D., Ph.D., Arthur L. Burnett, M.D., Daniel W. Chan, Ph.D., Jonathan P. Jarow, M.D., Joel Nelson, M.D., Jeffrey A. Cadeddu, M.D., Penny Marschke, R.N., Ph.D., Misop Han, M.D., Charles R. Pound, M.D., Terry E. Smith, Alice B. Baldwin, and Richard Howe.

We also acknowledge with deep gratitude the valuable contributions of these people: Peg Walsh, Mark Worthington, M.D., Barbara Downs, Ronald Farrar, Gayla Farrar, Bradley Farrar, Carole Farrar, Sally Worthington, Scott Worthington, Patty Worthington, Blair Worthington, Andy Worthington, Elizabeth Bibb, the Rev. John Brenneke, and Mount Moriah United Methodist Church in White Hall, Virginia.

We would like to thank the late Leon Schlossberg, for his original illustrations; David Rini, for his superb ability to tell a story with pictures; and Channa Taub, our literary agent, John Aherne, our editor, and Fred Chase and Bob Castillo, our copyeditors, for their unflagging patience and support.

And finally, we would like to honor Tom Worthington, who did not die in vain.

Contents

Preface

I hate prostate cancer. It's a devious adversary that can be mild-mannered in some men, percolating harmlessly for years or even decades, and vicious in others, steamrolling its way through the body, eroding bone, causing intolerable pain, and sucking away life at breathtaking speed. In 2001, an estimated 31,500 American men will die of prostate cancer. That's about one death, one family's heartbreak, every sixteen minutes. And nearly 200,000 will go to their doctor—maybe because they have such symptoms as urinary problems or unexplained back pain, or maybe just for a routine checkup—and get the bombshell that they, too, have been drafted into the "reluctant brotherhood" of men with prostate cancer.

Prostate cancer invaded my life in 1991, when I watched it attack my father-in-law, Tom Worthington, with a vengeance. His death was horrible: Within a year of his initial diagnosis, after fleeting success with hormonal therapy, his tumor spread like wildfire. He died in a nursing home, castrated, hooked up to a catheter, in agonizing pain, pitifully thin, his bones so riddled with cancer that his arm snapped in two when a nurse tried to move him. He was only fifty-three.

Until Tom got sick, I thought prostate cancer was an old man's disease. This was pre-Giuliani, pre-Schwarzkopf, pre-Dole, pre-Savalas, pre-Goulet, pre-Bixby, pre-Milken. Of course I was wrong. Then, as now, younger men had prostate cancer; they just didn't talk about it. Compared to today, most people knew little about it.

Needing to understand prostate cancer was my main reason for writing on the disease for *Hopkins Medical News* magazine, of which I was editor, in 1992. The heart of that article was Patrick C. Walsh, M.D., director of the Brady Urological Institute at Johns Hopkins and one of the most respected prostate disease specialists in the world. Walsh is the inventor of the revolutionary, now standard, operation called the anatomic radical retropubic prostatectomy, in which the prostate is removed but potency and continence are preserved. Today, most of the world—except Walsh himself—refers to that operation as the "Walsh procedure." Walsh's results, with the operation he devised, are the best of any surgeon in the world: One study recently found that, eighteen months after surgery, 93 percent of his patients have total urinary continence, and 86 percent were potent. His success is due to two main factors: One, he developed the operation only after years of intense, meticulous study of the anatomy of the prostate and male urinary and reproductive systems; if he were an athlete, he might be described as building on a bedrock knowledge of the "fundamentals." Two, he is a consummate perfectionist, always working to improve his technique and the operation itself. For example, he spent his free time during one recent summer watching hundreds of hours of videotape—of his hands performing the radical prostatectomy in dozens of patients. Why? He wanted to see whether some slight modifications in his technique could improve his patients' recovery of sexual function. I'm making a point of mentioning his excellence as a surgeon because—if it turns out that you require surgery to treat cancer of the prostate—it is essential that you, or your loved one, find the best surgeon you can. (This is discussed in Chapter 8.) There are many excellent surgeons out there. Unfortunately, there are also many surgeons who lack the expertise to perform the radical prostatectomy correctly; for some of them, it seems, continence and potency are happy by-products—but not expected outcomes—of surgery. (One respected surgeon, in fact, routinely implants a penile prosthesis at the time of surgery; he simply assumes that potency is not an option. Other surgeons routinely treat their patients' postoperative incontinence with one unsuccessful collagen injection after another—not knowing, apparently, when to seek a more durable solution.)

But surgery is only part of the complicated disease that is prostate cancer. And thus, although Walsh is most famous as a surgeon, he is also a global thinker whose determination to conquer this disease reaches far beyond the operating room. Building on a legacy of groundbreaking work at Hopkins, he has put together a world-class team of oncologists, molecular biologists, urologists, and geneticists who are tackling this disease from every angle.

When that article first appeared, Walsh's office was deluged with requests for reprints. To both of us, it was a clear reflection of the great and continuing hunger for information about this disease by people all over the country. So he and I decided to write a book together. That volume, *The Prostate: A Guide for Men and the Women Who Love Them*, was a best-seller in this country, and was translated into five languages. We wrote the book—and this one—for men *and* women. That's because, frankly, Tom Worthington probably wouldn't have bought this book for himself. Like most men—including my husband, father, and brother—he never wanted to dwell too closely on his health. This "guy philosophy" is simple: Ignore the subject, and it will go away. Chest pain? Probably indigestion. Back pain? Bursitis. Just the thought of a digital rectal examination makes these strong men cringe. Thus, it's often left to the women who love them—wives, girlfriends, sisters, daughters—to get these men to go see the doctor. Most men, Pat Walsh told me years ago, don't even know that they have a prostate until there is a problem. Thank goodness, that sad fact has changed somewhat over the last several years, as more men are getting the message that—just as their wives and sisters need regular Pap smears and breast exams—they, too, need a yearly physical, with a digital rectal exam (in which the prostate can be felt) and PSA blood test, which measures levels of prostate-specific antigen, an enzyme made by the prostate. Over the last several years, Pat Walsh and I have felt like missionaries preaching this gospel—or, if you will, like Paul Revere, trumpeting this message of hope: *Prostate cancer doesn't have to be fatal. If it's caught early enough, it is completely curable.*

A Word on This Book

So much has changed since Tom's death, even in the few years since our book was published! So much, in fact, that we felt that we should dedicate an entire book just to prostate cancer and the new advances in treatment and understanding of the disease (although other disorders of the prostate—BPH and prostatitis—are covered in Chapter 2). Now, for the first time ever, hope glimmers for the many men diagnosed too late for curative treatment—surgery or radiation therapy. Scientists are getting tantalizingly close to cracking prostate cancer, unscrambling its secret codes, devising ingenious ways to change and even fool cancer cells. We have done our best to put all of this—to include, in fact, everything that is known about prostate cancer—in this book.

"Read This First": For a small gland—the prostate is about the size

and shape of a walnut—the prostate is amazingly troublesome and complicated; its treatments are often just as intricate and difficult to understand. That's why we've started every chapter with a brief overview, called "Read This First." You may find these helpful, to cover the basic points, and then to fill in the details by reading the rest of each chapter.

What's new: The newest, most promising treatment strategies for advanced cancer are discussed in Chapter 12. In just the last few years, scientists have found genetic proof that prostate cancer can be inherited. Although only a small percentage of cases of prostate cancer are believed to be purely hereditary, many investigators believe that the defective gene or mechanisms involved are the same ones that somehow go askew in "sporadic" cancer—disease that develops over the course of a lifetime— the kind most men get. The information in Chapter 3 is particularly important for men—especially African-Americans—at high risk of developing prostate cancer. There is important new information that diet can delay or even prevent the onset of prostate cancer (see Chapter 4). Even men with established prostate cancer can benefit from certain easy dietary changes (see Chapter 12).

As before, we have written this book with the idea that patients and their families must be their own advocates. Once again, we have taken a journalistic approach: Although Pat Walsh is a top authority on prostate disease, we have also sought out experts in all important areas—radiation oncologists, medical oncologists, pathologists, nutritionists, specialists in pain management, and basic scientists. In an era of uneven medical care and an overwhelming abundance of information—unfortunately, much of it bad—on prostate cancer, we have done our best to provide the most helpful, detailed, state-of-the-art picture of the disease possible. There are tables and charts to help you understand your specific situation—whether or not you have cancer that needs to be treated, the odds that your cancer has spread, and your best options for treatment. We explain the results of relevant tests, tell you which tests and procedures are a waste of time and money, and talk a little about complimentary medicine, including prayer. We also tell you exactly what medications and symptoms to ask your doctor about, so you can help yourself or a loved one get relief from disabling pain. The book ends with some information on how to learn more, and where to get help.

Once Again, Too Close to Home

Our message has indeed saved lives. This I found out firsthand, as once again, prostate cancer hit too close to home.

"So, Dad," I said in 1992 as we were writing the first book, "you should get a physical and have a rectal exam." When my father stopped laughing, I continued: "And get this thing called a PSA blood test." And, because I knew he would not do these things, I added: "Mom, make him do it." She worked on him, and so did I, until finally he went to the doctor. He hated it, but he went. (Never underestimate the power of nagging and guilt.) He not only insisted on having the PSA test—which one doctor told him he didn't even need—but on knowing the result. That year, his PSA was 1.2, and there it stayed. In 1996, it was 1.3—still very low, still probably nothing. (PSA levels lower than 4 are generally considered in the "normal" range, and PSA is most useful as a diagnostic tool when doctors can monitor its rate of change over time. This is why it's so important for men over fifty to have both the yearly rectal exam and the PSA test. Men at higher risk—African-Americans and those with a family history of prostate cancer—should begin sooner, at age forty.) But Dad's internist felt a "rough spot" on his prostate during the rectal exam. He referred him to a urologist, who felt it, too. A transrectal ultrasound found prostatic calculi—little stones; many men have them. "What the heck," the urologist said, "let's do a biopsy, since we're here anyway."

I was playing Candyland with my little girl when the phone rang. It was my mom. In a small voice, she said: "Guess what?"

Cancer. Palpable cancer, moderately well differentiated. Pathologists use a classification system called the Gleason score, based on how cells look under the microscope, to rank cell differentiation. Basically, a low Gleason score—2, 3, 4—is good; these cells are the least aggressive, least likely to wander outside the prostate. A high score—8, 9, 10—is not. Scores in the middle are hard to predict. Dad's turned out to be Gleason 7, terrifyingly close to the kind of cancer cell that shows up in metastatic disease.

I called Pat Walsh about thirty seconds later. Then, in a totally surreal experience, I spent New Year's Day 1998 underlining key passages in my own book for my mother to read. The day before Valentine's Day, Walsh, my co-author and friend, in the operation he invented, took a scalpel and made an incision through skin and muscle in my sixty-one-year-old father's abdomen, extending from the pubic area to the navel. The knife cut through precarious terrain. The prostate nestles deep in the pelvis, surrounded by structures that are fragile and vulnerable to injury: the rectum, bladder, sphincter responsible for urinary control, some large blood vessels, and the bundles of nerves (discovered by Walsh and Dutch urologist Pieter Donker) that are responsible for erection.

As it turns out, my father's cancer had reached the wall of the prostate but, mercifully, had not yet moved beyond it. Walsh believes he got it all; the operation was in time. After the surgery Johns Hopkins pathologist Jonathan Epstein, M.D., who has probably looked at more radical prostatectomy specimens than anyone in the world and is an expert in interpreting how prostate cancer cells look (see Chapter 6), answered our prayers with this report: "Negative surgical margins. Negative seminal vesicles. Negative lymph nodes."

In May, we fidgeted for two days after Dad's first post-prostatectomy PSA blood test, waiting for this word: "Undetectable." The most beautiful word I ever heard. His PSA remains undetectable today.

My father's case is the best example I know of an ideal scenario: prostate cancer detected early, treated, and cured. But between my father-in-law's death and my dad's diagnosis, my husband's maternal grandfather died of complications from radiation therapy for—you guessed it—prostate cancer, at age eighty-five. My maternal grandfather died at eighty-four of a heart attack, perhaps caused by the heavy-handed regimen of hormone therapy (five times the dose Walsh recommends) he was taking for prostate cancer. That brings the tally in my husband's and my combined families to two grandfathers and two fathers. Three deaths, one save.

My husband, Mark, is the next one I'm worried about, and both our brothers. But I'm hoping that one day my four-year-old son won't have to worry about prostate cancer, and I won't have to dread it for him. Eight years of collaboration with Pat Walsh and the star team of scientists who surround him give me faith that by the time my little boy reaches his middle years, most cases of prostate cancer will no longer prove fatal. Or better still, they will be preventable.

—*Janet Farrar Worthington*

Dr. Patrick Walsh's
GUIDE TO
SURVIVING
PROSTATE CANCER

1

WHAT THE PROSTATE DOES:
A Brief Anatomy Lecture

Read This First

There's a "Read This First" in every chapter of this book. This is because prostate cancer—the last thing most men would ever choose to think about—is not just a scary subject to deal with, it's tough to understand. The disease itself is complicated, and the decisions about what to do next can be agonizing. Before you can chart your next course, you've got to sort through, and attempt to make sense of, many things.

If this were a potboiler novel, the kind of page-turner you start on page one and don't put down until you've savored the last word on the last page, you wouldn't need any guidance on how to read it; you'd just get going. If, on the other hand, this were an academic textbook, you might approach it with a highlighter in hand, emphasizing key points and "take-home messages" in bright yellow marker. This book falls somewhere in between, and people read it in different ways. They kick the tires, in effect—flip through the pages; maybe they head directly to a specific section, such as impotence, or biopsy, then backtrack and read about how prostate cancer gets started, or jump ahead to chapters on treatment.

With this in mind, in every chapter we've done our best to give you the highlights—what you really need to know—up front. Consider this your briefing. All of these overviews will familiarize you with the main ideas you'll be covering on the next pages.

That said, this is what you need to know about the anatomy of the prostate:

What is the prostate? The prostate is a small, and probably expendable, organ. Men can live quite comfortably without it. The prostate's biggest job, as far as we know, is to provide part of the fluid that makes up semen. But even this contribution does not appear to be crucial for reproduction—which is why some scientists think the prostate's main role may be to safeguard the reproductive tract from infection in the urinary tract. (In fact, its name in Greek means "protector.") It is not a vital organ. Thus, the major importance of the prostate is not what it does, but what goes wrong with it—the problems it causes to nearly all men who live long enough. These are:

- Cancer of the prostate, the most common cancer in men;
- BPH (benign prostatic hyperplasia, also called "enlargement of the prostate"), one of the most common benign tumors in men and a major source of misery as men get older; and
- Prostatitis, the most common cause of urinary tract infection in men.

If it's not a vital organ, why is it important? Although it's only as big as a walnut, the prostate is a miniature Grand Central Station, a busy hub at the crossroads of a man's urinary and reproductive tracts. It has a highly strategic location, right at the outlet to the bladder. Urine and semen cannot leave the body without passing through the prostate. It is also tucked away, deep within the pelvis, surrounded by vulnerable structures—the bladder, the rectum, the sphincters responsible for urinary control, major arteries and veins, and a host of delicate nerves, some of them so tiny that we've only recently discovered them. This is why *any* form of treatment for prostate cancer can produce side effects including incontinence, impotence, and rectal bleeding.

What else about prostate anatomy do I need to know? The prostate is like a complicated sponge, with five distinct parts, called "zones." The two most important here are the *peripheral zone*, which is located next to the rectum, contains most of the glands in the prostate, and is the main site where cancer develops; and the *transition zone*, which surrounds the urethra, and is the principal site where BPH begins. The prostate's growth and function are stimulated by hormones: Testosterone, produced in the testicles, is converted to another hormone, called dihydrotestosterone (DHT)—the most active male hormone—in the prostate.

The bottom line: In short, the prostate is a gland that does much more harm than good, located in a terrible area that complicates any attempt to treat it. Despite this, as you will learn in this book, there has never been more hope in the treatment of all prostate disorders— especially cancer.

The Prostate's Strategic Location

Welcome to Grand Central Station—the prostate, the bustling, walnut-sized hub at the crossroads of a man's urinary and reproductive tracts. What makes such a small, relatively obscure gland so important to men? The answer is not immediately obvious: The prostate is not, for example, a vital organ like the heart. Its biggest job, as far as we know, is to provide about one third of the fluid that makes up semen. But even this contribution does not appear to be crucial for reproduction— leading some scientists to theorize that the prostate's main purpose actually may be to safeguard the reproductive tract from infection in the urinary tract. (In fact, its name in Greek means "stands before," or "protector.") The prostate has few other redeeming features, isn't necessary for life or even for sexual function, and is known primarily for the clinical problems it causes to nearly all men who live long enough.

What the prostate *does* have, however, is a highly strategic location, right at the outlet to the bladder. Urine cannot leave the body without passing through the prostate, via a tube called the urethra. (Think of the urethra as an expressway, and the prostate as the Lincoln Tunnel.)

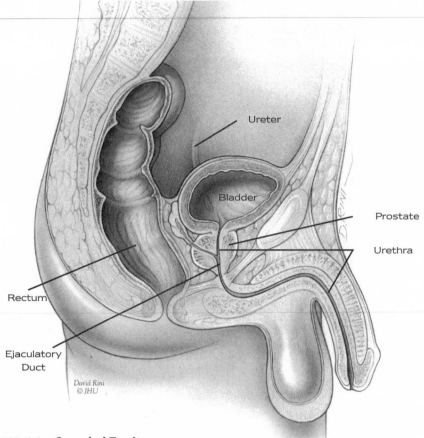

FIG. 1.1   Crowded Territory

There's the prostate, nestled deep within the male pelvis—at a highly strategic location, right at the outlet to the bladder. The prostate is surrounded by vulnerable structures—the bladder, the rectum, the sphincters responsible for urinary control, major arteries and veins, and a host of delicate nerves.

Nothing about the prostate is easy. From a urologist's standpoint, even a routine checkup—to feel for lumps or hardness in a digital rectal examination—is more complicated and takes more skill than many of our patients realize. (For a detailed discussion of diagnosing prostate problems, see Chapter 6.) The prostate is as tucked away—and as surrounded by booby traps—as any of the prizes sought by Indiana Jones in *Raiders of the Lost Ark*. It lies in the midst of vulnerable structures—the bladder, the rectum, the sphincters responsible for urinary control, major arteries and veins, and a host of delicate nerves, some of them so tiny that we've only recently discovered

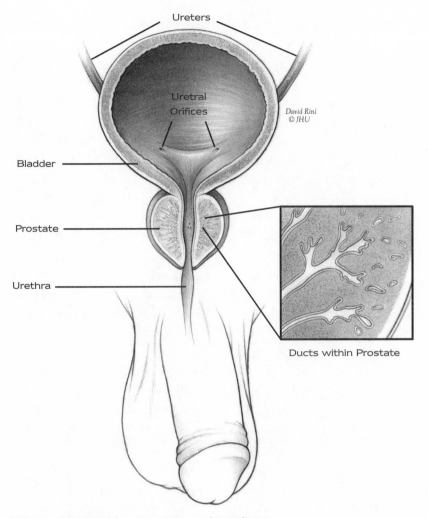

Ureters

Uretral
Orifices

David Rini
© JHU

Bladder

Prostate

Urethra

Ducts within Prostate

FIG. 1.2   The Bladder, Prostate, and Urethra

Urine flows from the bladder via a tube called the urethra—but it can't leave the body without passing through the prostate. Think of the urethra as an expressway, and the prostate as the Lincoln Tunnel. *Inset:* Like a sponge, the prostate is made up of tiny glands. These drain into ducts that, in turn, transport secretions to the urethra.

them—that can foil any physician who ventures into the area without exquisitely precise knowledge of the terrain. This is why *any* procedure to treat prostate cancer—surgery, external-beam radiation therapy or implantation of radiation "seeds," or attempts to kill cancer cells by cooling or heating the prostate—can produce side effects including incontinence, impotence, and rectal bleeding.

The prostate fits snugly within the pelvis; there isn't much "breathing room" here. Unfortunately, not only is the prostate packed tightly amid other structures, like pieces of a jigsaw puzzle, it is poorly insulated. The flimsy wall of tissue separating the prostate and the seminal vesicles is thinner than a piece of tissue paper—not much of a "buffer zone" for cancer. Consequently, once cancer reaches a critical size, it can easily penetrate the wall (also called the capsule) of the prostate, and escape into this overcrowded region of the body, spreading to the nearby seminal vesicles or lymph nodes, or even further, into the bloodstream.

This is why—even though treatment for prostate cancer is improving dramatically—a man's best protection against this disease is to have it detected as quickly as possible. For the American man at average risk of prostate cancer, this means, after age fifty, a yearly prostate checkup (a physical and digital rectal examination—see Chapter 5), and a blood test for PSA, prostate-specific antigen (also see Chapter 5). Men at higher risk—African-Americans, and men with a family history of prostate cancer—need to start screening for prostate cancer much sooner, at age forty.

In short, the prostate is a gland that does much more harm than good, located in a terrible area that complicates any attempt to treat it. Despite this, there has never been more hope in our field. At last, we are finding answers to the toughest questions of prostate cancer: Where exactly does it begin, and why? How does it spread? If we can't cure it, can we *contain* it—can we make advanced prostate cancer a *chronic* illness, like diabetes, instead of a fatal one? Can we change our thinking, and try drugs that were once considered "last-ditch" measures *sooner*—can we create adjuvant therapy? Can we actually prevent cancer, or somehow slow its progress with diet? If PSA comes back after surgery or radiation, what does it mean—and how much time do we have to find a more effective treatment? As for radical prostatectomy itself, can we make the operation even better, with fewer side effects and quicker recovery of potency and continence? How can we help men and their families get their lives back? How can we improve quality of life? All of these areas will be covered in detail in later chapters.

A Brief Anatomy Lesson

Although we've tried to keep it brief, this crash course in anatomy may still be more than you ever wanted to know about the prostate and anything even remotely linked to it. But we believe it's essential that you understand where the prostate is and what it does, the two main systems it influences—the reproductive and urinary tracts—and how they can be affected when something goes wrong.

The reproductive tract: For the reproductive organs, the basic act of sexual intercourse is as highly choreographed and synchronized as a NASA shuttle launch. First, the climate must be just right—in this case, the "weather" is a chain of coded chemical messages and hormonal signals. The equipment must be working properly, too. The main vessel, of course, is the penis, a remarkable construction that relies on hydraulic principles for erection, requires a delicate balance between arteries and veins, and is orchestrated by many intricate nerves. Orgasm, the climax of sexual intercourse, involves instantaneous, nearly simultaneous firings of fluid from the prostate, seminal vesicles, and testes (which make sperm). Because the prostate is the focus of this book, we'll begin there, although as you will see, sexual potency and intercourse really begin in the brain.

The prostate: The prostate is a complicated, powerful little factory. Its main products, manufactured in numerous tiny glands and ducts, are secretions—components of semen. During orgasm, muscles in the prostate drive these secretions into the urethra (where it is joined by sperm and fluid from the seminal vesicles), which pumps it out the penis. The prostate's fluid is clear and mildly acidic, and contains many ingredients, most of them designed to sustain sperm outside the body for as long as possible. (These include citric acid, acid phosphatase, spermine, potassium, calcium, and zinc.) Some prostatic secretions also protect the urinary tract and reproductive system from harmful bacteria that may enter the urethra. Here, the prostate truly lives up to its Greek name of "protector": Infections in this area can cause scar tissue to form in the ducts that drain the testicles, leading to infertility. If these infections were common, they would pose a serious threat to procreation—and this may be the major reason why all mammals have a prostate.

After ejaculation, the seminal fluid immediately coagulates—a key part of nature's "safety net" to maximize the odds of reproduction: If semen remained watery, it could not linger in the vagina. (In rats and other rodents, semen actually forms a pelletlike plug, which effectively blocks other rats from depositing their semen in the same female.) The semen is gradually broken down again by an important enzyme made by the prostate—*prostate-specific antigen (PSA).* PSA's other great value is that it can be detected in a simple blood test. In recent years, this PSA test has become a crucial addition to medicine's arsenal for detecting prostate cancer and monitoring the success of treatment. (For more on what PSA can do, see Chapter 5.)

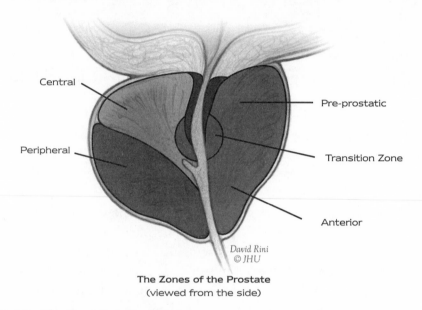

David Rini
© JHU

The Zones of the Prostate
(viewed from the side)

FIG. 1.3   The Prostate's Five Zones

The prostate is divided into five zones: *Anterior,* which is mainly smooth muscle tissue; *peripheral,* which contains three fourths of the glands in the prostate; *central,* which holds most of the remaining glands; *pre-prostatic* tissue, which plays a key role during ejaculation—muscles here prevent semen from flowing backward, into the bladder; and *transition,* which surrounds the urethra and is the epicenter of trouble in benign prostatic hyperplasia (BPH). *Most prostate cancer occurs in the peripheral zone.* Fortunately, this is the region most likely to be felt during a rectal examination and tapped in a needle biopsy of the prostate.

Like New York City, the prostate is divided into five zones: *Anterior,* which takes up one third of the space and consists mainly of smooth muscle; *peripheral,* the largest segment, which contains three fourths of the glands in the prostate; *central,* which holds most of the remaining glands; *pre-prostatic* tissue, which plays a key role during ejaculation—muscles here prevent semen from flowing backward, into the bladder;

and *transition*, which surrounds the urethra and is the epicenter of trouble in benign prostatic hyperplasia (BPH). For reasons not entirely understood, when a man reaches his mid-forties, the prostate tissue in the transition zone tends to enlarge, begins to push nearby tissue for room, and eventually starts to cramp the urethra. With this slow strangulation—think of a man's necktie slowly tightening around his collar—the prostate can make it exceedingly difficult for urine to get from the bladder through the prostate and out of the body. (For more on BPH, see Chapter 2.) *Most prostate cancer occurs in the peripheral zone.* Fortunately, this is the region most likely to be felt during a rectal examination and tapped in a needle biopsy of the prostate (see Chapter 6).

On a microscopic level, prostatic tissue is like a sponge, riddled with tiny glands. These are the micro-factories that produce the secretions, and they're connected by hundreds of ducts, which transport the fluid into the urethra. When these ducts become obstructed—as they do in BPH—PSA levels begin to rise in the bloodstream. Because prostate cancers don't make any ducts, glands in cancerous tissue become isolated. But these ducts still churn out fluid, which has nowhere to go— except into the bloodstream. That's why, gram for gram, prostate cancer contributes *ten times more* to blood PSA levels than BPH.

Prostate cells come in two basic models—*epithelial cells*, glandular cells that make the secretions, and *stromal cells*, muscular cells that hold the epithelial cells in place. The stromal cells aren't just passive scaffolding: They also help the prostate grow. From the stromal cells, in fact, spring many *growth factors*. And growth factors, we have learned, play a pivotal role in the development and function of the prostate when it is healthy, and when it is cancerous.

How do hormones affect the prostate? The prostate is very sensitive to hormones. In cancer treatment, this is a good thing: Cutting off the supply of these sex hormones, or androgens, can shrink prostate cancer and delay its progression. The hormones that control the prostate begin in the brain: The hypothalamus makes a substance called LHRH (luteinizing hormone-releasing hormone), which it transmits using a "chemical Morse code," or signal pulses, to the nearby pituitary gland. In response, the pituitary makes its own chemical signal, called LH (luteinizing hormone). LH, in turn, controls the testes, which make testosterone. Testosterone is the chief "male" hormone, the cause of—among other things—secondary sex

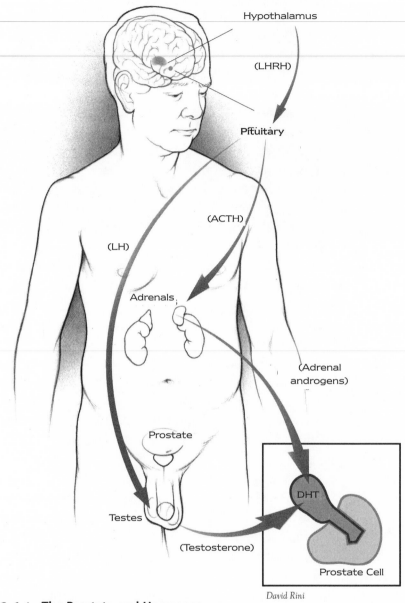

Hypothalamus

(LHRH)

Pituitary

(ACTH)

(LH)

Adrenals

(Adrenal androgens)

Prostate

DHT

Testes

(Testosterone)

Prostate Cell

David Rini

FIG. 1.4 The Prostate and Hormones

The hormones that control the prostate begin in the brain: The hypothalamus makes a substance called LHRH (luteinizing hormone-releasing hormone), which it transmits to the nearby pituitary gland. The pituitary then makes its own chemical signal, called LH (luteinizing hormone). LH, in turn, controls the testes, which make testosterone—the chief "male" hormone. Testosterone circulates in the bloodstream, and seeps into a prostate cell by diffusion—like water through a coffee filter. The prostate, using an enzyme called 5-alpha reductase, refines testosterone into another hormone called dihydrotestosterone (DHT). Soon, DHT joins up with a specific protein in the cell's nucleus, which acts like a key, switching on various genes within the prostate.

characteristics like body hair and deepening of the voice, and fertility. Testosterone circulates in the bloodstream, and seeps into a prostate cell by diffusion—like water through a coffee filter. To the prostate, testosterone is a raw material: The prostate, using an enzyme called 5-alpha reductase, refines testosterone into another hormone called dihydrotestosterone (DHT). Soon, DHT joins up with a specific protein in the cell's nucleus, and quickly becomes a powerhouse that switches on various genes within the prostate.

The prostate is not required for fertility or potency. Men and animals can remain fertile even if they have had their prostate—or their seminal vesicles, but not both organs—removed. This is surprising, considering that growth of the prostate clearly *is* linked to a man's sexual development: Starting at puberty, the prostate enlarges five times in size—from a weight of about 4 grams to 20 grams, the size of a walnut—by about age twenty. (For the rest of a man's life, the prostate continues to grow and become heavier, but much more slowly.)

The testes: The testes, or testicles, are a man's reproductive organs: They make the hormone testosterone, as discussed above. They also make sperm, in hundreds of tiny tubes and threadlike, winding tubules. (If these miniature pipes were straightened out, each would stretch to a length of two feet.) There are two testes, each less than two inches long and about an inch wide. The testes, attached to blood-supplying lifelines called spermatic cords, are covered by the scrotum. Have you ever wondered why the scrotum is suspended in such a vulnerable position, below the body? Wouldn't it make more sense—and provide better protection—if the testicles were inside the body? Yes and no. If the testes were tucked away inside the pelvis, they would indeed be better protected—but there wouldn't be much to protect. The testes are located in the scrotum for the simple but expedient reason that it's a more temperate climate down there, by a couple of degrees. Sperm are delicate; they fare poorly when the temperature is too warm. The scrotum, in effect, is nature's cooler. (In fact, men who have undescended testicles—which are located inside the abdomen—cannot develop sperm because the normal body temperature is just too hot.)

The epididymis: The sperm-making tubules in each testis converge to form the epididymis. Compared to the tubules, this is a river, as large and serpentine as the Amazon: Each tubule (one on each side), though only a millimeter wide, could be uncoiled to reach a remarkable length of fifteen to twenty feet. This is one continuous tube—thus, it's easy to see why an infection here could cause scar tissue and blockage that would result in infertility. These tubules are packed side by side, top to bottom, to form the epididymis, an elongated structure about the size of a woman's pinky finger. This is the greenhouse where sperm mature until orgasm, when they shoot from the tail of the epididymis during a series of powerful muscle contractions. The epididymis clings to one side of each testis before turning yet again and heading upward to meet still another tube, called the vas deferens.

The vas deferens: This impressive tube (again, one on each side; together they are called the vasa deferentia), now grown to 3 millimeters in diameter, is a hard, muscular cord, about 18 inches long. Its job is to pump sperm to the part of the urethra that lies within the prostate (the prostatic urethra). Because it is so thick, it can easily be palpated through the scrotum. (It can also be cut easily, in an outpatient procedure—a form of male birth control—called a vasectomy. When the cord is cut, sperm cannot exit the penis through ejaculation, and instead are reabsorbed by the body.) The vas deferens travels to a space between the bladder and rectum, then courses downward to the base of the prostate, where it meets with the duct of the seminal vesicle to form the ejaculatory duct.

The seminal vesicles: The lumpy seminal vesicles, each about 2 inches long, sit behind the bladder, next to the rectum, hanging over the prostate like twin bunches of grapes. Arching still higher over them, on either side, are the vasa deferentia, which meet the seminal vesicles at V-shaped angles; these form the ejaculatory ducts, slitlike openings that feed into the prostatic urethra. The seminal vesicles are made up of caves called alveoli, which make sticky secretions that help maintain semen's consistency. (The vesicles got their name because scientists used to believe they stored sperm; they don't.) Like the prostate, the seminal vesicles depend on hormones for their development and growth, and for the secretions they produce. However: Although the seminal vesicles are strikingly similar to the prostate in many ways, they're almost always free of abnormal growth—benign (as in BPH) as well as malignant. (This is covered in more detail in Chapter 3.)

Lately, scientists at Johns Hopkins have begun exploring the relationship between the prostate and seminal vesicles. What we have learned from their work is that the saga of human evolution is also a story of two male glands—both of which produce fluid that makes up semen. One gland, the prostate, is prone to cancer. The other, the seminal vesicle, is remarkably free of it. In nature, animals that are carnivores—meat-eaters like dogs and lions—don't have seminal vesicles. The only animals that have *both prostates and seminal vesicles* are herbivores—veggie-eating animals like bulls, apes, and elephants. There is only one exception to this rule: humans. Men have seminal vesicles, too. *In other words, man, a meat-lover, has the makeup of an animal that should be a vegetarian.* For more on this research, and what it means, see Chapter 3.

The penis: The penis—an engineering marvel built of nerves, smooth muscle, and blood vessels—has two main functions—sexual

---

SEMEN IS MOSTLY . . . NOT SPERM

Semen is the ejaculate, and it's made up of seminal fluid and sperm. (One third of the fluid originates from the prostate, two thirds from the seminal vesicles.) Sperm makes up just a tiny fraction of semen (which is why a vasectomy does not reduce the volume of the ejaculate). Semen is surprisingly rich. Its components, mainly secretions from the prostate and seminal vesicles, include prostaglandins, spermine, fructose, glucose, citric acid, zinc, proteins, and enzymes such as immunoglobulins, proteases, esterases, and phosphatase. These other ingredients probably serve as a buffer—to help sperm survive the trip and remain active—and, in the case of sugars such as fructose and glucose, as a snack "for the road," to provide energy for sperm's metabolism on its journey. Still other components—the zinc, for example, and proteases and immunoglobulins—may be cleansing agents, there to help fend off infections and other harmful substances in the urinary tract.

Semen undergoes extreme chemical transformations after ejaculation, metamorphosing from a viscous liquid to a semisolid and back again. A few minutes after ejaculation, semen coagulates into a gel-like substance; then, within about fifteen minutes, it becomes a sticky liquid. In most animals, a substance made by the seminal vesicles is the cause of the coagulation; then PSA, an enzyme made by the prostate (see above), makes semen runny again. The character of semen varies greatly among species. For example, in bulls and dogs (which don't have seminal vesicles), semen does not coagulate at all. But in rats and rabbits, semen quickly coagulates to form a pellet; for these animals, a PSA-like enzyme is crucial in helping the sperm reach their destination. Because semen is a bodily fluid, like blood, it is affected by drugs, and can be a carrier of sexually transmitted diseases such as AIDS.

intercourse and urination. (Note: There is no bone in the human penis, although this is not the case in dogs and some other animals.) The penis works like a water balloon. Its basic structure is that of a rounded triangle; all three corners have cylinders of tissue (called the *corpora cavernosa* and the *corpus spongiosum*) that fill and become engorged with blood. In erection, as arteries pump a steady supply of blood into the penis, the veins (which normally pump it back out again) clamp down—so the blood can't recirculate, thus keeping the penis "inflated" during sexual activity. All of this is made possible by the delicate nerves that lead to and from the penis. For years, these tiny nerves were poorly understood. The sad result was that removal of the prostate almost always meant impotence. (See Chapter 8.) That is no longer the case.

How the Urinary Tract Works

The kidneys are the body's main filters. With each heartbeat, they cleanse the blood of toxic wastes, excess water and salts, and (among many other chores) help maintain the body's balance of fluids and minerals. With more than a million tiny, wadded-up filters called nephrons, the kidneys sift through an incredible volume of fluid— about 45 gallons a day for a 150-pound man. (See Fig. 1.5.) Every sip of water we drink is refined, reabsorbed, and then processed again. (If the water and minerals weren't reabsorbed, our bodies would become seriously dehydrated within hours.) Not all of this material returns to the body, however; much of it passes out as urine. Every day, the average man excretes about two quarts of urine (a concentrated mixture of water, sodium, chloride, bicarbonate, potassium, and urea, the breakdown product of proteins).

Urine exits each kidney through a pipeline called the *ureter*. The ureters work like toothpaste tubes, squeezing or "milking" urine from the kidneys. Each ureter is about a foot long, and narrow—less than a half-inch wide at its broadest point. Ureters are one-way streets: Urine always flows the same way through them—straight toward the bladder.

The *bladder* is a big bag. Stretched to its fullest, this muscular tank can hold about a pint of urine. (See Fig. 1.2.) Unlike the kidneys and ureters, the bladder—in normal circumstances—allows us some voluntary control; it generally obeys our decision to eliminate or hold urine. (The inability to control urination is called incontinence.) With intricately woven layers of muscle and connective tissue, the

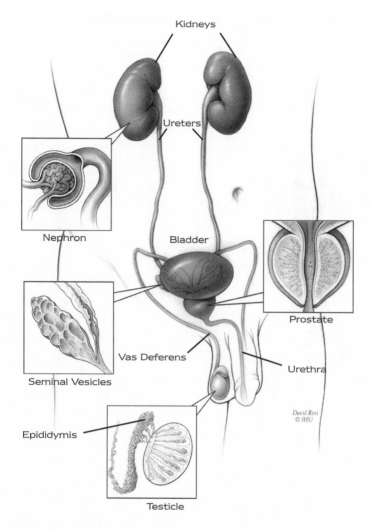

Kidneys

Ureters

Nephron

Bladder

Prostate

Seminal Vesicles

Vas Deferens

Urethra

Epididymis

David Rini
© JHU

Testicle

FIG. 1.5 How Urine Exits the Body

From the top: The kidneys are the body's main filters. With more than a million tiny, wadded-up filters called nephrons, the kidneys sift through an incredible volume of fluid—about 45 gallons a day for a 150-pound man. Every day, the average man excretes about two quarts of urine. Urine exits the kidneys through ureters, pipelines that work like toothpaste tubes, squeezing urine downward toward the bladder. The bladder is a big bag. Stretched to its fullest, this muscular tank can hold about a pint of urine. Unlike the kidneys and ureters, the bladder—in normal circumstances—allows us some voluntary control; it generally obeys our decision to eliminate or hold urine. The next stop is the urethra, another muscular tube, which begins at the neck of the bladder, then tunnels through the prostate and continues into the penis.

Also seen here are the seminal vesicles, made up of caves called alveoli, which make sticky secretions that help maintain semen's consistency, and the testes. The testes are a man's reproductive organs: They make the hormone testosterone; they also make sperm, in hundreds of tiny tubes.

bladder can collapse or expand, depending on the amount of fluid it's asked to hold at a given time. A sophisticated backup system protects the bladder from extreme distention and the risk of rupture: When the bladder is very full, it signals the kidneys to slow down the production of urine. At the neck of the bladder is a gate called the trigone. The purpose of the trigone is to make sure urine flows only one way—downward, away from the ureters and kidneys. The trigone's valve makes a tight seal that prevents urine from backing up into the kidneys, even when the bladder is distended.

The next stop of urine's downward passage is the *urethra,* another muscular tube, about 8 inches long. This one begins at the neck of the bladder, then tunnels through the prostate at a 35-degree angle and continues into the penis. The urethra is divided into three segments—*prostatic* (the part that runs through the prostate), *membranous* (in between the prostate and penis—this is where the external sphincter is located), and *penile.* Like the prostate, it plays a role in both the urinary and reproductive systems; it serves as a conduit not only for urine, but for sexual fluids. The prostatic urethra has its own gate to prevent fluid backup—a ring of smooth muscle that works with the bladder neck as a clamp during ejaculation. This keeps semen from flowing the wrong way—up into the bladder—and directs its course downward, out the urethra.

That's it for the anatomy crash course. Over the course of this book, as we describe diagnostic procedures, treatments, and complications, you may need to return to this chapter. That's what it's for—to give you a working familiarity with the territory we'll be covering in the next chapters. If it helps, think of these pages as your *Michelin Guide* to male anatomy. Now that we've discussed the context of the prostate—as a significant gland in both the urinary and reproductive systems—it's time to explain why this tiny gland is so important, and what can go wrong.

2

LITTLE GLAND, BIG TROUBLE

Read This First

At some point in their lives, most men are going to have to come to terms with the prostate, because this little gland is the source of *three of the major, common health problems that affect men*:

- Prostate cancer, the most common cancer in men;
- BPH (benign prostatic hyperplasia, also known as "enlargement of the prostate"), one of the most common benign tumors in men; and
- Prostatitis, a painful inflammation of the prostate, and the most common cause of urinary tract infection in men.

This news usually comes as an unpleasant shock, because most men don't even know that they *have* a prostate until something goes wrong. Worse, because there is no "statute of limitations" on prostate problems, some men are unlucky enough to endure more than one of these disorders. (In fact, some men find out they have prostate cancer during a routine procedure to treat BPH.) You may suddenly experience a bout of prostatitis, or develop urinary problems because of prostate enlargement. Or your "wake-up call" to the prostate may be an abnormal PSA blood test, or a suspicious lump felt during a rectal exam, raising the possibility that you have prostate cancer. Thus, even though this book is about prostate cancer, it's important for you to understand all of the "Big Three" prostate disorders:

Here's what you need to know:

Prostate cancer: This is the most common cancer in men, and, after lung cancer, the leading cause of cancer death in men. Because prostate cancer is the subject of this entire book, the only important point you need to know now is that *when prostate cancer is small, it is curable.* However, because is it "silent," and produces no early-warning symptoms, routine testing is very important. How can we save lives from prostate cancer? The rest of this book is devoted to answering this question. The key is a four-pronged approach—prevention, early diagnosis, better treatment for localized disease (cancer confined to the prostate) with fewer side effects, and better control of advanced disease.

BPH, or enlargement of the prostate: BPH is so common that most men, if they live long enough, will develop it. By age seventy, 70 percent of men have it, and one quarter of men with the disease require treatment. *BPH is not prostate cancer, and having it does not mean that a man is more likely or less likely to get prostate cancer.* BPH and prostate cancer are two different diseases, which develop in different regions of the prostate—almost as if the prostate were two glands rolled into one. Prostate cancer begins in the outer, *peripheral zone* of the prostate, and grows outward, invading surrounding tissues (that's why it rarely produces symptoms until it is far advanced). On the other hand, BPH begins in a tiny area of the inner prostate called the *transition zone,* a ring of tissue that makes a natural circle around the urethra, the tube through which urine and semen exit the body. In BPH, the growth is inward, toward the prostate's core, constantly tightening around the urethra and interfering with urination (which is why symptoms are almost impossible to ignore). BPH is a very common condition that affects most men. It is not cancerous, but it can mimic cancer. Today, there are many good ways to treat it, and most of them have few side effects.

Prostatitis: Prostatitis is the most common cause of urinary tract infection in men, and an estimated 25 percent of all men who see a doctor for urological problems have symptoms of prostatitis. There are five conditions lumped under the umbrella name prostatitis. The two least common, and easiest to treat, are caused by bacterial infection: *acute and chronic bacterial prostatitis.* These conditions are usually associated with fever, chills, severe burning on urination, frequency of urination, and, in some cases, a life-threatening infection in the bloodstream. Next, two forms of prostatitis fall into a category called *chronic prostatitis/chronic pelvic pain syndrome.* Nobody knows what causes these forms of prostatitis, and antibiotics do not help at all. The treatment here is largely aimed at relieving symptoms, with muscle relaxants such as alpha-blockers and other drugs, which ease muscle tension in the prostate and make urination easier. The final, mysterious category is *asymptomatic inflammatory prostatitis,* which produces no symptoms, and is usually found by chance, when inflammatory cells are found in the prostatic fluid, or inflammation is detected on a prostate biopsy.

The most important thing about prostatitis is that it is not cancer, and doesn't lead to cancer. The treatment for most prostatitis (except the bacterial kind, which responds to antibiotics) is often trial and error, and it helps if men and their doctors can work together—with much patience—to come up with the right plan. There is, however, some exciting new research that may help us find new ways to manage prostatitis. Many men have found that their symptoms improve when they change their diet and their lifestyle.

What Can Go Wrong with the Prostate:
Cancer, BPH, and Prostatitis

For most young men, the prostate falls in the category of obscure body parts that includes the spleen—that is, it's in there someplace, it probably does something useful, but it's best dealt with on a "need to know" basis.

Unfortunately, most men *are* going to need to know about the prostate sometime, because this little gland is the source of three of the major health problems that affect men: *prostate cancer,* the most common major cancer in men; *benign enlargement of the prostate* (BPH, for benign prostatic hyperplasia), one of the most common benign tumors in men and a source of symptoms for most men as they age; and *prostatitis*, painful inflammation of the prostate, the most common cause of urinary tract infection in men. Worse, because there's no "statute of limitations" on prostate problems, some men are unlucky enough to endure more than one of these disorders. (For example, having BPH or prostatitis doesn't mean a man has "had his prostate trouble" and won't have further difficulty—either a return of symptoms, or a new problem entirely, such as prostate cancer.) Although this is a book about prostate cancer, when it comes to making the diagnosis and planning treatment, the other prostate disorders must be considered, too. Thus, it's important that men know about all of the "Big Three" prostate problems—what they are and how they are treated, and telltale symptoms.

Fortunately, effective treatment—and relief of symptoms—is available for all of these prostate disorders. Even prostate cancer, when caught early, is curable—generally without causing loss of urinary control or sexual function. Better still, for the first time ever, we are very close to understanding how to keep advanced cancer in check, perhaps even for years.

Prostate Cancer

Prostate cancer is the most common major cancer in men and, after lung cancer, it's the leading cause of cancer death in men. Because prostate cancer is the subject of this entire book, we'll only use this space to make one point: When prostate cancer is small *and curable*, it is also silent—it produces no symptoms. That's why routine testing is so important, to detect cancer as early as possible. If it's caught too late, prostate cancer can be deadly, and if the disease is allowed to run its course, it can produce terrible symptoms and excruciating pain. *But: Prostate cancer is curable.* If caught in time, before the cancer spreads beyond the wall of the prostate, prostate cancer can be cured with surgery or external-beam radiation. For some men with small, slow-growing tumors, a process called "watchful waiting"—following the disease closely —may be a safe option (see Chapter 7).

Treatment of prostate cancer is better than ever: We are now able to cure prostate cancer in more men, and with fewer side effects, than ever before. And, for the first time, groundbreaking research and novel methods aimed at stopping advanced prostate cancer in its tracks are starting to pay off, with promising new drugs now being tested in patients. Even though in some men we may not be able to *cure* prostate cancer, we may be able to *stop* it from growing further—which makes it very likely that, within a few years, men with advanced disease will die *with* prostate cancer, but not *of* it. How can we save lives from prostate cancer? The key is a four-pronged approach:

- Prevention—to ward off prostate cancer entirely, or at least delay its onset for decades.
- Earlier diagnosis—with the help of highly sensitive tests and sophisticated models for analyzing the results, detecting prostate cancer at the earliest, and most curable, stages yet.
- Better treatment for localized disease—expanding and refining effective treatments, and working to minimize side effects even further.
- Better control of advanced disease.

Next, we cover the other two major prostate problems: benign prostatic enlargement (BPH) and prostatitis. Because none of the "Big Three" prostate diseases precludes the others, it is possible for a man to have more than one, even at the same time. However, if you don't have one of these problems you may wish to go on to Chapter 3 now, and refer to the rest of this chapter—just like those young men we mentioned earlier—on a "need to know" basis.

Benign Prostatic Hyperplasia (BPH)

Benjamin Franklin reportedly suffered from it; so did Thomas Jefferson. So will most men, if they live long enough. This almost inevitable condition is called benign prostatic hyperplasia (BPH), or enlargement of the prostate. The risk of BPH increases every year after age forty: BPH is present in 20 percent of men in their fifties, 60 percent of men in their sixties, and in 70 percent of men by age seventy. One quarter of men with BPH—more than 350,000 a year in the United States alone— eventually will require treatment (some of them more than once) to relieve the urinary obstruction BPH causes.

Before the 1990s, there was no effective *medical* (as opposed to surgical) treatment for this disorder. Men diagnosed with BPH were usually sent home, and told to return when their symptoms were severe enough to warrant surgery. Just a decade ago, an American man had a 25 percent risk of undergoing prostate surgery for benign disease at some point in his life. In fact, BPH is still a common cause of surgery in American men over age fifty-five.

In recent years, as medical therapy has become available, more men have sought treatment to relieve their symptoms. Based on the figures mentioned above, it's likely that after age sixty, a majority of men will either be taking medication for BPH or considering it. However, not all of these men will be helped by the medicine: For men with severe symptoms, or men who wait until the disease is far advanced before they seek treatment, surgery is still the best option.

Note: Growth is not the same thing as cancer. BPH is not prostate cancer, and having it doesn't mean a man is more likely or less likely to get prostate cancer. They're two different diseases—and in some ways the prostate is almost like two different glands rolled into one. Prostate cancer begins in the outer peripheral zone of the prostate (see Fig. 1.3), and grows *outward*, invading surrounding tissue. BPH begins in a tiny area of the inner prostate called the transition zone, a ring of tissue that makes a natural circle around the urethra. In BPH, the growth is *inward* toward the prostate's core, constantly tightening around the urethra (the tube that carries urine from the bladder through the prostate to the penis) and interfering with urination (see Fig. 2.1). This is why BPH produces such annoying, difficult-to-ignore symptoms, and why prostate cancer is often "silent," producing no symptoms for months or even years. *The key word here is benign.* (The word "hyperplasia" simply means an increase in the number of cells in the prostate, which causes it to become enlarged.) By itself, an enlarged prostate causes no symptoms and does no harm. If it weren't for the fact that the prostate encircles the urethra, BPH might never require treatment.

What causes it? The quick answer is, we don't know. Like wrinkles and gray hair, BPH just seems to come with the territory of aging. For reasons that are not clear, beginning at around age forty—in some men more than others—the inner zone of the prostate begins to grow. But even this is more complicated than it sounds. BPH involves two different kinds of tissue: glandular, made up of epithelial cells (the glandular factories that make the prostate's secretions), and smooth muscle cells (which contract to squeeze the secretions into the urethra). Somehow, BPH sets these two types of tissue at odds: It's the

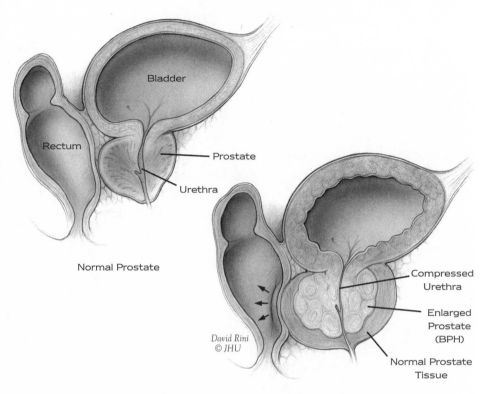

Normal Prostate

Bladder

Rectum

Prostate

Urethra

David Rini
© *JHU*

Compressed Urethra

Enlarged Prostate (BPH)

Normal Prostate Tissue

Prostate with BPH

FIG. 2.1   How BPH Squashes the Urethra

Here are two prostates—one with BPH, one without. What a difference! In the prostate with BPH, lumpy growths of glandular tissue plus tightening smooth muscle tissue act as a "double whammy" to choke the poor urethra and make urination increasingly difficult.

epithelial tissue that makes the lumpy lobes—but the smooth muscle tissue reacts to this buildup by tightening around the urethra.

Scientists suspect that the aging prostate becomes more sensitive to testosterone—even though there's less of it floating around in the bloodstream. Why? As men age, testosterone production starts to fall—but the body's levels of estrogen (which normally are very low in men) remain about the same. We know that even a slight amount of estrogen can make testosterone more powerful; it may be that this imbalance in androgen and estrogen levels contributes to the disease. Also, the tissue changes in BPH may be triggered by substances called growth factors, possibly those made by muscular cells in the prostate.

Curiously, even though the tissue is growing—which normally would mean a big increase in the number of cells being made—the enlarging prostate makes about the same number of cells as always. How can this be? In any tissue, the number of cells is a finely tuned balance between the number of new cells and the number of cells that are dying. Apparently, the population boom in BPH isn't due to an increase in cell birth, but a *decrease* in cell death. For some reason, the cells in BPH are living much longer. Some process—perhaps an increase in growth factors—has altered their normal life span, creating a "fountain of youth" for prostate cells. Although the growth is not malignant, the process is similar to what's happening in prostate cancer—which suggests that, once we understand the factors that control cell death in BPH, we may have a better approach for controlling it in cancer as well.

Does BPH run in some families? Several studies at Johns Hopkins suggest that it does. Hopkins scientists believe that for a small number of men—about 7 percent—age isn't the only major risk factor: These men probably have inherited one or more genes that somehow make them prone to BPH. In one investigation, scientists studied men aged sixty-four and younger with notable prostate enlargement. They also studied their relatives and family histories. They found that the male relatives of these men were four times as likely as other men to require a prostatectomy to treat BPH. And brothers of these men were six times as likely as other men to need surgery to treat BPH. Understanding how the disease works in these men—specifically, identifying the genes involved—may provide major insight into the far more common form of BPH, and one day may even help us prevent it. If you have a strong family history of BPH, scientists at Johns Hopkins would be very interested in hearing from you. (Send inquiries to the Hereditary Prostate Disease Study, James Buchanan Brady Urological Institute, Johns Hopkins Hospital, Baltimore, MD 21287–2101, Attention: Dr. Patrick Walsh.)

What does BPH feel like? How does what's happening on the inside translate to the outside—into symptoms and their impact on a man's life? It depends: BPH is a different disease in every man, depending on a delicate interplay of factors, including the shape of the growth, the specific tissue involved, and how these variables affect the bladder. As the cell growth progresses, the tissue becomes lumpy; bulbous nodules begin sprouting like mushrooms, forming characteristic clusters, or lobes.

These lobes tend to arrange themselves in one of three basic configurations: Lateral lobe enlargement features big knobs that sandwich the urethra. When a man urinates, these lobes can swing open and shut like double doors (think of a saloon in a cowboy movie) — so despite their size, they may not produce much urinary obstruction. In middle lobe enlargement, the lobe bobs around the bladder neck, plugging it like a cork in a bottle and causing great difficulty in urination. (Because this form of BPH is much harder to ignore than lateral lobe enlargement, men who have it are far more likely to seek medical relief for their symptoms.) And in trilobar enlargement, the obstruction can happen in the bladder neck as well as in the urethra.

As the prostate squeezes the urethra, it impedes urine flow. This may manifest itself as frequent urination, needing to go to the bathroom several times an hour; hesitancy, having to wait for the urinary stream to start; urgency, the sudden sensation of needing to urinate, which may culminate in involuntary urine leakage before you reach the bathroom; repeatedly awakening in the night to urinate; starting and stopping during urination; and a constant feeling of fullness in the bladder. BPH can also lead to urinary tract infections, and, rarely, can even cause damage to the bladder or kidneys. It is often frustrating, annoying, and disruptive.

Think of a man's necktie slowly starting to tighten around his collar. This is what happens, over time, as the prostate's inward growth toward the urethra takes its toll. At first, or in mild cases, this can mean an irritating, but still tolerable, change in the quality of life. However, when it progresses beyond the nuisance point—when the bladder is never completely empty, or when the kidney or bladder become damaged—it needs to be treated.

At first, BPH is invisible—it causes few symptoms, because the powerful bladder muscle compensates for the narrowed urethra by making more vigorous contractions and forcing urine through the prostate. But over time, this extra effort takes its toll on the bladder, making it less efficient (this is when a man may notice a decreased flow rate and obstructive symptoms). The bladder, after months of heavy duty, also becomes a victim of its own powerful muscles: The muscle-bound bladder wall thickens and loses its elasticity. With all that extra muscle, the bladder can't hold as much as it used to; it becomes unstable and overly reactive. When this happens, a man feels a need to urinate more often—unfortunately, sometimes sponta-neously. These are *irritative* symptoms: urge incontinence (when a man knows he has to urinate, but can't make it to the bathroom in time), and nocturia, the need to urinate often during the night. Noc-turia can also happen (or be made worse) if a man is unable to empty his bladder completely. If the bladder is always partly full with leftover urine, it doesn't take much—half a glass of water, even—to fill it all the way. Some of our patients joke that they've spent the first half of their life making money, and they're spending the second half making water. Imagine how disruptive, and frustrating, it is for a man who must go to the bathroom twice as often as he normally would.

How do you know if you have it? Some men go right to a specialty physician, a urologist, for help with their urinary problems, but most men start out with a generalist—their family doctor or internist. Most likely, all of these doctors will approach your symptoms the same way; there should be a digital rectal examination, and a PSA blood test. (These and other diagnostic tests are discussed in Chapter 5.) You should be referred to a urologist if your doctor suspects BPH (or, for that matter, prostatitis or prostate cancer).

Because other conditions can mimic BPH, your doctor will probably begin by taking a detailed medical history and performing a physical exam. It is very important for your doctor to know your entire medical history, even if you have what appears to be a classic case of BPH. For example: An injury to the urethra (from having a catheter inserted into the bladder during a surgical procedure, perhaps) can create a urethral stricture—scar tissue that narrows the urethra—that has nothing to do with the prostate, but does a great impersonation of BPH. Blood in the urine, or pain in the bladder or penis, could point to a bladder tumor, or mean that a stone has developed in the bladder, prostate, or kidney. If you have a history of urologic trouble—recurrent urinary tract infec-tions, for example, or prostatitis—it could be that an old problem has returned, but in disguise. BPH symptoms can also be produced by bladder cancer, prostate cancer, and neurogenic bladder (trouble with bladder function caused by a neurological problem, such as Parkinson's disease). You will also be asked to score the degree of your symptoms—and how much they bother you—on a questionnaire called the Interna-tional Prostate Symptom Score (I-PSS; the questionnaire appears below). This is a series of seven questions that can be scored from 1 to 5.

(Briefly, symptoms are considered mild if the score total is 0 to 7, moderate if it's 8 to 19, and severe if it's 20 to 35.) The last question is the most important of all: How much do the symptoms bother you? *This is critical, because BPH is not life-threatening.* All of its treatments are directed at relieving symptoms—which means this symptom score will be the main basis for selecting therapy. (Thus, it is essential that you be brutally honest—rather than stoic and long-suffering, or overly optimistic that this problem will go away by itself—in answering these questions.) The big question your doctor needs answered—and the one only you can decide—is, could you live the rest of your life this way? Are you changing your life to accommodate BPH—giving up seats to a basketball game, for instance, so you won't have to tough it out in the long lines at the men's room? Are you planning your day around trips to the bathroom? If not—if you can put up with it, for now—then you may choose to delay treatment. But if this problem is driving you crazy and disrupting your life, then it may be time to seek treatment.

The physical examination is discussed in detail in Chapter 5. With BPH—because the disease affects only the innermost core of the prostate—your doctor may not be able to feel anything out of the ordinary. It's important to keep in mind that the size of the prostate may have nothing to do with the degree of symptoms. Some men with major prostate enlargement have no urinary tract trouble, while other men with seemingly minor enlargement, or even a small prostate, can suffer terrible problems from obstruction. Again, it depends on where the trouble is (see above for the types of BPH).

You may also need other tests, including:

Uroflowmetry: This test measures the *speed* of your urinary stream and the *amount* of urine you pass, and is done as you urinate (while you're alone in a testing room) into an electronic machine. (It's a urological version of the radar gun used to measure professional baseball pitchers' throws.) To ensure an accurate result, it's important that you urinate at least five or six ounces. This test can identify men whose maximum flow rate is not noticeably diminished—and who may not benefit from treatment. (The normal peak urinary flow rate is 15 cubic centiliters or more per second.)

Ultrasound: This is a painless imaging technique. It works by creating a picture with high-frequency sound waves, like sonar on a submarine. It can be performed from the outside, through the abdomen, or transrectally, using a wand inserted in the rectum. Though not recommended for most men with BPH, ultrasound may be helpful in diagnosing such problems as obstruction of the kidney, stones, or a hidden tumor in the upper urinary tract, in estimating how well the bladder is emptying, and determining the size of the prostate.

Residual urine measurement: If you're not emptying your bladder completely, this important test will find out. Further, it will show how much urine you're leaving behind. This can be done indirectly, by an ultrasound examination of the lower abdomen immediately after you urinate, or directly, by inserting a small catheter into the bladder (like a dipstick) and measuring what's there. These measurements can be a helpful means of following the course of BPH, and showing any change for the worse. If it turns out that you have large amounts of residual urine, your doctor will probably suggest that you seek treatment to avoid chronic urinary tract infection or damage to your kidneys.

Urodynamic studies: Your urologist may want to do these studies if there is evidence that the primary problem is with the bladder, not the prostate. *Cystometry* is a way to measure bladder pressure and function. It's performed by threading a tiny catheter into the penis, through the urethra, and into the bladder to monitor pressure changes as the bladder is filled with water. *Pressure-flow studies,* using a small catheter, check bladder pressure as you urinate. (Note: Anytime a catheter is inserted into the urethra, there is a slight risk of a urinary tract infection developing a few days later. Be sure to tell your doctor if you experience any subsequent fever or discomfort.) In these tests, pressures within the bladder are compared to the rate at which urine is flowing. This can determine whether men with high peak urinary flow rates have obstruction. Imagine squeezing water out of a balloon with a small opening; if you can squeeze hard enough, you can make the water flow, not just trickle. Similarly, some men with significant obstruction can produce reasonable urinary flow rates because they can generate high bladder pressure. These men will have relief of symptoms if their obstruction is treated. However, in some men, low urinary flow rates are caused by diseased bladders that can't produce much pressure. Relieving the obstruction in the prostate won't help these men, because the true problem is the bladder.

Cystoscopy: This test, usually performed in an outpatient setting, is uncomfortable but not painful; it is often used to assess the situation before an invasive procedure. A cystoscope is a slender, lighted tube (often flexible) that works like a periscope. It is inserted in the tip of the anesthetized penis, and threaded through the urethra into the bladder; this allows the urologist to see the bladder, prostate, and urethra, and spot anything abnormal—such as a stone, stricture, or enlargement. With cystoscopy, your doctor may also be able to see thickened muscle bands in the bladder. Like rings in a tree trunk, these tell a story—that a condition of bladder obstruction has probably evolved over months or even years. (Note: As with insertion of a catheter in the urethra, this test carries a small risk of urinary tract infection. Some men also experience blood in the urine, or a temporary inability to urinate. Be sure to tell your doctor if you develop a fever or feel any discomfort.) Cystoscopy can also be used to rule out other conditions, such as the presence of a bladder stone or bladder tumor.

How is BPH treated? The first option is called "watchful waiting," and it doesn't mean "do nothing"; it means "wait and see." This is best chosen in men with mild symptoms—those who say they can live with it, for the time being. The course of BPH is often hard to predict. Your symptoms could stay the same, improve, or get worse. Men who choose watchful waiting must make an extra effort to avoid any condition (such as constipation) or medication (including over-the-counter cold remedies) that could aggravate the problem. Beyond watchful waiting, there are two basic approaches—medical and surgical.

For men with moderate symptoms, the initial treatment should be medical. Here, again, there are several approaches: One class of drugs is called alpha-blockers. Remember the two kinds of tissue involved in BPH? One is glandular, made up of epithelial cells, which secrete the prostate's fluids. The other is smooth muscle tissue—stromal cells, which contract and squeeze this fluid out into the urethra. As the glandular tissue enlarges and begins to narrow the urethra, the smooth muscle tissue tightens around it like a fist. In the normal prostate, there are two stromal cells for every epithelial cell. But in BPH, this ratio shifts—and it's five to one, leading some scientists to describe BPH as a "stromal process." In other words, it's a smooth muscle problem. Alphablockers (the same drugs often used to treat high blood pressure) counteract this by causing this muscle tissue to relax, and these drugs are helpful in men with small prostates and moderate symptoms.

For men who have a significantly enlarged prostate, it is reasonable to try another class of drugs, called 5-alpha reductase inhibitors. These drugs block 5-alpha reductase, the chemical that changes testosterone to DHT (dihydrotestosterone), the active form of male hormone within the prostate. (This is important because, scientists have learned, the trouble in BPH starts after testosterone is converted by 5-alpha reductase into DHT.) Chief among these is a drug called finasteride (Proscar), which shrinks the prostate and decreases obstructive symptoms. Finasteride causes a significant reduction in the tissue surrounding the urethra. But it may do even more: It may also halt the progression of BPH. Finasteride works by blocking a hormonal process without affecting a man's levels of testosterone (the hormone responsible for libido and sexual function). The problem with finasteride is that its effect is gradual and very slow—a significant change will come only after a man has taken it for several months to a year. Also, it only works well if the prostate is enlarged (men with smaller-sized prostates can have BPH symptoms, too); if the prostate is small, finasteride doesn't shrink it.

For men with severe symptoms, or men who do not respond to medical therapy, there are many effective surgical options. The "gold standard" of all of these is a procedure called transurethral resection of the prostate (TURP), also described by patients (although it makes urologists cringe) as a "Roto-Rooter" procedure. It is a proven, effective way to improve BPH symptoms quickly, and keep them at bay for years. The TURP is performed under anesthesia (usually spinal anesthesia); although it is a surgical procedure, the abdomen is not opened up. (Only in rare cases—usually in men with very large prostates—is it necessary to perform an open surgical procedure to remove the prostate tissue surrounding the urethra.) In a TURP, surgeons reach the prostate via the urethra by placing an instrument like a cystoscope through the penis. This instrument, called a resectoscope, shines a powerful light that allows surgeons to view the prostate as they chip away at excess tissue. The prostate's core is removed in fragments, by means of electrosurgical cautery. These tissue chips collect in the bladder, and at the end of the procedure they're flushed out, collected, and sent to a pathologist, who examines them and checks for prostate cancer. Because the resectoscope is threaded through the urethra, no skin incision is needed. In recent years, several promising new techniques have developed: They all channel a form of energy—heat, radio frequency, ultrasound, microwaves, and laser—to kill cells. Energy waves are generated, focused, aimed, and fired at the overgrowth of BPH tissue. Some waves work like a shotgun, blasting holes in the prostate. Others are as sensitive as a scalpel, delicately nibbling away at BPH tissue until the urethra is free.

To sum up: BPH is a common condition that affects most men. It is not cancerous, but it can mimic cancer. Today, there are many effective ways to treat it, and most of them have few side effects.

PROSTATE SYMPTOMS AND WHAT THEY MAY MEAN

Symptoms of urinary obstruction . . .
Weak flow
Hesitancy in starting urination; a need to push or strain to get urine to flow
Intermittent urinary stream (starts and stops several times)
Difficulty in stopping urination
Dribbling after urination
A sense of not being able to empty the bladder completely
Not being able to urinate at all
. . . could be caused by:
Benign prostatic hyperplasia (BPH)
Urethral stricture
Prostate cancer
Medication
Neurogenic bladder (bladder trouble caused by a neurological problem, such as Parkinson's disease)

Symptoms of irritation . . .
Pain or burning during urination
Frequent urination, especially at night
A strong sense of urgency in urination; inability to postpone urination
Sleep disrupted by the need to urinate
Urgency incontinence
. . . could be caused by:
Thickened bladder, caused by obstruction from BPH
Infection in the bladder or prostate
Bladder tumor
Bladder stone
Neurogenic bladder

INTERNATIONAL PROSTATE SYMPTOM SCORE (I-PSS)

	Not at all	Less than 1 time in 5	Less than half the time	About half the time	More than half the time	Almost always	Your score
1. Incomplete emptying Over the past month, how often have you had a sensation of not emptying your bladder completely after you finished urinating?	0	1	2	3	4	5	
2. Frequency Over the past month, how often have you had to urinate again less than two hours after you finished urinating?	0	1	2	3	4	5	
3. Intermittency Over the past month, how often have you found you stopped and started again several times when you urinated?	0	1	2	3	4	5	
4. Urgency Over the past month, how often have you found it difficult to postpone urination?	0	1	2	3	4	5	
5. Weak stream Over the past month, how often have you had a weak urinary stream?	0	1	2	3	4	5	
6. Straining Over the past month, how often have you had to push or strain to begin urination?	0	1	2	3	4	5	

	None	1 time	2 times	3 times	4 times	5 times or more
7. Nocturia Over the past month, how many times did you most typically get up to urinate from the time you went to bed at night until the time you got up in the morning?	0	1	2	3	4	5

Total I-PSS Score

	Delighted	Pleased	Mostly satisfied	Mixed; about equally satisfied and dissatisfied	Mostly dissatisfied	Unhappy	Terrible
Quality of Life Due to Urinary Symptoms If you were to spend the rest of your life with your urinary condition just the way it is now, how would you feel about that?	0	1	2	3	4	5	6

If your total score is:

0 to 7   your symptoms are considered mild

8 to 19   your symptoms are considered moderate

20 to 35   your symptoms are severe

Prostatitis

Prostatitis hurts. This painful condition—an inflamed, swollen, and tender prostate—can be caused by a bacterial infection, or by other factors. Men with prostatitis can experience aches, pain in the joints or muscles, lower back and area behind the scrotum, blood in the urine, pain or burning during urination, and painful ejaculation. In its own way, prostatitis is every bit as difficult and frustrating as BPH—not only because of the symptoms, but because there is not always an apparent cause. Prostatitis is a benign ailment—it is not cancer, and it does not lead to cancer. It is not always curable, but it is almost always treatable.

The National Center for Health Statistics estimates that about 25 percent of all men who see a doctor for urological problems have symptoms of prostatitis. An estimated half of all men will experience some of these symptoms during their lifetime. Prostatitis is the most common cause of urinary tract infections in men; in fact, American men make about two million trips to the doctor each year seeking help for the symptoms of prostatitis or its siblings, "irritative prostatic conditions."

What causes it? The answer here is, sometimes we know, sometimes we don't. As one urologist commented in a recent review of this disorder: "Prostatitis is one of the most difficult clinical problems for men who suffer from it, as well as for the families of those men and their physicians. It is a particularly perplexing problem for urologists, who see many men with prostatitis and have difficulties with diagnosis and treatment." Fewer than 8 percent of men with prostatitis actually have a urinary tract infection (symptoms caused by bacteria, which can be helped by antibiotics). What about the rest of these men? There are actually five conditions lumped under the umbrella name of prostatitis. Each one has distinct characteristics and responds differently to treatment; that's why getting the right diagnosis is so important.

The two *least common* forms of prostatitis are caused by bacterial infection.(Note: Although these are sometimes referred to as "infectious" prostatitis, neither form is contagious and neither form can be transmitted to your sexual partner.) *Acute bacterial prostatitis* is a severe, debilitating condition that hits with all the subtlety of a Mack truck. No mystery here—men who have it *know* something is wrong, and they require immediate treatment. In addition to the symptoms described above, acute bacterial prostatitis is usually distinguished by chills and fever, and extreme pain. It's difficult for a man to be stoic and try to "ride out" this condition. It's also a big mistake: If not treated, acute bacterial prostatitis can lead to more serious problems such as urinary retention (the inability to urinate); a life-threatening infection in the bloodstream (this is called sepsis); and development of an abscess (an accumulation of pus under pressure, like a pimple) within the prostate.

Acute bacterial prostatitis is really an acute urinary tract infection. Fortunately, because the inflammation is so intense, this enables certain antibiotics—which normally wouldn't be able to penetrate the blood-prostate barrier, a shield designed to protect prostatic fluid—to reach the prostate. (Usually, in keeping out bad things like infection, this barrier also blocks helpful agents.) Acute bacterial prostatitis responds dramatically to antibiotics. However, many men are under-medicated—they either don't think they need (and therefore don't take), or aren't prescribed, enough antibiotics to hit the infection hard and knock it out for good. A week to ten days of treatment may ease all signs of infection, and a man may even feel "back to normal" within a few days. But doctors have learned the hard way—from watching acute bacterial prostatitis return as a chronic infection—that it takes much longer, about six weeks of antibiotics, to get rid of the infection. In this sense, bacterial prostatitis is a lot like another stealthy infection—tuberculosis. The prostate is like a sponge, and if any trace of bacteria is not obliterated right away, acute bacterial prostatitis becomes much more difficult to cure. Eradicating acute bacterial prostatitis the first time around, by relentless treatment with antibiotics, is the best way to avoid developing chronic bacterial prostatitis.

Chronic bacterial prostatitis is also caused by bacteria, and also treated by antibiotics. It can be a recurring illness, coming back periodically for years after an initial episode of acute bacterial prostatitis. Its symptoms are usually milder versions of those in the acute form. Here, too, treatment with antibiotics should continue for six weeks. In many cases, the infection goes away *every time* with treatment; if, a few months later, it returns, it will vanish again after another round of antibiotics.

Both acute and chronic bacterial prostatitis are associated with urinary tract infections (UTIs), positive urine cultures that pinpoint the bacteria's location to the prostate, and the presence of inflammatory cells in prostatic secretions. (The hallmark of chronic bacterial prostatitis is that, when the infection returns, it's caused by the same type of bacteria that caused the previous infection.)

Chronic bacterial prostatitis, in fact, is so closely tied to urinary tract infection that many doctors believe that if you don't have a urinary tract infection, and if you've never had one, you probably don't have chronic bacterial prostatitis. One explanation for persistent bacterial prostatitis may be lingering infection in tiny stones, called calculi, in the prostate. Prostatic calculi (the prostate's version of gallstones or kidney stones) are harmless, and very common; about 75 percent of middle-aged men and 100 percent of elderly men have them.

The next category is called *chronic prostatitis/chronic pelvic pain syndrome,* and the cause here is a diagnostic puzzler: Nobody knows what causes the two forms of prostatitis in this group (which used to be named by what it was not, "nonbacterial" prostatitis), and antibiotics don't help at all. Men with chronic prostatitis/chronic pelvic pain syndrome may have many of the same symptoms as in chronic bacterial prostatitis. However, in some men, the prostate may not even be the problem—the pain and other symptoms may be a result of spasms elsewhere in the pelvis, rectum, or lower back. This category has two subgroups—inflammatory and noninflammatory, based on whether any white blood cells (also called inflammatory cells) can be found in the prostatic fluid.

Treatment here is largely symptomatic. Muscle relaxants such as alpha-blockers and other drugs have been helpful in easing the muscle tension in the prostate and making urination easier. Some doctors recommend anti-inflammatory drugs and sitz baths, and many men have been helped by changing their diet. Some foods—particularly spicy dishes, red wine, and caffeine—seem to make symptoms worse.

A final mysterious category is *asymptomatic inflammatory prostatitis.* This condition produces no symptoms, and is usually found by chance, when white blood cells are found in prostatic fluid, or are detected in a prostate biopsy.

How do you know if you have it? As described above, acute bacterial prostatitis leaves little room for guesswork. Other forms of prostatitis, however, have milder symptoms that may not immediately suggest that the prostate is to blame. The constellation of symptoms of prostatitis includes pain in the perineum (the area between the rectum and testicles), pain in the testicles, the tip of the penis, the lower legs and back, pain during or after ejaculation, blood in the urine, the need to urinate frequently, and incomplete emptying of the bladder.

You are at higher risk of developing prostatitis if you recently have had a urinary catheter or other medical instrument inserted in the penis; engaged in rectal intercourse or oral sex; have had a recent bladder infection; or have other urinary problems, including BPH or an abnormal urinary tract. Stress also seems to play a role in prostatitis. (Note: If you have undergone recent surgery or any other surgical procedure, be sure to tell your doctor.)

How is prostatitis treated? The easiest to treat is the most dramatic form, acute bacterial prostatitis. (The most likely cause of infection is *E. coli*, a form of bacteria that's common in the colon.) This can be cured with antibiotics—usually one of a class called fluoroquinolones, and for the full dose, of six weeks. Some patients have been helped by low, "maintenance" doses of antibiotics. This is called "chronic suppressive therapy" and, as its name suggests, it is designed to prevent new urinary tract infections from developing, instead of treating them after the fact. Other men have been helped by drugs such as alpha-blockers—often used to treat high blood pressure (described above in the BPH section), by antidepressants, and by antispasmodics (drugs that help calm muscle spasms). The treatment for most prostatitis is often trial and error, and it helps if men and their doctors can work together—with much patience—to come up with the right plan. New evidence suggests that some nonbacterial prostatitis may actually be caused by an autoimmune condition that mimics the symptoms. This exciting new research may help us find new ways to manage prostatitis.

Finally, many men with prostatitis have found that their symptoms improve when they change their diet—eating a good balance of fruits and vegetables, avoiding spicy foods, alcohol, caffeine, and soft drinks that contain saccharin, and drinking enough water to keep your urine running clear—and their lifestyle. A thirty-minute hot bath or sitz bath, twice a day, can relieve pain and make it easier to urinate. Getting daily exercise (but *not* riding a bike or even an exercise bike, which can irritate symptoms) and resuming normal sexual activity may also be helpful.

3

WHAT CAUSES PROSTATE CANCER?

Read This First

For American men—and men from all Western countries—prostate cancer is something to worry about, because so many of us get it: In the year 2001, almost 200,000 American men will be diagnosed with prostate cancer, and 31,500 will die from it. An American boy born today has a 16 percent risk of developing prostate cancer, and nearly a 3 percent risk of dying from it.

We expect these numbers to improve. Every year, we're getting better at spotting prostate cancer early. The average age of diagnosis has dropped from seventy-two to sixty-nine, treatments are better than ever, and for the first time we have hope of extending the lives of men with advanced disease. It is hard to make sense of statistics, and very easy to be scared by them. It may help for you to look at the numbers in terms of lifetime probability: Of men diagnosed with prostate cancer in 1991, and who did not die of other causes, 6 percent died from prostate cancer within five years. Of men diagnosed in 1986, 33 percent died from prostate cancer within ten years; and of men diagnosed in 1981, 48 percent died from prostate cancer within fifteen years.

So, nearly half of the men diagnosed with prostate cancer in 1981 had died from it fifteen years later. However: In 1981, prostate cancer was diagnosed at a more advanced stage. PSA testing didn't exist, and the only way of finding prostate cancer was to feel it during a rectal exam, or figure it out when a man developed other symptoms. Obviously, it's a different story today, and because of this, we expect these numbers to change dramatically over the next decade. The point of these hard facts is to emphasize the need to cure this disease. Because if it is diagnosed late in the game, or if men don't receive curative treatment, it does kill.

The three major risk factors for prostate cancer are age, race, and family history.

- *Age:* Prostate cancer takes time to develop. Mutations occur gradually, over time, as oxidative damage takes its toll. The incidence of prostate cancer rises dramatically with age—more so than any other cancer. An American man in his mid- to late seventies is about *130 times* more likely to develop prostate cancer than a man in his mid- to late forties. What a difference a few decades makes: In men aged forty to fifty-nine, the risk of developing prostate cancer is one in fifty-three. In men aged sixty to seventy-nine, it's one in seven.
- *Race:* African-Americans have the highest risk of prostate cancer of any ethnic group in the world. Worse, black men seem to get more severe forms of prostate cancer, are more likely to have cancer recur after treatment, and are more likely to die from the disease than white men. Exactly why this is remains uncertain, although it may relate to genetic susceptibility, diet, and inadequate exposure to vitamin D (see below).
- *Family history:* If your father or brother has had prostate cancer, your risk of developing the disease is twofold greater. If three fam-

ily members (such as a father and two brothers) have developed prostate cancer, or if the disease occurs in three generations in your family (grandfather, father, son), or if two of your relatives have developed the disease at an early age (younger than fifty-five), then you may develop a hereditary form of prostate cancer. The genes responsible for this are under intense investigation. When they are found, genetic testing will be available.

What about environment? Why is it that prostate cancer is common in Western cultures, and rare in Asia—but when Asian men migrate to Western countries, their risk of prostate cancer increases over time? Scientists believe environment—mainly diet—must play a large role in determining who gets prostate cancer.

Vitamin D, sunlight, and calcium: Vitamin D is a hormone that is known to protect us against cancer. We obtain vitamin D from two sources—from our diet, and from sunlight. When our skin is exposed to sunlight, vitamin D is synthesized from cholesterol. Next, it's transformed in the kidney to its active form—and the important thing here is that this metabolized form of vitamin D has been shown to keep cells *well differentiated;* that is, to keep their shape intact and healthy, and their growth slow and orderly. (When cells become cancerous, they become *poorly differentiated;* they lose their distinctive shapes and seem to melt together, and their growth becomes rampant.)

What about hormones? It makes sense that hormones must be a major cause of prostate cancer—after all, the male hormone testosterone is the major factor that causes the prostate to grow. Well, this correlation is still murky. It appears that it's not how much of a specific hormone a man has, but the way a man's genes respond to that hormone that makes the difference. It may well be that in some men, a little hormone goes a lot further, and has a much more powerful effect, than in other men. Studies of hormone receptor proteins in African-American men have shown increased activity, and this again may give us insight into why black men are so susceptible to prostate cancer. Another class of hormones, called *insulin-like growth factors* (IGF), also may influence the development of prostate cancer; one study found that men with elevated levels of IGF had a higher risk of developing the disease.

What else? There are a number of other factors that may or may not play a role in prostate cancer. The only occupation that has been found to be associated with a higher risk of prostate cancer is farming, and it is possible that this may be a result of farmers' increased life-time exposure to agricultural chemicals, particularly herbicides. Although this link between herbicides and prostate cancer is not absolutely certain, it's strong enough that the U.S. government has agreed to provide service-connected disability for any veteran who was in Vietnam and who develops prostate cancer. Factors that do not appear to increase the risk of prostate cancer include vasectomy, ciga-rette smoking, frequency of sexual activity, and having other prostate problems (prostatitis or BPH). Also, there is no strong proof that a man's exercise or occupational exertion, or lack of it, has an influence on the development of prostate cancer.

Who Gets Prostate Cancer?

If you are an Asian man who has lived all his life in, say, mainland China, you will probably not need this book. That's because, in your part of the world, few men ever get prostate cancer, and fewer still die of it.

This is not the case in America, as we will discuss in a moment. One of the most remarkable things about prostate cancer throughout the world is that there is a huge variability in the risk of getting it, and dying from it: The risk changes, from place to place and, in many ways, from man to man. The most common risk factor for prostate cancer is age; this is why most men don't need to begin screening tests for prostate cancer until they are fifty. But other factors are of major importance here, too, particularly: race, geographic location—where in the world you live—and family history. (There are others, but these are by far the most significant.)

Thus, as far as prostate cancer goes, Asian men are lucky: The dis-ease is not in the constellation of things they need to worry about. Men in Western countries—Europe and North America—do not have that luxury. Prostate cancer is a very real menace on our horizon.

The statistics are sobering: In the year 2001, nearly 200,000 Amer-ican men will be diagnosed with prostate cancer, and 31,500 will die because of it. Put another way, in the United States, every three min-utes or so, a new case of prostate cancer is diagnosed. And approxi-mately every sixteen minutes, a man dies from this disease. In men, it's the most common major cancer, and the second most common cause of cancer death. An American boy born today has a 16 percent risk of developing this disease, and a 3.5 percent risk of dying from it. Of all men who develop prostate cancer and live fifteen years, roughly half of them will die from it.

Despite these numbers, and despite all we've learned about this complicated disease over the years, many patients are glibly told by their doctors that "most men have prostate cancer, and few men die from it"—and thus, men shouldn't worry about prostate cancer. This is a gross, and dangerous, oversimplification. Some members of the medical community downplay the risk by fiddling with the numbers—dividing the number of new cases a year into the number of deaths. From this, they get the figure 18 percent: "Only 18 percent of men die of prostate cancer," they argue; "therefore, most men don't die of it." Tell that to the wife whose husband died within six months of his diagnosis. Tell it to the families of the 31,500 men who will die of prostate cancer in 2001. The truth is that some of these men—many of them in their eighties—found out they had prostate cancer, and died not too long afterward of other causes.

On the other hand, we're getting better at spotting prostate cancer early, the average age of diagnosis has dropped from seventy-two to sixty-nine, treatments are better than ever, and for the first time, we have hope of extending the lives of men with advanced disease. It is hard to make sense of statistics, and very easy to be scared by them. It may help for you to look at the numbers in terms of lifetime probability: Of men diagnosed with prostate cancer in 1991, and who did not die of other causes, 6 percent ultimately died from prostate cancer within five years. Of men diagnosed in 1986, 33 percent died from prostate cancer within ten years; and of men diagnosed in 1981, 48 percent died from prostate cancer within fifteen years.

So, nearly half of the men diagnosed with prostate cancer in 1981 had died from it fifteen years later. However: In 1981, prostate cancer was diagnosed at a more advanced stage. PSA testing didn't exist, and the only way of finding prostate cancer was to feel it during a rectal exam, or figure it out when a man developed other symptoms. Obviously, it's a different story today, and because of this, we expect these numbers to change dramatically over the next decade. The point of these hard facts is to emphasize the need to cure this disease. Because if it is diagnosed late in the game, or if men don't receive curative treatment, if they live long enough, prostate cancer does kill.

Now, if you are an American man, or someone who loves him, this doesn't mean you should panic. If you lived in a floodplain, or a hurricane-prone coastal area, or an earthquake zone, what would you do? You would learn what you could, be vigilant, and remain prepared—because your knowledge and actions could save your life. The same is true for prostate cancer: What you learn here, from this book (and from your doctor, and—if you develop the disease, from other men and their families), may save your life, too.

What Causes Prostate Cancer?

What, in fact, causes any cancer? The answer is very short, just three letters: DNA. We hear about DNA all the time—at infamous criminal trials, for instance, and as a plot device on TV—but what is it? DNA is short for deoxyribonucleic acid. It is our genetic blueprint, and it's in every cell in our bodies—the "chemical Morse code" that directs each of our cells to make specific building blocks. These blocks are actually strings of chemicals, which scientists identify with letters. Changing just one letter can change everything.

A gene is a particular sequence of DNA codes that directs the production of a single protein. This genetic code is precious. It is the body's greatest treasure, the secret to life itself, and the body guards it jealously. Each cell has its own security systems designed to protect the integrity of this code. Every time a cell divides, this genetic code must be replicated—perfectly. To guarantee that there are no errors in copying this vital information, every cell has a "spell checker," which examines the code and repairs any defects it finds. The genes given this particular job are called "mismatch repair" genes—more on them in a moment.

All cancers are caused by damage to the DNA. In this sense, all cancers are genetic. (Note: "Genetic" doesn't always mean "inherited," although some doctors use the terms interchangeably. For more on inherited, or hereditary, prostate cancer, see below.) Their development—sometimes sparked by *tiny damage to a single gene*—may be hidden deep within cells for years, or even decades. Like a pothole that grows from one little crack in the pavement, or a brushfire sparked by a lone bolt of lightning, cancer arises from one or a series of mutations in the DNA code. Incrementally, these changes create an environment that allows "bad" cells—cancerous or precancerous cells with hostile behavior and a disturbing tendency toward immortality—to flourish.

How does damage to DNA cause cancer? Actually, most of the time it doesn't: Damage to DNA is incredibly common. It happens all the time, often at random, and it's almost always repaired instantaneously by the most efficient "fix-it" crews in the world. However, when mutations happen to transform a pivotal gene, or several sensitive genes within a cell, the damage may overwhelm the body's normal defenses, and cancer may result. (Think of an old movie, in which a kid—like Mickey Rooney in *Boys Town*—"goes bad." Is there a genetic "Father Flanagan"—can the errant gene be saved? Yes it can, sometimes, if the damage is reversible. In fact, scientists are learning that some foods may help block or even salvage injured genes that otherwise might become cancerous—see Chapter 4.)

Here are three major types of genes that are involved in cancer:

Oncogenes: These genes encode for (provide the necessary information to make) growth factors, whose job is to make cells grow. They function as a chemical switch: Click—turn on cell growth; click—turn it off, and let the cells rest. However, when these genes are mutated, they become oncogenes, and normal cell replication can quickly turn into abnormal growth. Oncogenes speed up cell growth so much that this switch acts like a stuck accelerator in a car. If the switch can't be turned off, the cell's growth is out of control.

Tumor suppressor genes: These are checkpoint genes, and they, too, are normally present in all cells. Their purpose seems to be to put on the "brakes," to control cell division and prevent cancer from developing. Mutations here, too, can result in chaos: When these genes are disabled, the effect is like taking your foot off the brake of the car—giving oncogenes even more power, and allowing growth to hurtle along even faster.

Mismatch-repair genes: These are quality-control genes—the spell-checkers—that constantly monitor the genetic code as cells divide. If one or more of these inspector genes is mutated, widespread mutations can occur, with disastrous results.

What causes this DNA damage? Every day, our cells fend off countless threats from the outside—environmental factors as simple as sunlight (particularly, ultraviolet light), which can lead to skin cancer, or as complicated as the chemical cocktail packed into each puff of a cigarette, which causes lung cancer. For the most common cancers of all—prostate, breast, and colon—it is widely believed that our own cellular metabolism is at fault. Like Julius Caesar, the body is betrayed by an insider—one or more traitorous substances created within a man's own cells. The everyday metabolism, or processing of nutrients and other chemicals, produces a toxic by-product; even the name sounds dangerous—*oxygen radicals*, also called *free radicals*. These are highly reactive, unstable, electrically charged molecules that can surge with force enough to destroy tissue, melt membranes, and kill cells in an instant. Free radicals cause a toxic buildup that results in oxidative damage. Normally, they appear in small numbers as "hit men" for the immune system, wiping out bacteria and other foreign invaders; and normally, they are neutralized by "riot-control," or scavenger, enzymes within cells. However, if these enzymes are defective, or if they're overloaded by too many free radicals, then the free radicals can attack the DNA in cells, causing mutations that lead to cancer.

Glutathione-S-transferase-π (pronounced "pie"), which scientists call GST-π for short, is one of these scavenger enzymes. It serves as a genetic fire extinguisher, rendering free radicals into harmless, water-soluble products, and providing toxic cleanup on a cellular level. GST-π, or the lack of it, is crucial in the development of prostate cancer. This enzyme is as essential—and yet, as vulnerable—as the proverbial finger in the dike. Scientists at Johns Hopkins have discovered that although GST-π is present in normal cells, it's been knocked out of prostate cancer cells right next to them. It's absent, in fact, in all prostate cancer tissues, and even in the telltale "funny-looking" cells called PIN (for prostatic intraepithelial neoplasia), which are not cancerous themselves, but are strongly linked to prostate cancer and considered by some to be precancerous. This suggests that the normal oxidative damage that occurs in cells has much greater effects in prostate cancer cells because they lack this key enzyme. This is a terribly important scientific finding, because it helps us understand how normal prostate cells are turned into cancer. Now, Johns Hopkins scientists are searching for new ways to keep this enzyme from failing, and seeking alternate ways to detoxify the free radicals generated by cell metabolism. The best "drug" for this—allowing the body's defenses to stand up to prostate cancer—may be nature's own, one or more cancer-fighting dietary agents such as broccoli or tofu (both, coincidentally, present in the Asian diet), or an antioxidant (which neutralizes free radicals), such as selenium and vitamins E, C, and A. (More on cancer-fighting foods in Chapter 4.)

GST-π protects against these free radicals. So does selenium—a mineral found in the soil, present in some vegetables, many over-the-counter vitamins, and available as a dietary supplement. So does soy. In fact, in one series of experiments, the scientists found that rats given a soy-free diet were prone to prostate inflammation. Rats on a moderate soy diet developed very little inflammation—and rats on a high-soy diet developed none. Diet can control this inflammation of the prostate. Diet can also turn protective enzymes such as GST-π on and off. (This is covered in more detail in Chapter 4.)

DIET, EVOLUTION, AND PROSTATE CANCER

In the very big scheme of things—over the last four million years or so—prostate cancer is an illness of fairly recent evolution. Like heart disease, it is an apparent casualty of the sedentary Western lifestyle and its notoriously unhealthy diet—rich in animal fat, processed fare, fast and other junk food, and poor in fresh vegetables and fruits.

In other words, it's the dark side of progress. As resilient as we are, as remarkably adaptable as the human body is, there are some forces—the cheesesteak, for instance—that nature never equipped us to handle. How ironic that we, who have learned to defy gravity, can be brought down, incrementally, by years of supersized bacon burgers and meat-lover's pizzas. Today's man is far more likely to spend hours hunting for Web sites or TV channels than foraging for food, his fingers more likely stained by Cheetos than by the juices of nuts and berries.

We did not evolve to eat this way, says Johns Hopkins scientist Don Coffey, who has taken a four-million-year detour in his search to explain prostate cancer, and learned that somewhere along the way man took an evolutionary wrong turn. Consider, he says, two male glands, the prostate and the seminal vesicles. So similar in function (both provide fluid that makes up semen), but with one crucial difference: Cancer of the prostate is all too common. Cancer of the seminal vesicles is so rare that it almost doesn't exist.

Only mammals have prostates; by definition, only mammals have breasts as well. Breasts and prostates seem to have evolved on parallel tracks: The prostate appeared in the male at about the same time that the female developed the breast and fed her children by breast milk. Today, countries with high rates of breast cancer tend to have similar rates of prostate cancer; countries with low rates of prostate cancer have relatively few cases of breast cancer. When people migrate from areas with little breast or prostate cancer to places with high rates, their own odds increase over time.

In nature, meat-eating animals like dogs and tigers don't have seminal vesicles. The only animals that have *both prostates and seminal vesicles* are herbivores—vegetarians like horses. But men have both of these glands. Shouldn't we be vegetarians, too? The fact that men eat meat seems to be a mistake that nature never accounted for. How can this be? In exploring this question, Coffey looked a few rungs further down the evolutionary ladder and found the pigmy chimp, called the bonobo. Bonobos and humans have many things in common—except for diet. Bonobos are—as humans probably were, very long ago—vegetarians. They don't get prostate cancer.

Out of the four million years that humans have been around, it's only recently—within the last 600,000 years or so—that we even cooked. (Before that, the human diet was pretty much "scavenge and catch.") About twelve thousand years ago, humans took the next big step and started producing their own food. This brought about a major change in diet and lifestyle: Instead of chasing after animals, humans started herding them, and then breeding them in captivity. As this happened, we became increasingly sedentary. We quit eating a great variety of fresh vegetables and greens—from three thousand types down to about twenty. "We started smoking our meat, salting it, putting nitrates on it," says Coffey. "Now we get everything from the store, nothing from a farm. We call it fresh, but it's not fresh, especially our meat," which most of us prefer well done, not raw.

For decades, the American Cancer Society and National Cancer Institute have urged Americans to lower their cancer risk by changing their diet: Eat fewer animal fats and dairy products. Eat more fiber, fresh fruits, and vegetables. Exercise more.

If breast and prostate cancer have indeed developed from our evolutionary wrong turn, then how to prove it? Coffey pored over zoo records from around the world, and found that no animal in the zoo dies from prostate cancer or breast cancer. There are only three cases of cats dying of prostate cancer. Horses do not die of prostate cancer, bulls do not die of it, and only a very few primates have ever died of it. Yet one out of every six American men gets prostate cancer. And the only animal to develop clinical prostate cancer with any significant incidence is the dog—sedentary, like many humans, and the pet that eats most from our table.

What Does Environment Have to Do with It?

Environment, scientists have learned, has an awful lot to do with the development of prostate cancer. This we know—even though we're still not sure exactly why. The growing mountain of evidence that environment plays a key role in prostate cancer begins with a set of statistics that might be called "The Two Faces of Prostate Cancer." It is the case of significant cancer—the kind that kills, the subject of this book—versus its good twin, "insignificant," or *incidental* cancer—small clusters of the earliest stages of prostate cancer, in an apparently latent, or harmless, form that resides in millions of men.

Autopsy studies of men throughout the world have found that, by the age of eighty, this harmless cancer is present in between 30 and 50 percent of men of every race and culture—even Asian men, who hardly ever die from prostate cancer. These are minuscule spots of prostate cancer—most of them so small that they would never pose a danger. It is highly unlikely that these cancers would even be diagnosed—for example, they don't make enough PSA to warrant a biopsy. For all practical purposes, this cancer doesn't "count." The very fact that it's found only at autopsy tells us that: It means these men lived to a ripe old age and died and were never troubled by the presence of cancerous cells in their prostate. There are millions of men out there who manage to dodge the proverbial bullet. This is why some doctors erroneously conclude, and report to their patients: "If you live long enough, you will get prostate cancer." What they fail to say, or may not realize, is that these are cancers so small and insignificant that they are never diagnosed.

What makes these men different from the 16 percent of American men who develop clinically significant prostate cancer—the kind that needs to be treated? What's their secret? This "incidental" prostate cancer is found consistently, in so many men of every race and culture in the world—even in China. This means that whatever causes prostate cancer in the first place—the *initiating factors or events*—happens everywhere. The crucial difference is what happens next—whatever *promotes* these small cancers to grow and become potentially lethal. In the United States, for example, those cells seem to progress into cancer that needs to be treated in between 10 and 20 percent of men as they age. In Asia, the cancer-progression process seems to be arrested. The cancer stays put, stays benign, and rarely poses a problem.

Unless Asians change their lifestyle. It is well known that when Asian men migrate to the West, over time (twenty-five years), their risk of prostate cancer increases. So when Japanese men, people at low risk of developing prostate cancer, move to Hawaii or California, their risk balloons over the years—to approach the level of an American man's. (For more on this, see "Geographic Location: Where in the World You Live," below.) It is no longer a question of *whether* diet plays a vital role in the development of prostate cancer. We need to know *how* it does. More specifically, which foods are good—or bad—for the prostate? And is it possible, *through diet,* to change or delay the onset or progression of cancer? (For some promising candidates in the search for prostate-cancer-preventing foods, see Chapter 4.)

PROSTATE CANCER AND BREAST CANCER: TWO SIDES OF THE SAME COIN?

Just as Asian men hardly ever die of prostate cancer, Asian women hardly ever die of breast cancer. Autopsy studies have found that between 20 and 40 percent of all women have microscopic amounts—just like the incidental prostate cancer—of breast cancer. (These microscopic clusters might be even more common but for the fact that women go through menopause; the decrease in female hormones probably makes these microscopic cancers shrink, and become even more difficult to see. Men, however, keep making substantial amounts of male hormones until well into their eighties and nineties.) Both have benign forms of disease as well—in men, this is BPH (benign enlargement); in women, it's fibrocystic breast disease. (Neither of these benign diseases will progress to cancer.)

Risk Factors for Prostate Cancer

Of all the risk factors for prostate cancer, the three greatest are age, race (being African-American), and family history (which is discussed later in this chapter).

Age: Prostate cancer takes time. Why? As we discussed earlier, the process of transforming a normal cell into a cancerous cell—one that can divide, grow, escape the prostate, and invade other tissues—requires a number of genetic mutations that alter DNA. Scientists have estimated that the number of *mutations* necessary to transform a normal cell into a cancer correlates with the number of *decades* it

TABLE 3.1

PROSTATE AND BREAST CANCER: A COMPARISON

As these tables show, prostate and female breast cancer are remarkably alike. (Note: Men can get breast cancer, too; these statistics apply only to female breast cancer.) They share similar numbers of new cases and deaths per year, similar survival rates depending on when cancer is diagnosed—when it is localized, or when cancer has spread—similar responses to hormonal therapy, and similar geographic patterns of development.

	Prostate	Breast
Rank of all cancers	No. 1 in men	No. 1 in women
Lifetime risk of developing it	1 in 6	1 in 8
Number of new cases in U.S. in 2001	198,100	192,200
Deaths in the U.S. in 2001	31,500	40,200
5-year survival (all stages)	92 percent	87 percent
5-year survival if disease is diagnosed when it's localized (in men, this is T1 or T2 disease)	100 percent	96 percent
5-year survival if disease is diagnosed when it has spread, or metastasized	25 percent	21 percent
Average age of diagnosis	69	63
Responds to hormonal therapy?	Yes	Yes

takes, on average, for cancer to develop. For example, there is a highly malignant form of cancer that occurs in the eye in infants and children, called retinoblastoma. In those with the inherited form of this disease, only one mutation is necessary for this cancer to begin. In prostate cancer—where most men are not diagnosed until they are in their seventies—the number of genetic mutations may be seven or eight. These occur gradually, over time, as oxidative damage takes its toll. Even if a boy is born with the deck stacked against him—if he has a family history of the disease, for example, or if he is African-American—nothing will happen for many years.

Age is a risk factor for many illnesses, because—no matter how physically or mentally fit—the body of a seventy-year-old man is just plain different from the body of a twenty-five-year-old. In men, the incidence of prostate cancer rises dramatically with age—more so

TABLE 3.2

WHO GETS PROSTATE AND BREAST CANCER?

	Prostate	Breast
Least likely to develop in:	Chinese men	Chinese women
Most likely to develop in:	African-American men in Atlanta	Caucasian women in San Francisco
U.S. deaths per 100,000 African-Americans	54.8	31.4
U.S. deaths per 100,000 Caucasians	23.7	25.7
U.S. deaths per 100,000 Asian-Americans	10.7	11.4
More likely with migration from Asia to the West	Yes	Yes

than any other cancer. An American man in his mid- to late seventies is about *130 times* more likely to develop prostate cancer as a man in his mid- to late forties. Look at the difference a few decades makes: In men aged forty to fifty-nine, the risk of developing prostate cancer is one in fifty-three. In men aged sixty to seventy-nine, it's one in seven.

If you were just diagnosed with prostate cancer today, when did this cancer start? Scientists estimate that it takes roughly eleven or twelve years—about a year less in African-American men—from the *initiation* of prostate cancer—when those first few cells go bad—to its *clinical presentation*—when it causes a significant change in PSA, or when it's big enough for a doctor to feel during a digital rectal exam. There are, however, two circumstances in which prostate cancer strikes at an earlier age: African-Americans, and men with a family history of prostate cancer (this is discussed below).

Race: African-Americans, and Africans in Jamaica, have the highest risk of prostate cancer of any ethnic group in the world. If they get prostate cancer, they are more likely to die from it.

The number of black men per 100,000 who develop prostate cancer is about 40 percent higher than the number of white men, and of the men who get it, the number who die is almost double. The statistics would be even worse—except African-Americans also are at higher risk of other health problems, such as hypertension and coronary artery disease. Which means that, sadly, most black men in this country don't live long enough to make it to what we call the "peak incidence rates" that occur with old age. That's why the lifetime risk of prostate cancer is about 16 percent for white men, and 13 percent for black men—but these statistics are misleading; the black man's risk is actually higher. The only reason that the lifetime risk of developing prostate cancer is lower in black men is the sad likelihood that they will die of some other illness before they live long enough to get prostate cancer.

African-Americans—particularly, young black men—seem to get more severe forms of prostate cancer, and are more likely to have cancer recurrences and die from the disease than young white men. One reason for this may be that, in this country, black men delay seeking medical care—yet another reason that African-American men should start screening for prostate cancer at age forty. However, information from "equal-opportunity" health care studies—places such as military clinics, or HMOs, where availability of medical care seems to be equal—suggests that black men still seem to fare poorly when it comes to prostate cancer.

Why? A few years ago, scientists attributed this to environment. They believed that black men in Africa were at lower risk than black Americans—that somehow the African lifestyle was healthier, or the diet was better, or vice versa (that the American diet and lifestyle did not stave off cancer). Evidence from recent studies shows that this is not true. We now know that prostate cancer is probably the most common cancer in African men—and, in fact, the incidence of prostate cancer in Nigeria may be as great as that of black men in the United States. And Kingston, Jamaica (which has a high concentration of men of African descent), has the highest incidence of prostate cancer in the world—304 per 100,000 men, compared to 249 per 100,000 black men in the United States, and 182 white men.

Why are black men hit so hard by prostate cancer? We don't know yet, but there are a number of leads: genetic susceptibility, inadequate exposure to vitamin D (see below), and diet. The simple fact that the disease is so common in African and African-American men strongly suggests that genes play a role. (Men of different races are known to have genetic differences in how they are affected by male hormones. This is discussed below.) *Genetic susceptibility* refers to a complex of genetic factors that creates a more hospitable atmosphere for cancer. Briefly: The development of cancer is like a tumbling row of dominoes, in that a whole chain of genetic events must occur before a tumor can begin to grow. Inherited mutations in one or more genes probably speed up the process; presumably, in some men, a few of these dominoes are already knocked down at birth. (See "What Is Hereditary Prostate Cancer?," below.) Environmental variables— what men eat and drink and how they live—may topple the rest. Genetic susceptibility is somewhere in the middle of all this: not exactly a mutation that causes cancer, but a genetic makeup that creates a more hospitable atmosphere—which makes it easier for cancer to set foot in the door. In the domino analogy, maybe genetic susceptibility tilts the table slightly, making the dominoes more likely to fall, without actually knocking them over.

Hormones and race: Prostate cancer is affected strongly by hormones. For years, it was believed that the levels of male hormones in African-Americans were higher than those in Caucasian and Asian men. However, when scientists looked at the levels of male hormone in African-American men, they found no consistent difference. Recently, genetic research has shed new light: Hormones exert their effect on specific tissues by communicating with particular proteins within cells; these proteins are called *receptors.* A portion of the receptor for male hormones known as the *CAG repeat* (because it appears over and over), on average is larger in Asian men. It's intermediate in white men, and shorter in black men. The result of this slight variation is that for any given level of hormone, the shorter the CAG repeat, the more active the receptor. This short repeat makes testosterone more efficient in prostate cells, so that the same amount of testosterone goes further, and has more of an effect, than in other men. Men with longer repeats (such as Asian men) have less of this stimulation. In related research, Caucasian men with prostate cancer who turn out to have micrometastases—minuscule offshoots of prostate cancer in the lymph nodes (and thus, more aggressive and more advanced cancer)—also have this same type of overactive androgen receptor. This short CAG repeat may help explain why so many black men are more susceptible to developing prostate cancer, and particularly to developing more aggressive disease. One study by Harvard researchers concluded: "Men with shorter repeats were at particularly high risk for distant metastatic and fatal prostate cancer."

Another contributing factor for black men may be inadequate

exposure to vitamin D. As we discuss later in this chapter, vitamin D protects against prostate cancer; in fact, there is a suggestive correlation between *lack* of vitamin D and prostate cancer. Normally, vitamin D is transformed into a form that the body can use when sunlight hits the skin. Because black skin is more efficient at blocking out sunlight—and less efficient at absorbing it—black men are known to have lower levels of a form of the vitamin called 1,25-dihydroxy vitamin D. Again, this may make black men more susceptible to prostate cancer. Undoubtedly, scientists will discover other factors—and it is almost certain that some of them will be genetic—that will shed new light on this major racial difference in susceptibility to prostate cancer.

Geographic Location: Where in the World You Live

In general, the rate of prostate cancer is high in Western cultures and low in Asia. But that's about as straightforward as it gets. Chinese men have the lowest incidence of prostate cancer in the world. When Chinese men move to Western cultures, their risk of prostate cancer increases—but it is still only half that of a Caucasian American man, and even less than that of African-American men. This suggests that genetic factors continue to exert a protective influence. (One subtle but important racial difference may be in the CAG repeat, discussed above.)

When we break this down into specifics, the worldwide rates of prostate cancer get a lot more complicated. *The incidence of prostate cancer varies from place to place, and group to group, more than probably any other cancer in the world.* So, although China has the lowest reported rate of prostate cancer, for Chinese men elsewhere in Asia, particularly Singapore and Hong Kong, the rate is nearly five times higher—and for Chinese men living in the West, particularly Los Angeles and Hawaii, it's twelve to sixteen times higher. *Clearly, the risk of prostate cancer is more strongly tied to environment—diet and lifestyle—than to racial factors.* The prostate itself, interestingly, seems to react to a change in location or diet: The size of the prostate of men in China is significantly smaller than that of Chinese men who migrate to Australia. (For that matter, men of every race in Australia have larger prostates than men in China.) However, after a Chinese man has lived in Australia for ten or more years, his prostate increases to the same size as an Australian man's. What's going on here? Again, it's got to be the environment.

The risk of prostate cancer increases tenfold when native Japanese men move to Hawaii. Although scientists have recently noted a rise in prostate cancer in Japan, there has also been an increase in screening for the disease, and it's not clear whether prostate cancer is actually on the upswing there, or whether this is just an artifact of more intensive attempts to diagnose prostate cancer. Similarly, in Taiwan, the rate of prostate cancer has doubled over the last thirty years—but scientists attribute this mainly to the aging of the population.

It's also important to note that when Asians migrate to the United States, the increase in the development of prostate cancer doesn't happen overnight; it takes years. This suggests that whatever the environmental risk factors are that make a man more prone to cancer, they act late in life—and this, in turn, gives us great hope that once we understand just what these factors are, we may be able to prevent the disease.

CALORIES, EXERCISE, AND PROSTATE CANCER

What do caloric intake—the number of calories you eat a day—and exercise have to do with cancer? The answer may be, quite a lot. Studies have found that restricting caloric intake greatly reduces the development of breast tumors in animals. The impact can be profound: A 30 percent reduction in caloric intake can reduce the development of breast tumors by as much as 90 percent. But calories are just part of the picture: Just as important is "energy expenditure"—what happens to those calories in your body. Do they get burned up or turned into muscle, or do they just accumulate as flab? For example, a Marine in boot camp wolfs down about three thousand calories a day, and burns every one of them. But a sedentary man on the same diet would gain weight. Eating more calories than your body needs a day, and the resulting accumulation of body fat, can increase the risk of several major cancers, including prostate cancer.

Doctors use a measurement called body mass index to help them figure out, to put it bluntly, how fat a patient is (although very muscular men, who are not necessarily fat, can have a high body mass index, too). You can use it, too—see Table 3.3. In a study by the American Cancer Society, overweight men were shown to have a 30 percent greater risk of prostate cancer than men within 10 percent of their ideal body weight. Similarly, a study of Seventh Day Adventists found that the risk of fatal prostate cancer was elevated two and a half times in overweight men, and a study from Sweden showed that the risk of prostate cancer went up with increased food consumption, and with higher body mass index.

TABLE 3.3

WHAT'S YOUR BODY MASS?

Or, more precisely (perhaps too precisely), how fat are you? How much you weigh is only part of the equation: It's your weight in relation to your height that matters here. This chart will tell you if you are overweight (a body mass index between 25 and 29) or obese (a body mass index of 30 or above). (Note: Men who are very muscular may have a high body mass index as well.) To determine your body mass index:

- Multiply your weight in pounds by 704; then:
- Multiply your height in inches by itself.
- Divide the result of step one with the result of step two.

For example: If you are 5'10" (that's 70 inches) tall, and weigh 150 pounds: 150 x 704 is 105,600. 70 x 70 is 4,900. 105,600 divided by 4,900 is 21.55. Your body mass index, then, is 21.5, and you are not overweight.

BODY WEIGHT

Height	BMI=25	BMI=30
4'10"	119 lbs.	143 lbs.
4'11"	124	148
5'0"	128	153
5'1"	132	158
5'2"	136	164
5'3"	141	169
5'4"	145	174
5'5"	150	180
5'6"	155	186
5'7"	159	191
5'8"	164	197
5'9"	169	203
5'10"	174	207
5'11"	179	215
6'0"	184	221
6'1"	189	227
6'2"	194	233
6'3"	200	240
6'4"	205	246

Diet

What is it about Western countries that makes our men so susceptible to prostate cancer, and our women so prone to developing breast cancer? Why, in fact, are there such striking parallels between those two cancers—with countries having roughly the same high or low levels of both (see Tables 3.1 and 3.2). And why, in comparison, are those diseases so rare in Asian and some Middle Eastern countries? What are they doing right, and what are we doing wrong? *The answer must lie, in large part, in what we eat.* By unfortunate coincidence, the Western diet probably provides the worst of both worlds: Notorious for its overabundance of animal fat, it also lacks many substances— soy products, citrus fruits, vegetables (particularly tomatoes), and green tea—which may actually prevent cancer.

Are Americans and Europeans—whose rate of prostate cancer is ten times higher than that of many Asian countries—eating foods that cause these cancers? Or does the Asian diet somehow protect the prostate and breast against them? Are we dealing with sins of *commission*—eating too many french fries and hamburgers—or *omission*—not eating enough broccoli and carrots? Or is it an unlucky combination of both? As we will discuss later (in this chapter and the next), it is increasingly obvious that a poor diet triggers a specific, genetic chain of events. Each subtle mutation brings us one step closer to cancer. In Chapter 4, we will examine some possible acts of omission—foods that show great promise in protecting the body and *preventing* prostate cancer. In this chapter, we begin with the sins of commission.

Are there foods that weaken the body's defenses, and actually help *cause* prostate cancer? Scientific evidence strongly suggests that the answer is yes, and the greatest danger of all seems to come from animal (but not vegetable) fat. Many studies in the medical literature, of large groups of men followed for years or even decades, have shown a consistent link between consumption of fat-containing animal products— primarily red meat—and prostate cancer. For example, in one study of more than 51,000 health professionals, a positive association was seen between the intake of red meat, total fat, and animal fat and the risk of prostate cancer. A follow-up to the health professionals study showed that a high-fat diet appeared to be associated only with advanced cancer, and not with localized, slow-growing cancer. In that study, saturated and monosaturated fats were associated with advanced prostate cancer, but the strongest link was with alpha-linolenic acid—and the main sources of this are animal fats and vegetable oils (thus, it's found in a lot of fried foods). Another study of men in Hawaii found that the risk of prostate cancer went up with consumption of beef and animal fat. In one study, men who ate five or more servings of red meat a week had a 79 percent higher risk of developing prostate cancer. But again, this is complicated: Did those men also *not eat* very many vegetables?

We should emphasize that food studies are hard—tough to carry out, and tougher still to analyze. A finding that red meat is associated with an increased risk of prostate cancer, for researchers, easily raises as many questions as the ones it attempts to answer. For example: Is it the meat itself that raises the risk of cancer? Or some specific fat within that meat? Or maybe it's the way the meat is cooked—are carcinogens, or cancer-causing agents, created when the meat is fried or charred? We know, for instance, that charred meat is bad. Every time we fry a pork chop, grill a steak, or cook a hamburger, we generate a few unwanted extra ingredients—carcinogens. One of them is PhIP. PhIP is what scientists call a "pro-carcinogen." It's benign enough by itself—like a werewolf before the full moon comes out—but when it's metabolized, it becomes something far more dangerous. In the liver, PhIP is transformed into a chemical called N-hydroxy PhIP. For some cells in the body—including prostate and breast cells—this new chemical is far more dangerous, because it attacks DNA. In laboratory animals, the PhIP carcinogen can even cause breast cancer and prostate cancer. Johns Hopkins scientists are working to use PhIP as a marker: PhIP causes telltale changes, or adducts, to the DNA—picture barnacles on a sailboat—that can be monitored. If scientists can figure out which foods protect against prostate cancer, these adducts should decrease. Among other things, a test using these adducts could confirm that scientists are on the right track in preventing prostate cancer.

We know that diet can have an effect on hormones such as testosterone. A diet that's low in fat and high in fiber lowers the amount of testosterone in the blood, and hormones such as testosterone play a big role in the growth of prostate cancer. Although much about hormone levels and race remains unclear, one study several years ago found blood testosterone levels in young black men to be about 15 percent higher than those of young white men; a similar study found that Dutch men had higher levels of male hormones than Japanese men. Is the difference racial, or cultural—due largely to diet? Also, studies of American men have found that they have higher levels of DHT (dihydrotestosterone, the active hormone in the prostate) metabolites than Japanese men. Some scientists speculate that having more DHT may contribute to prostate cancer. However, DHT is produced by the secondary organs of reproduction (such as the prostate), and Asian men tend to have smaller prostates. Which is the cause and which is the effect? The lower DHT may simply reflect the fact that Japanese men have inherently smaller secondary organs of reproduction, which contribute less DHT to the bloodstream.

Other studies have found that black and white American men have higher amounts of these male hormones in their urine than black South African men, and that the level of these hormones has a lot to do with diet. When the black South African men ate a Western diet, instead of their usual vegetarian fare, their hormone levels went up. And when black American men ate a vegetarian diet, their hormone levels went down.

There is also evidence from animal studies that dietary fat may not just *cause* cancer, it may affect the way that cancer *progresses* —among other things, the rate at which cells proliferate, the ability and likelihood of cancer to invade other tissues, and the body's ability to defend against this invasion. For example, scientists have found that a specific type of fatty acid called linoleic acid (found in corn oil, safflower oil, soybean oil, and other polyunsaturated fats) can stimulate the most dangerous prostate cancer cells—the ones that do not respond to hormones, and thus, to hormonal therapy. Of all the dietary fats, scientists consider linoleic acid to be the most powerful stimulator of tumor metastasis. Increased intake of saturated fat also has been suggested to raise the risk of prostate cancer. Another undesirable class of fats, usually described on food packages as "partially hydrogenated oil," can be found in foods that remain more solid at room temperature. These and similar oils— often hidden in cakes, doughnuts, cookies, and many packaged snack foods—can also increase free radicals, and thus damage DNA.

In Chapter 4, we will talk about carotenoids (the most famous of these is beta-carotene), which are metabolic precursors of vitamin A. Some studies have associated vitamin A with an increased risk of prostate cancer, but—like so many issues in diet—it is more complicated than it sounds. In Asia, vitamin A in the diet comes almost entirely from green and yellow vegetables. But Americans get most of their vitamin A from animal fat—and this correlation between vitamin A and prostate cancer, as one Canadian study concludes, "may be due solely to increased fat intake."

Caution: Not all fats are bad. In fact, some of them are downright good for you. Because this issue is so complicated, and because there is such a variety of fats and fatty acids, some patients wonder if they should "throw out the baby with the bathwater," and shun fat altogether. (In fact, many diets simply advise, "reduce total fat," without making the distinction between "good" and "bad" fats.) But some "good" fatty acids—particularly, some present in vegetables and fish—may slow or even inhibit the growth of prostate cancer cells. Thus, simply emphasizing these "good" fats may make a big difference in your body's ability to fend off cancer. In one Finnish study, men aged forty to forty-nine reduced their total fat consumption from 40 to 25 percent of total calories, and increased their ratio of dietary polyunsaturated to saturated fats. Although the men did not change their total caloric intake, or otherwise alter the diet (to add more fiber, for example), this simple change produced significant decreases in the total level of testosterone. (More on "good" fats below.)

One large Harvard study, looking for connections between intake of fat and specific fatty acids (including total fat, animal fat, saturated, polyunsaturated, and transunsaturated fats) and breast cancer in thousands of women, couldn't find a specific link—even in women with a family history of breast cancer. "In this large prospective study, we found no evidence that higher total fat intake was associated with an increased risk of breast cancer, even though the relationship was assessed many different ways," the researchers said. "These findings suggest that reductions in total fat intake during midlife are unlikely to prevent breast cancer, and should receive less emphasis. Rather, women's decision about fat intake should be guided primarily by risk of heart disease, which is strongly influenced by the type but not total amount of fat."

In another study, these Harvard scientists made an important point: "The lack of association of total dietary fat with breast cancer, and probably other cancers as well, should not be confused with the relation of excess body fat to cancer risk. Higher body weight has been associated with increased risks of cancers of the endometrium, colon, and (among post-menopausal women) breast." Dietary fat, the researchers note, doesn't necessarily determine a person's body fat, which "is largely determined by the balance between physical activity and total caloric intake, which in almost all diets derives mainly from carbohydrates."

DIETARY FAT: HOW DO YOU KNOW WHAT'S WHAT?

The words are long, and even worse, they all sound alike. Try using "linoleic acid" and "linolenic acid" in the same sentence and keeping them straight. And who can tell the difference between saturated, polyunsaturated, and monounsaturated fats? And yet, somehow you're supposed to make sense of these nitpicky words, decipher the labels on packaged foods, seek out the good fats, and avoid the bad. Does your fat consumption really have anything to do with prostate cancer?

Yes, it does, although scientists are still learning exactly how it all works. Fats are complicated, and although these terms can be frustrating, you can learn enough about them to get by in the grocery store. Here's a quick primer, starting with the worst:

Saturated fats: We should call these the "All-American" fats, because the average American diet is full of them. These are the ones in red meats, and in dairy fats. The Asian diet has hardly any saturated fat in it.

Polyunsaturated fats: These are found in vegetable oils (corn oil, safflower oil, and other cooking oils), nuts and seeds, fish oils, and margarine. There are a lot of these polyunsaturated fats, and some are worse than others. Some, called *omega-3 fats,* are found in fish oils, and may be helpful in preventing coronary artery disease; in any event, nobody has suggested that fish oils have anything to do with prostate cancer. (The main source of these, obviously, is the fish themselves; however, you can also buy fish oil supplements at health food stores.) *Alpha-linolenic acid* is in the omega-3 class of polyunsaturated fats, but it's not in the benign category with fish oil. It's a bad one, it's found in red meat, margarine, cooking oils, and mayonnaise, and is discussed above. Others are called *omega-6 fats* (these names simply refer to the chemical makeup of these fats). One of these is *arachidonic acid,* which is found in red meat, whole milk and cheese, and egg yolks. Another is *linoleic acid* (discussed above), found in corn oils, baked goods, and many snack foods.

Food processors use a preservation method called *hydrogenation,* and the most annoying thing about this, for our purposes, is that it introduces a whole new set of terms, all of which sound alike, for us to learn. Hydrogenation helps keep Crisco solid at room temperature. Unfortunately, the process seems to have a similar effect in your arteries, and people seeking "heart-healthy" food are learning to avoid words like "partially hydrogenated," or "hydrogenated," or even "transhydrogenated," because these foods raise your cholesterol level. What do they do to the prostate? Well, they're known to damage DNA, and may contribute to oxidative damage.

Monounsaturated fats: Finally, some of the safe ones. Olive oil is a monounsaturated fat; so is canola oil. Neither is linked to prostate cancer. In fact, the Mediterranean diet is rich in olive oil, and Mediterranean men have a much lower risk of prostate cancer than American men.

The bottom line? Basically, the message is the same: Avoid red meats, whole dairy foods, and limit your intake of processed, hydrogenated snack foods, cake mixes, and the like. Eat more vegetables and fruits. And become a "label-checker." Read what's in there before you buy anything, even a candy bar. You may be surprised at the hidden fats you're putting into your body every day—and how easy it is to cut fat and calories simply by watching what you eat.

Vitamin D, Sunlight, and Calcium Intake

The vitamin D story: Where you live determines, in large part, how much vitamin D you get. Vitamin D is a hormone, known to protect the body against cancer. In the body, it's metabolized into a form called 1,25 dihydroxy vitamin D, which has been shown to keep cells well differentiated—to keep their shape intact and healthy, and their growth slow and orderly. It's in milk and some fish (actually, the Japanese diet is rich in fish that contain vitamin D), but the main source of vitamin D is the sun—everyday exposure to the sun's ultraviolet rays.

Sunlight: People who live in southern climates get a lot more sun than people in the north. Several years ago, researchers looked at geographic distribution of the sun's ultraviolet rays and the number of prostate cancer deaths throughout the United States. After adjusting the data to account for the south's higher concentration of older men, the scientists uncovered a striking north-south pattern, with the highest areas of prostate cancer death in the north, and the lowest in the south. But when they looked at sunlight exposure, they found just the opposite—the heaviest exposure in the south, and the least in the north. Areas getting the least UV radiation had the most prostate cancer, and vice versa. They concluded that ultraviolet radiation may protect men from getting clinical prostate cancer—and that vitamin D somehow slows or prevents incidental prostate cancer from becoming clinical. This might explain why prostate cancer death rates are highest in Scandinavian countries, Canada, and the United States, and lowest in Asia. Also, it may explain a key racial difference. Vitamin D is mostly formed in the skin: When our skin is exposed to sunlight, vitamin D is synthesized from cholesterol. People with dark skin absorb less sunlight, and are known to have lower levels of vitamin D. In one study, African scientists compared blood levels of vitamin D in black men in Zaire (now Congo) with Zairian black men living in Belgium and found significantly lower levels of vitamin D in those who had left sunny Zaire.

The best way to help your body produce vitamin D is to spend some time outside in the sunlight every day for at least half an hour. Note: Be cautious about trying to duplicate the sun's rays with mega-dose supplements from the health food store; too much of anything, including vitamin D, can be toxic. If you do take supplements, the recommended dose is 400 to 800 IU (international units) daily.

Yet another explanation—one that deserves further study—for the observation that prostate cancer risk correlates with sunlight may be quite simple: Where do fruits and vegetables grow best? In the sunlight. Fifty years ago (before greenhouses and hydroponic gardening, and before world markets and widespread importing of foods), it was much easier for an Italian man to eat fruits and vegetables year-round than a Scandinavian man. Today there is much less prostate cancer in Italy than in the Scandinavian countries.

Calcium intake: Remember Elsie the cow? Picture a whole herd of happy-looking black and white cows just like her, grazing in the countryside in a field full of buttercups, little bells tinkling around their necks. In the list of things that are considered wholesome and good, dairy products rank right up there with apple pie. How is it, then, that milk, which according to the ads "does a body good," could possibly be linked to cancer? This makes the following all the more surprising: In a series of case-control and cohort studies, there was a direct association between dairy intake and the risk of prostate cancer. Furthermore, it may be that calcium—stalwart preserver of strong teeth and bones—is in large part to blame. Scientific evidence has linked a higher daily diet of calcium with advanced prostate cancer—and, more commonly, with metastatic disease. It seems that calcium interferes with the anti-tumor effect of 1,25 dihydroxy vitamin D (discussed above). Normally, your kidneys take vitamin D and convert it to its active form, 1,25 dihydroxy vitamin D. But the kidney's ability to transform vitamin D is regulated by the amount of calcium in the bloodstream: If you have low levels of calcium, your body makes more 1,25 dihydroxy vitamin D; if you have high levels of calcium, your body makes less of it—which means that vitamin D doesn't get the "oomph" that it should. Thus, calcium can effectively block vitamin D from becoming a helpful cancer-fighter in your body, and make it more likely for prostate cancer to develop. But here's something interesting: Fructose (the sugar found in fruit) may help counteract the calcium. Fruit is a major source of phosphorus. Phosphorus binds calcium—it ties it up, reducing its "bio-availability"—in other words, making it inactive in your body. A study from Harvard found that a high fructose intake was associated with a decreased risk of prostate cancer. "We hypothesize," the Harvard researchers said, "that diets high in dairy products and meat and low in fruits are associated with increased risk of prostate cancer *because these diets tend to be high in calcium . . . and low in fructose, and thus associated with lower circulating (1,25 vitamin D) levels.*"

WHAT IS HEREDITARY PROSTATE CANCER?

Of all the men who will be diagnosed with prostate cancer this year, about 9 percent of them will be men born with a head start—one or more bad genes, such as HPC1 and HPX (discussed below), that greatly increase their odds of developing cancer, and of developing it at an earlier age. Although purely hereditary cases of cancer make up only a small percentage of all the men with prostate cancer, we believe understanding hereditary prostate cancer may help us crack the genetic code of how this disease works. The defective gene or mechanisms involved in hereditary cancer are almost certainly the same ones that somehow go wrong in the far more common "sporadic cancer," which develops over the course of a lifetime.

In most men, cancer probably happens because of an unfortunate chain of events—at least one genetic aberration, plus one or more things environmental, such as a poor diet. Say it takes three "strikes" in order for cancer to begin: Being born with a faulty gene might be worth one or two strikes; add a lifetime of eating the wrong foods (or not eating the right ones); and bingo—strike three.

An estimated 250,000 American men may carry one of these defective genes, which can be inherited from *either parent:* Briefly, if your father or brother has prostate cancer, your risk is two times greater than the average American man's, which is about 16 percent. It goes up from there: Depending on the number of affected relatives you have and the age at which they develop the disease, your risk could be as high as 50 percent if you are in a family that meets the criteria for hereditary prostate cancer— if you have at least three close relatives, such as a father and two brothers affected, or two relatives if both were younger than fifty-five years old when diagnosed; or if your family has disease in three generations—a grandfather, father, or brother. In hereditary prostate cancer families, men should have a digital rectal examination and PSA test every year, beginning at age forty.

Family History

About 25 percent of men with prostate cancer have a family history of it. But only about 9 percent of men have hereditary prostate cancer—an inherited, genetic form (involving mutated genes that can be passed on from either parent) of the disease that develops at a younger age. Simply having a family history of prostate cancer raises your own risk of developing the disease—but it doesn't necessarily mean you have the hereditary form of prostate cancer. How can this be? How can prostate cancer run in families and *not* be inherited? We see this in other forms of cancer (breast cancer, for example), and the explanation is complicated—or, as scientists put it, "multifactoral." In other words, there are several reasons. One is that there could be shared environmental factors—such as eating the same foods, or living in the same geographic location. Another is that if a man's brother, uncle, or father develops the disease, he may be more likely to get his own PSA tested and begin regular screening.

However, there are some aspects of a family history that make it more likely that a family is dealing with the inherited form (see "What Is Hereditary Prostate Cancer?" above). We now understand that men with a hereditary tendency to prostate cancer actually *inherit a mutated gene* (one of the same genes that, in "regular" prostate cancer, mutate over the course of a lifetime). This has two important implications: First, because a man inherited one of these faulty genes, he is more likely to develop prostate cancer, and—*because he has a head start*—to develop it at a younger age. (Thus, as we've noted before, men with a family history of prostate cancer need to start yearly screening earlier, at age forty.) Second, because prostate cancer can be inherited from either your mother or your father, it is crucial that you know the medical history of both sides of your family.

Note: Just because hereditary prostate cancer starts earlier doesn't mean that it isn't *every bit as curable as "regular," or sporadic prostate cancer.* In a Johns Hopkins investigation, patients with hereditary prostate cancer and patients who had *no* family history of prostate cancer were matched based on the pathology of their cancer (all of these terms, signposts for cancer that pathologists look for when they examine the surgically removed tumor, are discussed in Chapter 6). The scientists compared the Gleason score, lymph node status (whether or not cancer had penetrated the lymph nodes), seminal vesicle status, extracapsular penetration (whether cancer had gone beyond the prostate wall), and surgical margins of the men in both groups; then studied the men's follow-up data for ten years after surgery, looking for a detectable PSA level, or any other evidence that cancer had returned. They found no significant difference in either group. Thus, if you have a family history of prostate cancer, you are more likely to develop the disease—but not more likely to die from it.

Scientists didn't always know this much about hereditary prostate cancer. In fact, it took the medical community a long time to recognize that prostate cancer could be inherited at all. In this chapter, we've discussed the various risk factors—including simply getting older—that can make men more prone to prostate cancer. We've seen that prostate cancer is very common—confoundingly so, as a matter of fact. That's why, for decades, researchers downplayed the idea that (just like more conspicuous illnesses such as hemophilia) it could be inherited—even though it was known to run in families. Thirty years ago, genealogists in Utah noted that prostate cancer seemed to "cluster" in families. They found that if a man's father died of prostate cancer, his own risk of dying of prostate cancer was two- or threefold greater. Even more striking, they found that, among familial cancers, this clustering of prostate cancer was actually more common than breast or colon cancer—yet both of these diseases were recognized much earlier to have a hereditary predisposition. In order of "familiality" (an index of how likely it is for a cancer to run in families), the common cancers are ranked in this order: melanoma, ovarian cancer, prostate cancer, colon cancer, and breast cancer. This observation was reinforced recently in a large Scandinavian study of identical twins; researchers found that hereditary factors were highest for prostate cancer, explaining 42 percent of the risk of developing the disease, and lower for colon and breast cancer (35 and 27 percent, respectively; for more on twins and prostate cancer, see below).

Yet for some reason, prostate cancer got lumped in the category of ailments that happen to come with old age—part of the baggage of aging, in effect. With this perception muddying the water, these observations went relatively unexplored for a couple of decades; scientists just couldn't get past the commonness of prostate cancer. In the 1980s, I began to see increasingly younger men with prostate cancer, and was struck by how many of them had a family history of the disease. Then, in 1986, I met a forty-nine-year-old man with an unforgettable legacy: Every male member of this man's family had died of prostate cancer—his father, his father's three brothers, and his grandfather. At that time, virtually every physician in the United States could reel off the statistics for breast cancer—that a woman's risk increased twofold if her mother or sister had it. It seemed odd to me that there was no similar information available on prostate cancer.

These questions launched the first of a series of studies at Johns Hopkins. The first question: Would the observations that had been pretty much limited to Utah Mormons hold true with a larger, more diverse group of men? A study of 691 patients, who had come to Hopkins for radical prostatectomy, confirmed that having a family history of prostate cancer did indeed increase a man's risk of developing the disease. Next, we ruled out environmental factors; further, our results strongly suggested that increased susceptibility to prostate cancer could be inherited from *either parent* (which we have since proven—see below). We then went on to define and characterize hereditary prostate cancer, showing the clear link between family history and a man's probability of developing prostate cancer (see box, page 65).

Next, out of a pool of 2,500 families that met the criteria for hereditary prostate cancer came an elite group of seventy-nine families—handpicked and rigorously screened. Sadly, these families were the ones hardest hit by prostate cancer—so there could be no mistaking hereditary cancer for terribly bad luck, in which several men in the same family happened to develop the disease. The families filled out detailed questionnaires about their health, occupations, and family history, and sent blood samples, from which the scientists extracted their DNA.

Scientists from Johns Hopkins and colleagues at the National Human Genome Research Institute began scrutinizing these blood samples, using a technique called "linkage analysis," looking for patterns of association between certain portions of chromosomes and the presence of cancer in multiple members of a family or families that couldn't possibly happen just by chance. In this way, they can link cancer to a small segment on a chromosome.

Evidence of at least two defective genes: Slowly but surely, the hard work of the last decade is paying off: Scientists at Johns Hopkins and colleagues at the National Human Genome Research Institute, along with investigators from Sweden, Finland, and the Mayo Clinic, have found good evidence that at least two defective genes do exist: One is located on the long arm of Chromosome 1, and the other, most recently discovered, lies on the X chromosome—a milestone in cancer research, this is the first time the X chromosome (which sons inherit only from their mothers) has been definitively linked to a major cancer.

Although we haven't yet pinpointed the faulty genes on either chromosome, we have identified certain characteristics that suggest which mutation a family may have: In families with a mutated HPC1 gene:

- At least five men in the immediate family, or multiple men in multiple generations, have prostate cancer.
- The average age of diagnosis is younger than sixty-five.
- There is evidence of father-to-son transmission.

In families linked to a mutated HPCX gene, the defect is always passed on from the mother: In this case, a father cannot pass the disease to his son. (X and Y are the "sex" chromosomes, and they have distinct patterns of inheritance. Fathers always pass along the Y chromosome to their sons. A man inherits the X chromosome from his mother—so every man has one X and one Y chromosome. Women have two X chromosomes.)

In an X-linked family, there is no way for a father to pass on a mutated gene on the X chromosome to his son. However, he can pass it on to his daughters, who can then transmit it to their sons—to the man's grandsons. In such families, prostate cancer might seem to skip a generation. On the other hand, HPC1 can be transmitted from *either* the mother or father.

Eventually, as many as a half-dozen different genes will turn out to play a role in HPC. Scientists elsewhere have reported linkage to other sites on Chromosome 1, one of which may also be associated with brain tumors.

This exhaustive search for "the gene" or genes probably won't turn up some weird-looking mutant that instantly calls attention to itself as a cause of cancer. The genes involved here are genes that everybody has: For example, everybody has a BRCA-1 and BRCA-2 gene, both of which are involved in breast cancer. However, everybody *doesn't* have the same sequence of those genes. The sequences fluctuate, like ingredients in a recipe—just as bread and salt dough have the same ingredients; but, depending on the recipe, one is edible and one is not.

What's the next step? Once the precise location of the mutation is pinpointed, we will be able to sequence the gene. At this point, we know that in the families with the mutation on Chromosome 1, *every man who inherited this gene ultimately developed prostate cancer.* Once we have the exact sequence, we can develop genetic tests—so that, for example, if a man with prostate cancer has a strong family history of the disease and he tests positive for this sequence, his male siblings and children could also be tested. If these men are found to carry the mutation, their doctors could follow them very closely. Eventually, we hope, scientists will be able to use the information about what these genes do and how they cause cancer to develop strategies to treat or prevent prostate cancer.

Although it's not always clear when scientists talk about genetics, there are *two kinds of genetic influences.* One of them is what we've been talking about here—true hereditary prostate cancer, which is relatively rare, and accounts for only about 9 percent of all cases of prostate cancer. Hereditary prostate cancer and other inherited diseases are what geneticists call "highly penetrant": If you inherit a specific gene or genes, that's it—you get the disease. But there's a second type of hereditary influence, which is much more common, much more subtle, and leaves the door open to *not* getting cancer. In this case, your genetic makeup may have one or two chinks in it that may have a bearing on whether you get a disease, may increase your susceptibility to it somewhat—but cancer may not be a predestined conclusion. One example of this increased susceptibility—scientists call this a "polymorphism"—we discussed above, a specific "short repeat" of CAG, a protein sequence most likely to be found in African-American men and in Caucasians with metastatic cancer. Another is a variation in the vitamin D receptor gene, which can affect the body's response to vitamin D, and still another is a variant in 5-alpha reductase type II, an enzyme in the prostate that converts testosterone to DHT (dihydrotestosterone), the active male hormone in the prostate. The 5-alpha reductase-II enzyme seems to be more active in white and black American men than in Japanese men. Some scientists have speculated that levels of male hormones correlate with a man's risk of prostate cancer. These studies by and large have been disappointing, with no consistent conclusions. Instead, a more likely explanation is that it's not *how much* of a specific hormone a man has, but the way a man's genes respond to that hormone. It may well be that in some men, a little hormone goes a lot further, and has a much more powerful effect, than in other men. This is how variations in the androgen and vitamin D receptors and 5-alpha reductase enzyme may influence risk of prostate cancer.

What we can learn from twins: One of the best examples of how genetic makeup and environment interact comes from studies of twins. Identical twins have the same DNA; nonidentical, or fraternal, twins are no more alike than brothers. If being born with the same DNA were the only factor that made a man susceptible to prostate cancer, then we would expect that every time one identical twin developed prostate cancer, his brother would soon follow. Fortunately, that is not the case. There have been two major studies of twins and prostate cancer, one from Sweden, and the other a study of U.S. World War II veterans. These studies found that in the vast majority of cases, *both* identical twins did not get cancer. The likelihood of both identical twins developing prostate cancer was 19 percent in one study, and 27 percent in the other. In both studies, the likelihood of non-identical twins both developing cancer was much lower—only 4 percent in one study, and 7 percent in the other. These studies showed that DNA isn't everything: Although identical twins were four to five times more likely to develop the same disease, it was by no means inevitable. Other factors, presumably environmental, must play a stronger role: Indeed, these studies concluded that the relative role of genetic versus environmental factors was 50/50.

Why, if these men had the same DNA environment—basically, the same body—didn't genetics count for more? Because what happens to that body—the influence of environment—is critical. This means that, if you are an identical twin, and your brother has cancer, you are not destined definitely to get the disease. If you and your brother have not made exactly the same lifestyle choices, then your risk for getting prostate cancer is not exactly the same. This message is extremely important: It emphasizes the role of environment in the risk of developing prostate cancer. If, in future studies, scientists could determine how the twins' lifestyles were different, we might be able to understand why the disease occurs in the first place. Studies like this, and of men who inherit the susceptibility genes (in hereditary prostate cancer) but who *do not* get the disease may tell us much about prostate cancer.

Association with other tumors: Cancer researchers have known for years that some families don't just have a higher risk of a particular cancer, but a "cancer syndrome," such as hereditary breast/ovarian cancer syndrome, in which cancer develops at more than one site. (Note: This is different from cancer that starts in one place and then metastasizes, or spreads, throughout the body.) There is no evidence to suggest that hereditary prostate cancer is strongly associated with cancers at other sites, or that it is part of a significant hereditary cancer syndrome. In hereditary breast cancer families, the story is somewhat different: Men who inherit defects in the two breast cancer genes BRCA-1 and BRCA-2 do seem to be at a slightly higher risk of prostate cancer; however, these are not genes involved in hereditary prostate cancer, and their influence is not nearly as strong.

What About Hormones?

Scientists have known for a long time that prostate cancer is under the control of hormones—that men who are castrated before puberty rarely develop prostate cancer, and that men with advanced prostate cancer can be helped by hormone therapy (shutting off the supply of male hormones to the prostate). The complicated relationship between hormones and prostate cancer is discussed in much greater detail above.

Having said that, there is no good evidence that the level of testosterone in the blood can be used to estimate whether a man is more likely or less likely to develop cancer. Instead, as we discussed above, the way the body responds to hormone levels may be more important.

Another class of hormones, called *insulin-like growth factors,* may also influence the development of prostate cancer. These growth factors—which can make prostate cancer cells grow and proliferate—are found in the prostate's epithelial and stromal cells, which have specific receptors for insulin-like growth factor type I (IGF-I). IGF-I receptors are found in advanced prostate cancer cells that can function without help from hormones (these are called androgen-independent cells). IGF can be counteracted by particular proteins that bind to it and block its action in the cells. One study found that prostate cancer risk was higher in men with elevated levels of IGF-I. (For more on IGF as a possible predictor of prostate cancer, see Chapter 5.)

DHEA: If there is no association between hormone levels and the development of prostate cancer, is it okay for a man to "pump up" his testosterone levels? The answer here is categorically *no!* DHEA (dehydroepiandrosterone) is a dietary supplement; you can buy it at any health food store. Many men do—because DHEA levels drop as a man ages, and the hope is that boosting DHEA will be the proverbial fountain of youth. It isn't. Worse, there's a risk involved in taking hormones. If a man has latent prostate cancer (the "incidental" kind discussed above), it is possible that this could be like pouring kerosene on a fire. It should go without saying that any man who has had prostate cancer should *never* take any form of male hormone supplementation. As a recent review of DHEA concluded: "There is no convincing evidence that DHEA has any beneficial effect on aging or any disease. Patients would be well advised not to take it."

But what if your testosterone is low, and your doctor wants to treat you with supplemental testosterone? Is this okay? Again, it's probably not a good idea unless you are tested first, to be sure you don't have cancer. Having low testosterone doesn't mean you won't get prostate cancer; one study, in fact, showed that a number of men with low testosterone *did* have prostate cancer. Thus, if you are a man at risk of developing prostate cancer because of your age or family history, and if a doctor tells you that you need extra testosterone because your own levels of this male hormone are low, you should probably have a needle biopsy of the prostate first, just to rule out cancer. PSA levels are driven by testosterone, and if your testosterone level is low, your PSA level could be falsely low—low enough to "fake out" your doctor. Although there is not a wealth of scientific information on this subject, there are enough red flags raised here to suggest extreme caution when tampering with hormones.

Other Risk Factors

This section is a compilation of loose ends that scientists haven't figured out what to do with. For example:

Occupation: The only occupation that has been found to have a higher risk of prostate cancer is farming. This has been shown in a number of studies. For example: One University of Iowa study found

TABLE 3.4

PROSTATE CANCER RUNS IN MY FAMILY:
WHAT'S MY RISK OF HEREDITARY PROSTATE CANCER?

Just because you have a family history of prostate cancer, this doesn't mean that you are definitely going to develop the disease. After all, prostate cancer affects millions of men worldwide, and it may just be coincidence that your father or brother develops the disease. However, the likelihood of this happening goes up if one of your family members develops it at a younger age, or if several members of your family have prostate cancer. For example: Say your father developed prostate cancer at age seventy, and nobody else in your family has the disease. Although your risk is probably somewhat greater than someone without a family history of prostate cancer, in this example we'll set your *relative risk* at one. *Note: These risks are "relative." They are not absolute, but designed to give you an approximation.* Now, if your father developed prostate cancer at age sixty, your risk would be 50 percent higher; if he developed it at age fifty, your risk would now be twice as high.

What if your father developed prostate cancer at age seventy, but your brother also developed it? Your risk would now be four times higher. And if your father developed it when he was fifty, and your brother has it, your risk is seven times higher. This is why it's so important to know not only who in your family has had prostate cancer, but how old he was when he developed it. And remember, increased risk of prostate cancer can be passed on by both sides of the family—so it's important to know the health history of your mother's father and brothers, too.

Age at Diagnosis	Additional Relatives	Relative Risk
70	None	1.0
60	None	1.5
50	None	2.0
70	1 or more	4.0
60	1 or more	5.0
50	1 or more	7.0

Iowa farmers to be at a higher risk of dying from certain cancers, including prostate cancer. The question, however, is why? Is it due to lifestyle? It is very hard to know what to do with information from this type of study, because it is so difficult to separate what people *are*—their family history—from what they *do*—their eating habits. For example, in some studies farmers have been shown to have more fat in their diet, and to eat fewer fruits and vegetables. (The Iowa study found that farmers had a higher total energy intake, consumed higher levels of protein, fat, and saturated fat—and ate more red meat—than other men; in addition, older farmers ate fewer fruits and vegetables than other men their same age.)

Nonetheless, one plausible explanation for a link between farming and prostate cancer may be an increased lifetime exposure to agricultural chemicals, particularly herbicides (some of these concentrate in fat; also, some affect body chemistry by causing a drop in estrogen levels). Researchers from the National Academy of Sciences looked at agricultural exposure to herbicides, and concluded that there was some evidence that this made men more susceptible to prostate cancer. As a result of this study, the U.S. government agreed to provide service-connected disability for any veteran who was in Vietnam and who develops prostate cancer. According to the Department of Veterans Affairs, "Vietnam veterans who believe they have health problems that may be related to their exposure to Agent Orange while serving in Vietnam or their survivors should contact the nearest VA medical center or regional office. VA's nationwide toll-free number is 1-800-827-1000." Vietnam veterans interested in finding out more may also want to contact the Vietnam Veterans of America, 1224 M Street, N.W., Washington, D.C. 20005-5183; or call 1-800-VVA-1316, or 1-202-628-2700; internet address: http://www.vva.org. The VVA is a nonprofit, congressionally chartered, veterans service organization dedicated to helping veterans and their families receive benefits and services.

Things That Do Not Increase the Risk of Prostate Cancer

Vasectomy: Why is it that so many men who are diagnosed with prostate cancer are men who have had a vasectomy? One reason is that vasectomy is very common; a lot of men have had one. It is felt that these men, having established a professional relationship with a urologist, are more likely to go back to a urologist—and urologists are probably more likely than other physicians to look for prostate cancer.

Cigarette smoking: Although several studies have suggested that smoking cigarettes raises a man's risk of developing prostate cancer, there is no solid evidence that proves it. However, because each puff of a cigarette injects nicotine and a bunch of toxic chemicals into every cell of your body, it's probably a safe bet that smoking doesn't *lower* a man's odds of getting prostate cancer. A panel of scientists recently concluded that smokers who have prostate cancer are more likely to die from it. However, smokers apparently are no more likely to *develop* it in the first place than anybody else.

Sexual activity: Some people worry that increased sexual activity can cause prostate cancer, because of the mistaken belief that ejaculation causes an increase in testosterone levels. This is not true. There is no good reason to believe that having an active sex life would stimulate the prostate to grow, or cause prostate cancer. In fact, at least one conclusive study has shown that priests have the same risk of prostate cancer as married men.

Other prostate problems: There is no evidence that having prostatitis or BPH (benign prostatic hyperplasia, or enlargement) increases a man's risk of developing prostate cancer. However, the good news here is that having other prostate problems makes it more likely that a man's cancer will be diagnosed as early as possible.

Physical activity: No strong proof has been found to link a man's exercise or occupational exertion—or the lack of it—to prostate cancer. In fact, the evidence is simply contradictory; one recent study stated that cardiorespiratory fitness and physical activities may protect against the development of prostate cancer, while another study found that physical activity may increase the risk. If being sedentary or the opposite, very active, plays a role in the development of prostate cancer, it is a bit part at best.

Now that we've talked about what causes—and doesn't cause—prostate cancer, the next step is to turn this around, and see how we can *prevent* it. The main focus of prevention is diet: not only avoiding those "sins of commission"—keeping away from foods that probably encourage cancer—but reversing those "sins of omission," by identifying and eating foods that actually fight cancer. On to Chapter 4.

4

CAN PROSTATE CANCER
BE PREVENTED?

Read This First

Ultimately, the way we'd prefer to treat all cancers is to prevent them from happening in the first place. One day, in the not too distant future, we hope to look back on the era of cancer—just as we now reflect on the eras of polio and smallpox—as a plague of the past. It sounds like wishful thinking—an ideal right up there with eliminating poverty and crime. And yet, scientists firmly believe that one day this will happen. Until then, what do we do?

In the last chapter, we talked about what most likely *causes* prostate cancer—oxidative damage to DNA. It's a domino effect—a cascade of genetic changes, in which a normal cell is transformed into a cancerous cell. These changes can happen before birth, in men with hereditary prostate cancer, or—as is the case with most men who get prostate cancer—they can happen over the course of a lifetime.

When we talk about the environment causing cancer, mostly we mean diet—the high-fat, low-vegetable-and-fruit Western diet that clogs our arteries and also, it seems, makes us more prone to cancer.

Thus, if a man's diet—every bite of cheeseburger, or hot dog, or sausage-bacon-biscuit—can contribute to these incremental changes that somehow push a cell over the edge and make it cancerous, is it possible that changing what he eats can also lower his risk of developing prostate cancer? Yes. The problem now is, what do we eat instead? And how long do we have to eat these other things for it to show an effect?

This is what scientists are trying to do now, determine the specifics of a cancer-fighting diet.

Scientists worldwide are working to isolate specific cancer-fighting substances in the hopes of making "nutraceuticals," or drugs extracted from specific nutrients. This is very exciting work. And yet, to put it in perspective, much of this research is simply confirming something scientists have known for decades, an inescapable finding so basic that it easily could be put into the category called "Duh!" *The best way to prevent cancer is to eat more fruits and vegetables, eat less red meat—consume fewer calories in general—and burn off a few of those calories with regular exercise.* This is why the American Cancer Society, for years, has made the following recommendations: Make sure most of what you eat comes from plants. Eat five or more servings of fruits and vegetables a day, and other foods from "plant sources," including breads, grains, rice, pasta, or beans, several times a day. Eat foods low in fat, and limit your consumption of meats, particularly meat high in fat. Stay within your healthy weight range (see the body mass index in Chapter 3), and get at least moderate exercise for thirty minutes or more, most days of the week.

Finally, eating all of the broccoli and good things in the world—though it may well make a difference in the long run—doesn't take away your risk of having prostate cancer right now. If you are age fifty or older, you need more than a good diet can guarantee. If you have a family history of prostate cancer, or are African-American, you need it sooner—a yearly rectal exam and PSA test, beginning at age forty.

How Food Can Help Your Body Fight Cancer

We've talked about the things that cause prostate cancer, including such environmental factors as food. But could it be that foods can actually help prevent prostate cancer? Can we use food as preventive medicine? Yes: In fact, many scientists believe this is what Asian men do every day, and why these men—who develop the same "incidental" prostate cancer that's found in all men (see Chapter 3)—so rarely develop prostate cancer that needs to be treated.

How can diet help your body fight prostate cancer? There are two main ways: The first is in *preventing or delaying onset of the disease.* Cancer that is big enough to be diagnosed today probably started growing at least ten years ago (this is discussed in Chapter 3). Most men are diagnosed with prostate cancer in their late sixties. This means that even men in their fifties and early sixties should be able to make a significant difference in their body's ability to fight off cancer. The second area of promise is in *slowing the growth of cancer that has already begun.* Here, diet is one of several avenues being explored to lengthen the life of a man with established or advanced prostate cancer—with the ultimate goal of managing it as a chronic disease, like diabetes or even AIDS, which may not be possible to cure, but which can be controlled for many years.

Compared to research in other aspects of medicine, the idea of altering the course of cancer with diet is relatively new. As a urologist at Memorial Sloan-Kettering Cancer Center recently commented, Western medicine has been characterized by a search for the "magic bullet," a "unidimensional attempt to find a single answer to the cause of the disease. We are continually looking for the *one* antibiotic to cure the infection, the *one* agent to cure cancer." Fortunately, this is changing, and so is this idea of medicinal "one-stop shopping." If you were to spend an afternoon in a library reading the medical journals published during the last decade, you would notice that the number of scientific articles pertaining to nutrition, nutritional supplements (vitamins, herbs, and minerals), and disease has skyrocketed in recent years. Now, scientists worldwide are working to isolate specific cancer-fighting substances—some of which we'll discuss in a moment—in the hopes of making "nutraceuticals," or drugs extracted from specific nutrients. This is very exciting work.

And yet, to put it in perspective, much of this research is simply confirming something scientists have known for decades, an inescapable finding so basic that it easily could be put into the category called "Duh!" *The best way to prevent cancer is to eat more fruits and vegetables, eat less red meat—consume fewer calories in general—and burn off a few of those calories with regular exercise.* This is why the

American Cancer Society, for years, has made the following recommendations: Make sure most of what you eat comes from plants. Eat five or more servings of fruits and vegetables a day, and other foods from "plant sources," including breads, grains, rice, pasta, or beans, several times a day. Eat foods low in fat, and limit your consumption of meats, particularly meat high in fat. Stay within your healthy weight range (see the body mass index in Chapter 3), and get at least moderate exercise for thirty minutes or more, most days of the week.

Although this message obviously makes good sense, it seems to be one that doesn't stick, or resonate, with the general public: Way back in 1898, in the medical journal *The Lancet*, a scientist wrote a scathing condemnation of Victorian dietary excess and its negative effect on health: "In England, four and a half times as many people die now from cancer as half a century ago. Probably no single factor is more important in determining the outbreak of cancer in the predisposed than high feeding. Many indications point to the gluttonous consumption of meat as likely to be especially harmful. Statistics show that the consumption of meat has reached the amazing total of 131 pounds per head per year, which is more than double what it was half a century ago. No doubt other factors co-operate, among these I should be inclined to name deficient exercise and deficiency in fresh vegetable food." More than a century later, what's the most popular crash diet craze in America? One that eschews balance, a high-fat diet that relies heavily on meats and protein.

Recently, in an editorial in an American medical journal, the president-elect of the American Cancer Society and other leading scientists stated flatly: "Cancer is largely a preventable illness. Two thirds of cancer deaths in the U.S. can be linked to tobacco use, poor diet, obesity, and lack of exercise, all of which can be modified." Eating a poor diet, these scientists added, is quantitatively as big a risk factor for cancer development as smoking tobacco. They cited evidence that eating a lot of fruits and vegetables reduces the risk of many forms of cancer, "including cancers of the lung, stomach, colon, esophagus, and larynx." Studies suggest that eating more legumes and grains lowers the risk of stomach and pancreatic cancer. Finally, "total fat intake and saturated animal fats are linked to the occurrence of hormone-related, lung, and colorectal cancers." Prostate cancer and breast cancer, both hormone-related, fall into this last category. A recent study published in the *Journal of the American Medical Association* suggests that women who eat a diet rich in fruits, vegetables, whole grains, and low-fat meat and dairy products may lower their risk of dying from cancer, heart disease, and stroke by a significant amount—as much as 30 percent. These results, the investigators said, suggest a "simpler approach" to achieving good health.

The foods discussed in this chapter are part of this simpler approach, they make good sense, and most of them have been put to practical use for centuries—in Asia, where clinical prostate cancer hardly exists. As we take a look at the most promising of these candidates for prostate cancer prevention, remember one final caveat: *Moderation in all things* (see "Don't Overdo It, Especially with Herbal Remedies," below). The Asian diet isn't all soy, all the time—or all

---

THE COMPLICATED BUSINESS OF FOOD RESEARCH

Think, for a moment, of the many nutrients you ingest every day—hundreds of them, in varying portions. Look at the labels of prepared foods—your morning cereal, a box of cake mix, a package of frozen lasagna, even a slice of bread—and consider just how many different things you're putting into your body with every meal.

Now imagine you're a scientist exploring the link between diet and prostate cancer, trying to figure out exactly what's wrong with the Western diet, or what's right with the Asian diet. Where do you begin? How many Americans eat one-ingredient meals? In the U.S., even a pet goldfish consumes more than a dozen nutrients in a single flake of fish food. But even the simplest meal—a plain potato, with no butter, salt, or pepper, for example—raises a host of questions: What is it about that potato that might raise or lower cancer risk? Is it (as many believe) selenium, a nutrient abundant in potatoes and other root vegetables? Or is it something else? Is it something found in all potatoes, or does it vary, depending on the mineral content of the soil in which *that particular potato* was grown?

Get the picture? Food research is intensely complicated, frustrating—because what seems obvious in lab studies, in petri dishes and test tubes, doesn't always pan out when those same tests are attempted in humans—and time-consuming. Say the scientist isolates a food or nutrient that actually seems to prevent prostate cancer. What's the dose? How much of it, in other words, does a man need, per day, per week, to achieve the desired effect? Will he have to take it forever? These aren't short-term questions, and it will take several years, at minimum, before we can find the answers.

green tea, or all anything in particular. It's a variety of foods, eaten in a balanced way. Because all of this research is still unfolding, take the findings from any of these early studies with—continuing the food metaphor—a big grain of salt. Remember, it is possible to overdose on just about *anything*. The most harmless substances can make you sick if you eat or drink too much of them. Even water—if you drink huge amounts of it in too short a time—can be harmful, causing toxic imbalances in the body's electrolytes. This is why you must resist the "more is better" approach: "If 200 micrograms of selenium are good for me, then 1,000 must be even more beneficial." Such thinking is dangerous. The body is a delicate thing, and no matter how tough yours may be, you can easily get too much of a good thing, and defeat the purpose of trying to stay healthy.

A Word on Oxidative Damage

Remember the foods in the category of "sins of commission"— red meat loaded with animal fat, plus charred meat? They're bad, as far as cancer goes, because they hamper the body's ability to fend off *oxidative damage.* In oxidative damage, cells are injured by free radicals—volatile molecules that cause a buildup of toxic by-products in cells. (See Chapter 3.) Normally, free radicals are helpful things— rushing like the local militia to a scene of unrest, fighting bacteria and other foreign invaders. And normally, the body makes substances that are able to control free radicals and limit their damage. The most important of these substances is the enzyme we discussed in the last chapter, with the difficult name of glutathione-S-transferase-π(pronounced "pie," called GST-π for short), which provides toxic cleanup in cells.

Johns Hopkins oncologist William G. Nelson, M.D., Ph.D., was the first to figure out GST-π's role in prostate cancer. He showed that in all cancers, and even in the cells that are not yet cancerous, but well on their way (these cells are called PIN, discussed in Chapter 6), GST-π is knocked out—it is simply not there to prevent oxidative damage. If cancer is a chain reaction—one genetic mistake, or mutation, that leads to another, and so on—then what happens to this enzyme, he believes, is probably among the very earliest events.

The attack against GST-π—apparently all that stands in the way of prostate cells and potentially toxic agents—happens first. It's the preemptive strike. If you were planning to break into a bank, your first move would be to take out the security system. The theory is the same here: Without this cancer-fighting enzyme, prostate cells are far less able to detoxify carcinogens—and thus are more vulnerable to prostate cancer.

Several years ago, Nelson began to wonder: If GST-π can be knocked out by bad environmental agents, can the reverse happen? Can it also be *stimulated*? Is there some dietary equivalent to Charles Atlas that can build up the wimpy hero before it's too late, so it can fend for itself—and perhaps deter prostate cancer? In other words, is it possible to use food, or some particular nutrient, as preventive medicine?

Nelson, a pioneer in this area, is not alone: All over the world, scientists in many disciplines are studying diet as never before—for the first time, trying to understand exactly how specific foods work in the body, right down to which particular enzymes (like GST-π) are helped or hurt by what we eat and drink. Where are the smoking guns—the cancer instigators? Again, the basic "omission versus commission" question: Is it something we eat too much of, or something we routinely omit from our meals?

How much fat? If too much animal fat is bad, how much fat is not bad? How much fat is it okay to eat? The answer from several studies seems to be that *no more than 20 percent of your total calories should be in the form of fat.* In interesting research from the Memorial Sloan-Kettering Cancer Center, scientists investigated how dietary fat influenced mice with palpable prostate cancer. In animals that had a 40 percent fat diet, the tumor grew as the scientists expected it would. But in one group of mice, the fat content was cut in half—to 20 percent—and their tumors were smaller, and grew at a much slower rate. "To our knowledge," said the researchers, "this is the first demonstration that changing the fat composition of an animal's diet could alter the growth rate of already established prostatic tumors, and raises the possibility that nutritional changes may be worthy of consideration as a means of augmenting the effectiveness of other therapies in the treatment of prostate cancer."

What does a 20 percent fat diet mean for you? If you weigh about 150 pounds, your caloric intake should be about 2,000 kilocalories (when doctors talk about "calories," they really mean kilocalories) a day. There are 9 kilocalories in each gram of fat. Thus, you should have no more than 44 grams a day of fat.

FRUITS AND VEGETABLES? WHY EAT "FIVE A DAY"?

What exactly is it about fruits and vegetables that makes it so important for the American Cancer Society to recommend that we eat at least five servings a day? Well, some of them contain known antioxidants, such as selenium and lycopene. Others—cruciferous vegetables such as broccoli, brussels sprouts, and cauliflower—contain an ingredient called sulforaphane, which acts by increasing the amount of GST-π in cells. The result: Your cells make more of their own natural antioxidants, so they can do a better job of fighting off cancer.

Note: One study suggests that, for prostate cancer at least, vegetables do more than fruits (although fruits are just plain good for you in general, and you still need to eat them, or drink fruit juice, every day). This study, published in the *Journal of the National Cancer Institute*, found no link between fruit intake and prostate cancer risk, but confirmed what other studies have shown—that eating a lot of vegetables, particularly the cruciferous kind, lowered the risk.

Note: It is not clear that a percentage of fat lower than 20 percent would be even more successful, or whether there would be a point of diminishing returns. That's just as well, because in the United States it is virtually impossible to avoid fat altogether. At almost any restaurant, if you eat a typical menu item—a jumbo beef burrito, or a bacon-cheese omelet, for instance—you could blow several days' worth of fat content in a single meal. Look at what we Americans like to eat: french *fries, fried* potato chips, *fried* chicken (notice a theme here?), multiple-*meat* pizzas, ice *cream*—they're all loaded with fat. Even the vegetable offerings at many eateries—such as *fried* zucchini, or onion rings—are not designed with cancer prevention in mind. Your best bet is to check the labels of packaged foods, and the fat content of food in restaurants (many big restaurant chains provide this information).

Selenium

Selenium is a mineral in the soil. It appears in fruits and vegetables, and also in meats and fish. The average American probably eats about 70 micrograms of selenium a day. However, this can vary, depending on where we live—and, more importantly, where the food we eat has been grown—because some soils are far richer in selenium than others.

THE FIZZLE OF BETA-CAROTENE

Beta-carotene was a milestone in dietary research, and it's important for you to know about it for the simple fact that here was a substance, extracted from vegetables, that sounded good, seemed promising in every way, but shocked everyone when it turned out to be a dud. This has had a profound impact on scientists who study diet and cancer, whose great fear is to end up with "another beta-carotene."

A few years ago, in several case-controlled studies, scientists noticed that smokers who ate a lot of fruits and vegetables seemed to be protected against lung cancer. What, in particular, was it about fruits and vegetables that warded off cancer? The scientists homed in on beta-carotene, a nutrient that's rich in vegetables. They wondered if beta-carotene could be a biomarker—a sort of barometer in the bloodstream—hypothesizing that people with high levels of beta-carotene would have a lower risk of lung cancer. Sure enough, in early studies with lab animals, beta-carotene performed like a champ, seeming to protect against several kinds of cancers. Suddenly, beta-carotene was the hot new scientific flavor of the month, the focus of three separate studies. But then look what happened: "*All* of them showed not only that beta-carotene did not do what it was predicted to do and prevent lung cancer development—in two of the trials, it actually made things worse," explains Johns Hopkins scientist William Nelson. In one study, men who received beta-carotene had an 18 percent increase in the incidence of lung cancer. Also, their rate of prostate cancer was 23 percent higher, and the death rate in these men was 15 percent higher than in men who did not receive the beta-carotene.

Beta-carotene turned out to be a cautionary tale, which confirmed the perils of leaping before looking—and on the wrong bandwagon, no less. There may be several explanations for these results—whether the men continued smoking, for instance, and how beta-carotene affected their lungs. In any event, the story of beta-carotene highlights yet again the trouble of trying to pinpoint an element of diet and determine whether it has the power to prevent cancer.

In a large study several years ago, people who had been treated for skin cancer were given selenium supplements, in hopes of preventing the cancer from coming back. During the course of the study, the researchers noticed that the patients getting selenium developed fewer other cancers—prostate, lung, colon—than patients in the placebo group. The incidence of prostate cancer in these men, in fact, was two-thirds less than that of the men in the placebo group.

Their intriguing results prompted Johns Hopkins researchers to design their own case-control study of selenium's beneficial role in prostate cancer, using the valuable database of the Baltimore Longitudinal Study of Aging (a study begun more than forty years ago and involving about 1,500 men, who return every other year for physical examinations and medical tests). In this study, the Hopkins scientists studied fifty-two men with prostate cancer and ninety-six "age-matched controls," men of the same age who did not have cancer. Their findings were exciting: For one thing, they discovered that in *both* of these groups—men who developed prostate cancer, and men who did not—the level of selenium in the blood dropped over time. In other words, selenium apparently decreases in everybody, with age. "Yet, no other cancer increases more rapidly with age than prostate cancer," notes Johns Hopkins urologist H. Ballentine Carter, M.D. "For all we know, selenium levels are playing a role in that." This investigation also confirmed what the skin cancer study had suggested—that selenium seems to protect against prostate cancer. *In the Hopkins study, men with the lowest levels of selenium were those most likely to develop prostate cancer, and men with the highest levels of selenium were almost 50 percent less likely to develop it.* Other studies have shown that people living in regions of the U.S. with selenium-rich soil have fewer deaths from many kinds of cancer—including cancer of the lung, colon, esophagus, pancreas, breast, and ovary. One recent study looked at the level of selenium in toenails (the idea being that toenails—like rings on a tree—tell a story of the body's intake of minerals over the last year or so). This study, too, found that men with the highest levels of selenium were significantly less likely to have prostate cancer.

How does it work? It turns out that selenium is an essential component of an antioxidant—glutathione peroxidase, an enzyme like glutathione-S-transferase-π that helps the body fight off potentially toxic substances. One of the most exciting things about selenium is that it seems to make a difference in the body within just a few years—which encourages scientists to think that a man can take it later in life, and still potentially change the course of prostate cancer. A large, nationwide trial of selenium supplementation is now under way.

Some scientists speculate that in the future, when men go to the doctor for a PSA blood test, they will also have their selenium level checked. If it turns out to be low, just taking a selenium supplement (already available where most vitamins are sold) a day, for several years or maybe a lifetime—may help prevent prostate cancer. It may be that selenium and vitamin E work better together than either separately; some studies have suggested that these two antioxidants act synergistically—that is, each makes the other work better. For this reason, the National Cancer Institute is sponsoring a twelve-year nationwide trial, in which 32,000 men will be given either vitamin E alone, selenium alone, both vitamin E and selenium, or a placebo. The scientists in this study will be looking to see which of these men develop prostate cancer—and which of these supplements, if any, seems to have a protective effect. Biopsies will be performed on men who develop an elevated PSA, or cancer that can be felt in a rectal exam.

In the meantime, should you take selenium, and how much? See "Now What Do I Do?" below.

Vitamin E

Vitamin E may turn out to be the silver lining in the cloud that was the beta-carotene phenomenon (see "The Fizzle of Beta-Carotene," above). In one beta-carotene study in Finland, more than 29,000 men—all of whom smoked—were given either supplements of vitamin E alone, beta-carotene alone, or both compounds, or a placebo, for five to eight years. The men in both vitamin E groups (with or without beta-carotene) had a death rate from prostate cancer that was 41 percent lower than that of the other men. (Another benefit of the vitamin E: Men taking it seemed to be less troubled by symptoms of BPH, benign enlargement of the prostate.) Another study of male smokers had similar findings—men with low levels of vitamin E in their blood were found to be at higher risk of developing prostate cancer. In laboratory studies, vitamin E—an antioxidant, a free radical fighter—has been shown to slow down cancer growth; it also may have a boosting effect on the body's immune system, to help it battle cancer more effectively.

Is vitamin E protective against prostate cancer? Is it more protective in smokers than in other men? These questions are still being answered, and debated. One Harvard study, published in *Cancer Epidemiology: Biomarkers and Prevention*, found no overall decrease in prostate cancer in men who took vitamin E supplements (of 100 IU a day), and a questionable decrease even in men who smoked. However, many scientists believe vitamin E has great potential, perhaps in combination with selenium (see above).

How much should you take? See "Now What Do I Do?" below. Note: Too much vitamin E can be dangerous, especially if you are taking aspirin or a blood-thinner such as warfarin. Like aspirin and warfarin, vitamin E reduces the blood's ability to clot. Before you jump on the vitamin E (or any) bandwagon, talk to your doctor to make sure this is safe for you. Also, you must stop taking vitamin E before you undergo any surgical procedure, to avoid the risk of excess bleeding. (Find this out from your surgeon at least three weeks ahead of time, so your blood will be back to normal well before surgery.)

Soy: Isoflavones, Phytoestrogens, and Genistein

Is soy really a wonder drug? Or does it simply prevent cancer because of all the things soy-eaters are *not* eating instead? (Back to the old "sins of commission" versus "sins of omission" argument.) For example, there aren't many Big Macs in the Asian diet.

Increasingly, scientific evidence suggests that it's more than what soy eaters *don't* eat. In fact, although advertisements proclaim bananas as "quite possibly nature's most perfect food," the many proponents of soy as a cancer-fighter have good reason to disagree. In laboratory studies, an extract of soy has been shown to inhibit growth of prostate cancer. It doesn't prevent it from forming altogether, but the slow-growing cancer is much more like that "incidental" cancer found in Asian men (see Chapter 3)—the kind that is rarely big enough to diagnose, and rarely causes a problem.

What, exactly, is soy? It's soybeans, and the many products made from them: tofu (which comes in various forms and textures), soy sauce, soy tempeh (blocks made from cooked soybeans), soy milk, flour, and a host—rapidly expanding—of other products. "Phytochemicals" are chemicals that come from fruits and vegetables ("phyto" means vegetable matter). There is a particular class of phytochemicals in soy called *isoflavones*, and the biggest of these—and the one stirring up the most scientific interest—is called *genistein.*

In the late 1980s, genistein entered the field of potential anticancer agents when laboratory studies showed that it could inhibit a key enzyme—the epidermal growth factor tyrosine kinase, which speeds up cell division (thus, it could slow tumor growth). Since then, genistein has also been found to block proliferation of glandular cells (such as those found in the prostate), and to thwart a process called *angiogenesis*. Angiogenesis (which we'll discuss further in Chapter 12) is the laying down of new blood vessels, and this is a major way that cancers spread—paving the road ahead of themselves. Cancer needs a ready blood supply. If this process is blocked—by something called an angiogenesis inhibitor—then the cancer can't go anywhere. It doesn't die, but it doesn't grow. Some scientists believe that isoflavones such as genistein could prevent tumor promotion or progression simply by blocking formation of new blood supplies. Genistein is also what's called a *phytoestrogen;* it has the properties of a weak form of estrogen. It has been found to inhibit breast cancer cells in laboratory studies. Other studies have shown that newborn rats given genistein had a lower incidence of breast cancers, that genistein can restrain the growth of prostate cancer cells and lower PSA.

For most Asians, soy is a mealtime staple. For most Americans—although this is slowly changing—it's barely a blip on the dietary horizon. Consider these statistics: Most American men eat only 1 to 3 milligrams of isoflavones a day. In contrast, the average Japanese man consumes an estimated 12 milligrams a day. The blood levels of isoflavones may be at least seven times higher in Japanese men than in men on the typical Western diet—and maybe much higher.

Et tu, tofu? Remember, the key to all of this, even soy, is: Moderation in all things. This was suggested yet again by the unexpected results of one long-term study, the thirty-five-year longitudinal Honolulu-Asia Aging study, of the effects of different foods on rates of disease, aging, and death. In this study, 3,734 surviving participants over age seventy answered questions about their eating and drinking habits, including their consumption of rice, fish, meat, soy products, milk, green tea, and coffee.

Surprisingly, the researchers found that elderly Japanese-American men who ate tofu regularly during midlife showed more cognitive decline in their later years than those who didn't eat so much tofu. The increased rates of cognitive decline were "roughly of the magnitude as would be caused by a four-year difference in age," said the Honolulu researchers, who reported their findings in the *Journal of the American College of Nutrition.* Only tofu, they found, could be linked to this decline: 96 percent of the men who "almost never" ate tofu had normal cognitive function (based on screening tests, adjusted for age and education)—compared to 80.7 percent of the men who ate tofu more than four times a week.

These results have engendered much speculation as to how this could be, that tofu might have an adverse effect on the aging brain. One theory is that tofu is high in glutamate, a neurotransmitter (a chemical messenger in the brain), and elevated levels of glutamate can cause free radical damage to brain nerve cells, called neurons. However, as with any study of diet, it's tough to be certain. For example, researchers noted, it may be that the men who ate large quantities of tofu were from poorer families, and the lower cognitive ability was due to inadequate nourishment in childhood. In any event, we can be sure that many scientists will be seeking answers here. What does this mean for you? Again, moderation.

Carotenoids: Vitamin A and Lycopene

There are two main types of vitamin A: One, called "preformed vitamin A," comes from animals. This is the kind of vitamin A that most Americans get. The other is a carotenoid—a pigment, found in green and yellow vegetables. Guess which kind is found most in the Asian diet? Yes, the carotenoid. It's hard to know what to make of vitamin A (see "The Fizzle of Beta-Carotene," above), because there is conflicting evidence: Although one group of researchers, in laboratory experiments with mice, found that vitamin A could reduce the incidence of prostate cancer, other studies suggest that not only does vitamin A *not* protect against prostate cancer, it might even increase a man's risk of getting it.

And yet, vitamin A is known to help cell differentiation. Cell differentiation is discussed more in Chapter 6, but the idea here is that normal tissue, and even slow-growing and "incidental" cancers, are well differentiated. Well-differentiated cells, as seen under the microscope, have distinct, clearly defined borders and clear centers, and their growth is relatively slow and orderly. Poorly differentiated cells are murkier, not so well defined, and as cancer progresses they seem to melt together into aggressive, malignant blobs. In the Gleason grading system, well-differentiated cells are given a low grade, and the more dangerous, poorly differentiated cells are given a high grade. The advice here is to keep eating carrots and other vegetables—which we know are good for you, even if we haven't yet pinpointed the exact reason why they are.

Lycopene: Today, the most exciting member of the group of carotenoids (although this one can't be converted to vitamin A) is another antioxidant—a free radical fighter that combats oxidative damage—called lycopene. In laboratory studies, lycopene has been found to slow the growth of endometrial cancer cells, certain breast cancer cells, and some forms of lung cancer and leukemia.

Lycopene, found in tomatoes, red grapefruits, watermelons, and berries, entered the world of potential prostate cancer preventers a few years ago, as scientists studied results of a food frequency questionnaire (an analysis of diet). Of the men who had a lower incidence of prostate cancer, the common theme seemed to be food with cooked tomatoes—tomato sauce, like pizza or spaghetti. (Cooking appears to release more of the lycopene in tomatoes, so that tomato-based pasta sauces and soups may be especially beneficial.) The scientists zeroed in on lycopene as the likely reason for this decrease in cancer. However, although this idea is very popular—a great excuse to eat pizza and spaghetti—it remains to be seen whether or not lycopene can protect the body against prostate cancer. In fact, in one set of laboratory experiments, lycopene made no difference in tumor growth in mice with prostate cancer. So here again, the jury's still out. Before doctors can recommend lycopene as a probable cancer preventative, there are several "next steps" in this research that need to happen. Do men with prostate cancer have less lycopene in their prostates than men who don't have it? (The prostate seems to like lycopene. For one thing, lycopene—unlike many substances, including some medications—actually is absorbed by the prostate; for another, levels of lycopene are higher here than anywhere else in the body.) Are there lower levels among people who are *going* to get prostate cancer?" (This could be tested in a study such as the Baltimore Longitudinal Study of Aging, which has decades' worth of data already stockpiled, monitoring the levels of lycopene in the blood samples of men as they age.) Then, what do lycopene supplements actually do in men? One problem with studying any potential preventive treatment in prostate cancer is that such outcomes can take years. On the plus side for lycopene is the simple fact that—unlike many substances, including some antibiotics—it does manage to reach the prostate. Theoretically, it could work. In any event, it certainly won't hurt you to eat more tomato sauce.

Green Tea

In Asia, many people drink more green tea than they do water—and many scientists believe the tea (like the other two nonherbal teas, black tea and oolong) has healthful, healing properties. Scientific evidence suggests that tea may help prevent cancer of the esophagus, and maybe other cancers as well, including cancer of the pancreas, colon, and liver. It also may be beneficial to the heart.

The key is in the brewing: Interestingly, green, black, and oolong tea are all harvested *from the same plant.* The difference is in what happens to the plant next. If it's processed (by heating the leaves) right away, the leaves stay green and produce green tea. If the leaves are heated a bit later, the result is oolong tea; heating the leaves even later than this produces black tea. Despite their differences in taste and appearance, black and green teas (iced or hot) contain many of the same chemicals—including polyphenols, chemicals that are known to have cancer-fighting properties. Both black and green teas (less is known about oolong) are antioxidants. How much of a prostate cancer-fighter is green tea? Nobody knows yet. However, results from studies involving other types of cancer are encouraging: In one National Cancer Institute study in China, nine hundred patients with esophageal cancer were compared with 1,500 healthy people. Looking at the patients who *didn't* smoke or drink alcohol, the study found that green tea drinkers were about 60 percent *less likely* to develop cancer than others. In another study, of fourteen thousand older Americans in California, the risk of developing pancreatic cancer decreased in those who drank tea, and in an eight-year study of 35,000 postmenopausal women in Iowa, women who drank at least two cups of tea a day were much less likely—some 40 to 70 percent—to develop cancer of the digestive system or urinary tract than women who drank little or no tea.

Some components of green and brown teas, including catechin,

EGCG (epigallocatechin gallate), and epicatechin, are being studied now. They are known to be "biologically active," but the big question remains: Is consumption of large amounts of green tea the reason that people in Asia—who also consume a lot of soy, eat more vegetables and less red meat—get less prostate cancer? Nobody knows yet.

Note: In addition to all the good things it has, tea also has caffeine, and can make some people feel jittery or anxious. If you have heart problems—irregular heartbeats, or high blood pressure—drinking a lot of tea may not be good for you. Tea can also heighten symptoms of gastroesophageal ulcers, colitis, and Crohn's disease, and—because it is rich in oxylates, a common ingredient of kidney stones, and potassium, which is sometimes difficult for people with kidney disease to process—may also increase the risk of kidney disease.

DON'T OVERDO IT, ESPECIALLY WITH HERBAL REMEDIES

Herbs are natural. They're nature's healers—and that's a good thing, right? Well . . . the message we've been saying all along certainly applies here, too: Moderation is the key to any dietary agent. Herbs can make you feel better; they can also make you sick. Even though they're "natural," a single herbal remedy may contain thousands of active chemicals, and you can have a reaction to herbs just as you can to other drugs or foods.

A few examples:

• Long-term use of comfrey (*Symphytum officinale*) can cause significant liver damage.

• Ginkgo biloba, feverfew, and vitamin K should not be taken by people who are also taking blood-thinners such as Coumadin. Also, ginkgo biloba can react with MAO inhibitors (found in many antidepressants).

• St. John's wort can also interfere with MAO inhibitors, can interact with chemicals found in certain types of cheese, red wine, and cured meats, and can make your skin more sensitive to sunlight (and thus, more likely to burn).

• Ginseng and ephedra can raise blood pressure, and should not be taken by people with high blood pressure, diabetes, heart disease, or a blood-clotting disorder.

There's something else you should know about herbs, and the message here is, caveat emptor—"Buyer beware." The U.S. Food and Drug Administration (FDA) makes sure that any drug sold in this country is safe, and that it lives up to the manufacturer's claims. It takes its job very seriously— in fact, a common criticism of this agency is that its exacting standards often require years of testing before a drug can be made available to patients who need it. But the FDA doesn't apply these same rigorous testing policies to herbs, or the labels on herbal products. Many people don't realize this; they are too trusting, and think, "It must be safe, or they couldn't sell it at the health food store." Or: "It's natural. How could it hurt you?" Wrong. Because of the 1994 Dietary Supplement Health and Education Act, "dietary supplements"—a murky category that includes vitamins, minerals, herbal remedies, amino acids, and other herbal derivatives—are not only exempt from most federal regulation, they don't even have to file reports when someone has an adverse reaction to one of their products. How responsible is that?

Further, even though the law requires that an herb's label tell you how much each dose contains, these are often inaccurate. If this happens, at best you'll be spending your money for a product whose benefit you're not fully receiving; at worst, you could get sick, or even cause permanent damage to your liver or kidneys.

Your best bet is to buy herbs—even herbal teas—from a reputable company. Your odds of getting a contaminated product, or substandard quality—such as some Asian herbals found by California investigators in 1998, which were tainted with lead, arsenic, or mercury—are much greater if you buy herbs or teas packaged in loose form, without manufacturer's packaging or detailed labels. And make sure your entire knowledge of the herb's benefits is greater than just the list of claims on the box or bottle. Even if the label says it's "clinically proven," it may be referring to study results involving another brand—and there may be a difference in quality and effectiveness. Try to choose brands with the words "standardized extracts" on the label.

If you start to have any side effects—such as dizziness or nausea, or symptoms of allergic reaction—stop taking the drug, and talk to your doctor. If you develop more urgent symptoms—especially heart palpitations, or trouble breathing—call your doctor, or seek medical help right away.

Finasteride

Finasteride is not a food, but a drug—Proscar, currently used to shrink the prostate and ease the symptoms of BPH (benign prostatic hypertrophy, or enlargement). To understand how it works, remember that the active form of male hormone in the prostate is not testosterone, but dihydrotesterone, or DHT. (See Chapter 1 for more details.) It is the job of an enzyme called 5-alpha reductase to make this transformation—to turn testosterone into DHT. Finasteride is a 5-alpha reductase *inhibitor:* It blocks this enzyme, and stops testosterone from changing to DHT. As a result, the amount of DHT in the bloodstream and in prostate tissue drops—but because testosterone is not affected, and testosterone levels in the blood remain the same, impotence is generally not a problem for men who take finasteride. Over time, the drug causes a substantial reduction in prostate tissue surrounding the urethra.

What does this have to do with prostate cancer—which, as we have described in Chapter 2, involves different processes, and is, in fact, a different kettle of fish altogether? The National Cancer Institute (NCI), in hopes that finasteride can somehow stop malignant growth in the prostate, has launched a multimillion-dollar, seven-year study to find this out. This massive project will follow eighteen-thousand otherwise healthy men aged fifty-five and older. Half of these men are receiving finasteride, half a placebo. The men have regular physicals, including a digital rectal exam and a PSA test, and will have a biopsy when the study ends.

Why does the NCI think a BPH drug can have an effect on prostate cancer? One reason is that finasteride lowers a man's levels of PSA. Another assumption is that, because finasteride alters the prostate's normal hormonal pattern—and prostate cancer is intrinsically linked to hormonal activity—then maybe prostate cancer can be stopped before the disease gets a foothold.

A few problems with this thinking: One is that there is no evidence that DHT is the hormone responsible for the growth of prostate cancer. In fact, the levels of 5-alpha reductase activity are actually lower in prostate cancer than in normal tissue. There is no supporting evidence from laboratory experiments to suggest that finasteride will work; in one animal tumor model, finasteride has no effect at all. In another animal, DHT itself helped *prevent* the disease. And finally, finasteride's effect in men who already have prostate cancer is marginal at best—which makes it questionable that it will have any effect in preventing the disease. In fact, in one study of finasteride on PSA in 3,040 men, the men in the finasteride group actually had a slightly higher rate of positive biopsies than the men in the placebo group. We should know the outcome of the NCI study in a few years. Until then, finasteride should not be used as a means of preventing prostate cancer from developing.

Now What Do I Do?

So what does the concerned man—who reads about lycopenes and selenium and vitamin E and soy, and wants to change his diet somehow—do to reduce his risk of prostate cancer? The good thing about many of the foods we've discussed here is that they have very low toxicity. Eating more soy is not going to hurt you; it may help, not only in terms of preventing cancer, but if eating more soy means that you eat less red meat and high-fat foods, this will benefit your cardiovascular system, too. Besides soy, the two most promising of these nutrients are selenium and vitamin E. Taking daily supplements of one or both of these may well have a protective effect against prostate cancer, and more importantly, it probably won't hurt you. Beyond that, eat plenty of fruits and vegetables—at least five times a day—and avoid red meat. And beyond that, remember: Moderation in all things. Sobering evidence from a report by the Institute of Medicine, part of the National Academy of Sciences, warns the health-conscious against taking "megadoses" of vitamins and dietary supplements. There's not a direct correlation between the amount of antioxidant you take and the beneficial effect you get; there is, instead, a point of diminishing returns. Not only does a jumbo-sized portion of selenium, for example, not provide jumbo-sized cancer protection, it can make you sick. The consequences of selenium toxicity, or poisoning, to the body include loss of hair and even fingernails. What about vitamin C? Many people think, "It's impossible for the body to overdose on Vitamin C; you just excrete what you don't need." Not true, says the institute's report; even vitamin C, in excessive quantities, can cause diarrhea and other gastrointestinal side effects, and, among other things, may lead to false readings on blood and urine tests. (The institute's scientists' recommended daily dose of vitamin C: 90 milligrams for men, 75 milligrams for women. And nobody, the report says, should consume more than 2,000 milligrams of vitamin C a day.)

Selenium: Now, how much selenium is good, and how much is too much? The Institute of Medicine recommends 55 micrograms a day, with an upper limit of 400 micrograms a day. Note: Scientists studying selenium's role as a possible means of preventing prostate cancer recommend taking a 200 microgram pill a day. Although more than the institute's recommended daily dose, it is still well within the institute's upper limit.

Vitamin E: How much vitamin E do you need? The institute recommends 15 milligrams, or 22 IU (International Units) a day, with an upper limit of 1,000 milligrams. Scientists studying vitamin E's preventive effects on prostate cancer recommend a higher dose (still within this limit), of 400 IU. However: *Natural vitamin E is more potent than the synthetic stuff.* A recent nutrition study found that the body absorbs natural vitamin E, called "d-alpha tocopherol," about twice as well as it does the synthetic form, called "dl-alpha tocopherol." Thus, to achieve the same dose as 400 IU of natural vitamin E, it takes about 600 IU of the synthetic product. (The institute's panel recommends a daily limit of 1,000 milligrams, or 1,500 IU, of d-alpha tocopherol, and 700 milligrams, or 1,100 IU, of dl-alpha tocopherol.) But remember: As noted above, vitamin E can increase the risk of excess bleeding. Before you begin this supplement, talk to your doctor. And it is essential that you stop taking vitamin E well in advance of any form of surgery.

Other advice: Eat an apple a day. Better yet, an apple, an orange, a bowl of vegetable soup, and maybe some corn on the cob. Try nature's packaging of phytochemicals instead of the health food store's. Findings from a Cornell University study, published in *Nature,* suggest that simply eating an apple gives your body far more antioxidant and cancer-fighting help than taking megadoses of vitamins.

Think about it: When a scientist isolates a single chemical from a piece of fruit or a vegetable and a laboratory churns out huge doses of the compound, and you buy it, you're gambling that the scientist got it right. There may be hundreds of phytochemicals that were overlooked—and maybe one of these is the magic ingredient. Nobody knows yet. The best way to hedge your bets is to diversify: Eat the real thing, if you can. In a study funded by the New York Apple Research Development and the New York Apple Association, scientists found higher free radical–scavenging ability in apples with the skin than in those without the skin. And a single fresh apple packed a wallop of antioxidants—equal to 1,500 milligrams of vitamin C.

Finally, eating all the broccoli in the world—though it may make a difference in the long run—doesn't take away your risk of having prostate cancer *right now.* (By the way, there is absolutely no evidence that drinking alcohol changes the risk for prostate cancer.) If you are age fifty or older, you need more than a good diet can guarantee. If you have a family history of prostate cancer, or are African-American, you need it sooner—a yearly rectal exam and PSA test, beginning at age forty. Which brings us to Chapter 5: "Do I Have Prostate Cancer? Screening and Detection."

5

DO I HAVE PROSTATE CANCER?
Screening and Detection

Read This First

At its earliest stages, prostate cancer is silent. There are no early warning signals—no symptoms at all, in fact, until the cancer grows outside the prostate and progresses to the point where it's rarely curable. Thus, if a man wants to maximize his odds of surviving prostate cancer, he needs to find out he has it when the disease is easiest to cure. The best way to detect prostate cancer early is through regular screening.

Although scientists are working hard to prevent prostate cancer, we're not there yet. So we're doing the next best thing—reducing deaths from prostate cancer through what's called "secondary prevention." This means diagnosing the disease when it's at a curable stage, and going after it with curative therapy.

Twenty years ago, this would have seemed like science fiction; back then—not so long ago—the words "surviving" and "prostate cancer" didn't often appear in the same sentence. Because there were no early, effective ways to detect it, by the time most men were diagnosed, the cancer had already spread beyond the prostate. The last two decades have seen a revolution in prostate cancer detection and treatment. Today, with the "one-two punch" of PSA testing and the digital rectal examination of the prostate, most men are diagnosed at a curable stage, and the last decade has seen thousands of lives saved by this effective screening combination.

As successful as routine PSA screening has turned out to be, there still may be room for improvement. Recently, using a highly sophisticated computer model, which mathematically simulated the progression of prostate cancer in a hypothetical group of men, Johns Hopkins scientists found that men at normal risk should have their first digital rectal exam and PSA test at age forty, then again at age forty-five, and then, beginning at age fifty, be tested every other year, until old age or ill health suggest that a man's life expectancy is less than ten or fifteen years. If the rectal exam is positive, the man should undergo a biopsy. If the rectal exam is negative, a biopsy should be performed in men in their forties who have a PSA greater than 2.5; in men in their fifties who have a PSA greater than 3.5, and men sixty or older who have a PSA higher than 4 (these numbers will be explained below). These recommendations do not include free PSA (which means having more blood drawn for a second test). Do you need a free PSA test? (Free PSA will be discussed below.) The decision may come down to what bothers you and your doctor the most—the thought of missing cancer at the earliest possible diagnosis, or having an unnecessary biopsy because of a false alarm. If your PSA is in an abnormal range, but you are worried about having a biopsy, you should have a free PSA test. If your free PSA is greater than 25 percent, you could avoid a biopsy for now. On the other hand, if you're worried about having prostate cancer, even if your PSA is in the normal range, if your free PSA is less than 25 percent, you should undergo a biopsy.

Why You Should Be Tested

Tomorrow, we may be able to prevent prostate cancer. Today, the best we can do is work to catch the disease early—at a point where the tumor is curable in men who are going to live long enough to need to be cured (more on this below). Over the last decade, thousands of lives have been saved by the highly effective "one-two punch" of the *PSA blood test* and the *digital rectal examination*. ("Digital" here simply means that this exam is performed using the doctor's finger, or digit).

As much as scientists have learned about PSA (prostate-specific antigen, an enzyme made by the prostate that can be checked in a simple blood test), it's still a pretty new tool. A decade ago, the test was virtually unheard of by patients, and used by doctors mainly to monitor already diagnosed prostate cancers. But the 1990s were, in effect, the "PSA decade." We learned that simply checking a man's blood regularly, and watching for a rise in his levels of PSA, can predict cancer years before it can be diagnosed by any other means. Any recurrence of PSA after treatment for prostate cancer—even more specifically, how soon it comes back, and how fast it rises—can give important clues about the nature of the cancer (whether it's aggressive or mild-mannered, for instance, and how best to attack it). Despite all these advances, there are still some basic questions about PSA—which, by the way, still rattles or just plain stumps many physicians, who discourage use of the test because they are unsure how to interpret it, or because they cling to the persistent but obsolete belief that prostate cancer screening will never work.

This is the problem: *Prostate cancer is easiest to cure early on, before it spreads outside the prostate. But unfortunately, it generally doesn't produce any symptoms* until *it spreads outside the prostate.* Thus, if a man wants to maximize his odds of having prostate cancer detected when it's most curable, he needs to catch it early, and the best way to do that is with regular screening.

A simple idea—and one that's been proven to save lives (see below). And yet, not everyone agrees that screening with the PSA blood test as well as the rectal exam is the best way to go—or that it's even a good thing. In fact, some doctors hate PSA. They're determined to hate it, despite the evidence that fewer men in the U.S. are dying of prostate cancer—unlike other countries such as Sweden, where there has not been a push for early detection. Recently, a policy statement of the American College of Preventive Medicine appeared in the *American Journal of Preventive Medicine:* "Screening can detect prostate cancer early, and early detection has the potential to decrease both morbidity and mortality, but these benefits are unproven and may not be realized because of the characteristics of this disease (e.g., prevalence of latent, clinically insignificant prostate cancer, indolent growth rate, and treatment-associated morbidity). For now, there is no convincing evidence that early detection and treatment improve outcomes. When cancers are well or moderately differentiated, expectant management may be as effective as surgery and only palliation is possible for cancers that have spread beyond the prostate capsule. While early detection of some tumors may translate into decreased mortality, it is difficult to predict definitively which men will die of prostate cancer and which will die with it."

In conclusion, the American College of Preventive Medicine recommended against routine population screening with the digital rectal exam and PSA. Instead, the college recommends that men age fifty or older with a life expectancy of greater than ten years *be given information* about the potential benefits and harms of screening, and be allowed to make their own choice, in consultation with their physician, based on personal preferences about whether they're interested in making an early diagnosis of prostate cancer.

Other critics have contended that the PSA test could prompt thousands of men to have unnecessary and expensive diagnostic procedures, which might lead to unnecessary surgery. One leading magazine told its readers that PSA "could do more harm than good by leading to premature biopsy or treatment"; that the biopsies it prompts are "an infection waiting to happen" (actually, this is not the case; see Chapter 6); and that the PSA test can be wrong "four times out of 10."

Several years ago, doctors at a National Cancer Institute meeting took the PSA arguments several steps further. Many men over age fifty have cancerous cells in their prostates, they said, but just a small percentage of men die from prostate cancer. Most prostate cancer, they argued, is slow-growing and causes no problems. As one doctor told a *New York Times* reporter: "There are millions and millions of American men who have this cancer and are never ill, yet these powerful tests [PSA] are going to detect them. . . . If the PSA is elevated, the chance that it is prostate cancer is relatively small. But even if it does represent prostate cancer, there is no way to know whether testing and treatment change the outcome or improve the health of patients." Some doctors went so far as to state that men should sign informed consent agreements before getting a PSA test. "The information you get back can lead you down a cascade of interventions that can be deadly," one doctor said, citing controversial statistics from a Medicare study for incontinence, impotence, rectal injury, and death resulting from surgery to remove prostate cancer.

Whew! After such strong denunciation, why should anyone still want a PSA test? *Because it is saving lives.* It's true, a lot of men out there *do* have prostate cancer that doesn't do a whole lot—that just seems to percolate in the prostate, but not spread. Are you one of those men? Are you willing to gamble, with your life, that you are? Or that you won't live long enough for your prostate cancer to spread? Currently, scientists are working to predict which tumors are harmless and which will be aggressive—with the goal of treating only the "bad" kind of cancer. However, until this predicting technology is perfected, as one urologist said in a recent study: "One must assume that any prostate cancer identified in a man with a life expectancy of ten years or more is potentially life-threatening, and should therefore be treated." This doesn't mean, as some would argue, that surgery—and particularly, unnecessary surgery—is the automatic next step; it isn't, not by a long shot. (For more on treatment decisions, see Chapter 7.)

Although some skeptics contended that routine PSA testing would lead doctors to spot those incidental cancers that are present in 30 percent of all men over age fifty (the argument being that, because these cancers are incidental, they don't require treatment or even diagnosis), this is not the case. A number of studies have confirmed that most cancers diagnosed as a result of PSA testing are indeed significant, not incidental.

The most heated criticism of PSA is that it is not specific enough—that, because not every man with an elevated PSA has cancer, it forces some men to undergo further tests, such as a needle biopsy, that are unnecessary. For perspective, let's look at the accuracy of mammography. Which test do you think is more of a bull's-eye for cancer? Say a fifty-year-old woman learns that her mammogram is positive, and on the same day her fifty-year-old husband finds out he has a PSA greater than 4. Which spouse is more likely to harbor cancer? It turns out to be the husband. In the U.S., the odds that a woman with a positive mammogram will have cancer vary with her age. The likelihood of having cancer is 19 percent for women over age seventy, 17 percent for women in their sixties, 9 percent for women in their fifties, 4 percent for women in their forties, and 3 percent for women in their thirties. For a man in his fifties with a PSA greater than 4, the likelihood of having prostate cancer is 25 percent.

Now that the dust has settled: undeniable statistics. Imagine a seismograph: the calm before the earthquake, then the huge jolt of the quake, aftershocks, and then, gradually, a return to the normal baseline. In the world of prostate cancer, the introduction of PSA testing in the late 1980s was the equivalent of an earthquake. The number of new cases diagnosed increased sharply—by a staggering 83 percent— between 1988 and 1992. Was there a sudden epidemic of prostate cancer? No, the number of men with the disease was the same then as it is now. It's just that, for the first time, we could catch it earlier, in men who had not yet developed symptoms. And there were a lot of them—ticking time bombs, in effect. After this "bubble" of not yet symptomatic men was diagnosed, the number of new cases has fallen steadily. Today, the number of new cases is still somewhat greater than it was in the days before PSA testing, as one would expect after a new diagnostic test is introduced (the same is true for breast cancer after the introduction of mammography). If, as the critics warned, this increase were due to the diagnosis of the small, "incidental" cancers, the number of new cases would keep on rising. But again, the cancers diagnosed with PSA testing have proven to be significant, not harmless. And even more exciting: There has been a decrease in the detection of advanced cancers at the rate of 18 percent a year since 1991—to the point where today, *only about 8 percent of men who are initially diagnosed with prostate cancer are found to have distant metastases.* This is a dramatic improvement from the pre-PSA era: In 1988, sadly, 20 percent of men had metastatic cancer by the time it was diagnosed. In 1995, the American Cancer Society estimated that 40,400 men died from prostate cancer; by 2001, the estimate will be down to 31,500. In short, what was supposed to happen, has happened.

Ultimately, for any new cancer treatment strategy to prove its worth, it must demonstrate that it is saving lives. Before 1991, deaths from prostate cancer in the United States were on the rise, increasing by 1 to 2 percent a year. But starting in 1991—and continuing today—the number of deaths from prostate cancer has been falling, on average, 1.6 percent a year. Now, in 1986—two years before PSA testing began to be widespread—the number of men dying from prostate cancer began to rise. (Although we're not entirely sure why, this may be because fewer men were dying of cardiovascular disease—and, as the average life span lengthened, men were starting to live long enough to die from prostate cancer.) Some skeptics cite this increase, and say that the decrease in deaths from prostate cancer over the last decade won't mean anything until the number drops below the 1986 death rate. A recent study by scientists at the National Cancer Institute showed that this has finally happened: In 1997, the researchers found, the number of men between the ages of sixty and seventy-nine who died from prostate cancer *was lower than in any year since 1950.* This study is especially meaningful, because its senior author, for years an outspoken critic of PSA testing, seems to be changing his mind about the test's value, and told the *New York Times,* "We are starting to have evidence that there may be a positive to prostate cancer screening and treatment."

Clearly, we're doing something right. What is it? Because PSA testing began in the late 1980s and this trend was first spotted in 1991, it is just too soon to attribute this decrease in deaths to PSA testing alone. So we've got to look for other trends, starting about a decade earlier. Beginning in the 1980s, there was greater medical interest in diagnosing prostate cancer early, through such efforts as transrectal ultrasound. At about this time, the technique of radical prostatectomy underwent its own revolution: It used to be that every man who underwent surgery to treat prostate cancer bled heavily during the operation, and wound up impotent; many men had severe incontinence as well. But the drastic bleeding that once was routine could now be controlled with the advent of an "anatomic approach," and the radical prostatectomy gained widespread acceptance: For example, in 1980, only 7 percent of men with localized prostate cancer had the operation. By 1990, that number had increased to 35 percent. Critics originally pointed to this rise in radical prostatectomy as a troubling trend. However, it may well prove that this, too, is something we were doing right: For the first time, men with prostate cancer were being treated aggressively—by surgeons aiming for a cure—in large numbers. So: Why are fewer men dying from prostate cancer? The answer may well be the fortunate combination of early diagnosis plus better treatment.

Regardless of the cause, the most important message here is that we are on a winning streak. In America, fewer men are dying from prostate cancer. The disease is being diagnosed earlier, and treated at a more curable stage. But unfortunately, this is not an across-the-board drop in deaths. What about countries that do not provide early diagnosis and treatment? Sweden is such a country. In Sweden and parts of northern Europe, death rates from prostate cancer are where American death rates were more than a decade ago—still increasing, by 2 percent a year. Worse, in Sweden, 50 percent more men die of prostate cancer than women die of breast cancer. In the United States, today 25 percent fewer men die of prostate cancer than women die of breast cancer. Is this because Sweden does a better job of treating breast cancer than the U.S.? Or is it because Swedish doctors don't attempt to cure prostate cancer, believing the disease will "percolate" for years, and men will die of other causes? (More on this in Chapter 7.) This "wait and see" philosophy may be changing, slowly, in parts of Europe. A study from the Tyrol region of Austria, where early, free screening for prostate cancer has been introduced, shows that death rates from prostate cancer in this area have fallen dramatically—by 42 percent from 1993 to 1998—compared to the rest of Austria, where wide screening is not yet done, and death rates have remained steady.

How Do You Know if You Have Prostate Cancer?

No early warning signs: If prostate cancer started where BPH does—right by the urethra—then the disease would almost announce itself: "Hey! Something's wrong, I'm having trouble urinating! I need to get this checked out!" But it doesn't. Instead, the disease begins in a different part of the prostate, relatively far away from the urethra, in the peripheral zone (see Fig. 1.3, in Chapter 1) and grows silently for years. As a result, there really aren't any clear-cut, telltale symptoms of prostate cancer—signs that men notice and worry about, signs that make a doctor say, "Aha! This must be prostate cancer!"

Every single symptom of prostate cancer can be attributed to another cause. Say a tumor becomes large enough to encroach on the urethra and block the urinary tract: It produces classic symptoms of BPH: frequent or urgent urination, hesitancy, interrupted or weakened flow, dribbling, trouble urinating at all, or even blood in the urine. In the past, valuable time was wasted as these BPH-like symptoms were pursued, while the real trouble remained hidden. (Fortunately, this is changing as more doctors are using the PSA test.) A less common symptom is the development of impotence or of less rigid erections, which can happen in advanced tumors as cancer invades the nerves involved in erection. But this, too, is accepted as something else—a normal sign of aging (and the subject of Viagra ads, which describe "erectile dysfunction" as a commonplace problem in men of a certain age), but certainly not a cause for alarm. Similarly, a decrease in the amount of fluid ejaculated, a problem that results when the ejaculatory ducts become blocked by the tumor (this blockage can also cause blood in the semen), can be written off as normal aging. Still other manifestations, such as severe pain in the back, pelvis, hips, or thighs (which can develop as the cancer begins to attack the bone), also might be mistaken for other problems such as arthritis or fibromyalgia.

Obviously, if you have any of these symptoms, see a urologist right away—even if you think it's "just" BPH or prostatitis. As we have seen, prostate cancer is an excellent mimic. But better yet, *don't wait until you have any symptoms to get tested for prostate cancer*. Men can have palpable cancer—a tumor big enough to be felt during a rectal exam— and never even feel a twinge, or experience the slightest change to suggest that something is wrong. Look at it this way: If you haven't had a PSA test and a digital rectal exam, how do you know that you're *not* harboring potentially lethal cancer?

Why You Need the Rectal Exam

Why do men over fifty (or over forty, if their risk of prostate cancer is increased—see below) need a yearly rectal exam? Why not get the most painless one—PSA—by itself, and then have a rectal exam if the blood test suggests cancer? Because the PSA test is not foolproof. About 25 percent of men with prostate cancer have a low PSA, one that doesn't get flagged as suspicious. For this and other reasons (including the way some tumors make PSA), the PSA test does not detect every cancer early. Then again, neither does the digital rectal exam: In more than half of men with prostate cancer, the tumor is growing in an inopportune spot just out of finger-reach, where it simply cannot be felt by a doctor. In other men, the cancer is "multi-focal"—there are several patches of cancer, not just one—and the prostate feels uniformly firm. It's a deceptive feeling, but the doctor's finger doesn't have a microscope on it, and doesn't always know when it's being fooled. A firm prostate doesn't necessarily mean cancer; although most normal prostates feel soft, some don't—so this alone might not call attention to itself as something that warrants further investigation. Similarly, not all prostates feel smooth: In some men, the balance between muscular (stromal) and the smoother glandular (epithelial) tissue tilts toward muscle; these men have small, dense prostates. Finally, the cancer may simply be too small to feel yet—even though it's growing, and dangerous.

SYMPTOMS IN MEN WITH ADVANCED PROSTATE CANCER:

- Blood in the urine or ejaculate.
- BPH-like symptoms: trouble urinating, frequent or urgent urination, interrupted or weakened flow, hesitancy, dribbling.
- Severe pain in the back, pelvis, hips, or thighs.
- Less rigid erections or impotence.
- A decrease in the amount of fluid ejaculated.

Also, the PSA test may spot *different* cancers than the digital rectal exam—another reason why doctors can't rely on an either-or approach for early detection. (It's like using breast exams and mammograms together to find breast cancer in women.) This was confirmed in one study of 2,634 men; investigators found that PSA and digital rectal exam were nearly equal in cancer-detecting ability, but that they didn't always find the same tumors—that if only one technique had been used, some cancers would have been missed. Together, these two tests make a formidable team.

If you are an American man, you should begin testing for prostate cancer at age fifty—unless your risk is higher than average: that is, if you are an African-American man, or if you have a strong family history of the disease—especially if more than one man in your family has had prostate cancer, or if anyone developed it before the age of fifty-five. (For more on risk factors, see Chapter 3.)

The digital rectal exam can tell an astute clinician many things about prostate cancer—whether it encompasses part of one lobe, an entire lobe, or both lobes of the prostate; whether it has spread outside the prostate, into the pelvic side wall or seminal vesicles. (For a description of the prostate's anatomy, see Chapter 1.) But as good as this exam can be, the digital rectal exam is not an ironclad guarantee that cancer will be found in its earliest stages. Frankly, the digital rectal exam is only as good as the doctor performing it. It is a subjective test. In this area, urologists probably have some advantage over general practitioners simply because diagnosing prostate cancer is a major part of this specialty. In some cases, a general practitioner has felt a suspicious area on a rectal exam, but not pursued it because the PSA was in the "normal" range (less than 4)—not realizing that one quarter of men with prostate cancer have a low PSA.

THE RECTAL EXAM: AN INSIDER'S GUIDE

This is the test that men dread. In fact, some men hate the idea of a rectal examination so much that they jeopardize their health by avoiding it like the plague. The rectal exam is certainly not fun; in fact, it's downright awkward and uncomfortable. But it shouldn't hurt, it's generally brief, and—most important of all—this little exam can provide essential information that simply can't be gotten any other way. (Note: If what you feel during the exam goes beyond the obvious discomfort of having someone's finger in your rectum and is clearly pain, this could be an important signal of another problem, such as prostatitis or inflammation. If the exam is excruciating, don't be stoic—tell your doctor.)

Unfortunately, many men hate this test for another reason—their doctor's bedside manner, or lack of it. Many doctors are not as thoughtful as they should be; they fail to position the patient correctly, and then perform a hasty, rough examination. From a medical standpoint alone, this is a mistake: A soft touch can detect areas of suspicious firmness much better than a rough hand. Worse, because some men learn—from their doctor's brutish technique—to perceive the exam as dehumanizing, or just generally unpleasant, they put off going to the doctor because they don't want to deal with someone who is rude, gruff, disrespectful, or uncommunicative, and this is a terrible shame. Good doctors know how to make their patients feel at ease. They talk to their patients, and treat them with respect. If your doctor's unfortunate bedside manner is keeping you away from this or any other exam, find another doctor. There are plenty of good ones out there.

Now, from your standpoint, what can you do to make the rectal examination as painless and productive as possible? First and foremost is how you "assume the position": The best way for the doctor to feel the prostate is for the patient to bend over the edge of the examining table. (Some doctors perform the examination by having the patient lie on his side. This is not as good: At best, the doctor can feel only the lower edge of the prostate.) For most men, the worst part of the exam is the first—the introduction of the doctor's finger through the rectum, and past the muscles in the pelvic floor. Although the examining finger is gloved and well lubricated, if these muscles are tense (a very normal reaction, especially in men who are undergoing this exam for the first time), the doctor must exert more pressure—which adds to the discomfort, which then makes the man even more tense.

How can you relax these muscles? Don't even try; let your position do it for you. First, don't rest your elbows on the examining table—even though it feels more comfortable. Instead, put all your weight on your upper torso: Bend your knees, so that your feet are just barely touching the floor. *Your feet should not be supporting any weight.* This way, your buttocks muscles will be completely relaxed, permitting the doctor's finger to be introduced easily—and ideally, slowly, giving the muscles a chance to relax ahead of time.

To understand what the doctor is looking for, feel your hand. The normal prostate usually feels like the soft tissue in your palm—the fleshy part at the base of your thumb. Now, slide your fingers around to the other side, and feel the knuckle of your thumb. This is how cancer often feels—like a knot, or hard lump.

BEFORE THE PSA TEST

• Don't ejaculate for at least two days before you have your blood drawn (this can raise your PSA level).

• Be sure to have this test *before* your digital rectal exam (the trauma from the physical exam can raise PSA, too).

• Remind your doctor if you are taking Proscar for BPH, or Propecia for hair loss (Proscar lowers PSA; Propecia is a lower dose of Proscar).

• If the PSA reading indicates a borderline elevation, or a significant increase since the last reading, repeat the test in the same laboratory. If there is a clear-cut elevation, ask your doctor about prescribing antibiotics to rule out a possible infection. (Often, men receive ciprofloxacin or levofloxacin for three to four weeks, and have the PSA measured again.) If it is elevated again, you should have a biopsy.

Why You Need the PSA Test

No other cancer is diagnosed strictly by trying to feel it. Why? Just think how much a cancer must grow—how many times those early cancer cells must divide, what a tremendous head start this gives the tumor—before it becomes big enough to be felt. This is why, for years, doctors searched for a man's version of the Pap smear—an early-warning cancer detector that could spot a tumor long before it is clinically evident.

In this area, no development has been more promising than the PSA test. PSA is an enzyme, called prostate-specific antigen, that's made by the prostate in large amounts. It is secreted through the prostate's network of ducts, and it forms a major part of the ejaculate (for more, see Chapter 1). Although the enzyme PSA is prostate-specific, it doesn't just stay in the prostate: It leaks into the blood-stream, and can be detected in a simple blood test.

The PSA test is not new. In years past, however, its purpose was limited; it functioned mainly as a means of monitoring already diagnosed prostate cancer. Could it do more? Could it detect cancer that had not yet been diagnosed? The answer, doctors found a few years ago, was yes—that elevated levels of PSA can indeed point to the presence of cancer. However, although our knowledge of PSA has grown exponentially over the last decade, the basic PSA test is not a magic wand, pointing with resolute certainty toward prostate cancer—and that's the problem. Even now, doctors aren't exactly sure how best to use the test, and how to make sense of the information it provides.

PSA is *prostate-specific, not cancer-specific.* This is why a blood test alone isn't enough, why a digital rectal exam is also a must. You can have prostate cancer and still have a low PSA level. And, just because you have a high PSA does not necessarily mean you have prostate cancer—many men with high PSA levels don't. About a quarter of men who turn out to have prostate cancer have a low PSA level, less than 4 nanograms per milliliter. About 25 percent of men with a PSA between 4 and 10 turn out to have cancer. In men with a PSA over 10, about 65 percent are found to have cancer. Many conditions can cause PSA to rise; see "My PSA Is Elevated? What Else Could It Be?" below.

Gram for gram, cancerous tissue results in PSA levels in the blood that are about ten times higher than levels in benign tissue. The reason for this is that, normally, PSA is secreted and disposed of through tiny ducts in the prostate. But prostate cancer doesn't have a working ductal system; its ducts are "blind"—dead-end streets. So instead of draining into the urethra, PSA builds up, leaks out of the prostate, and shows up in the bloodstream. That's why it has proven to be such a good marker for cancer.

Still, there is much we can do to make the PSA test even more meaningful and specific. Some of the most promising approaches to PSA include:

Bound and Free PSA

Chemically speaking, a PSA molecule is like a tiny pair of sharp scissors (the main function of PSA is to break down coagulaged semen after intercourse—see Chapter 1). Now imagine millions of these tiny scissors clanking around in the bloodstream—each pointed blade slicing tissue to ribbons. If PSA circulated in the blood in its native form, it could be devastating to everything it touched. But the body is smarter than that: Normally, PSA is packed in a protective case—a chemical straitjacket, which keeps it from harming innocent tissue. In this form, PSA is "bound"—tied to other proteins, rendered harmless. But sometimes, PSA inactivates itself: Imagine a pair of scissors with one broken blade. These scissors don't fit in the case anymore, but they don't need it; they are chemically passive. This form of PSA is called "free." Like the wings of the ravens at the Tower of London, it's clipped. It circulates freely in the bloodstream on its own.

In a regular, or "total PSA," blood test, both of these forms are lumped together—the dangerous scissors in the case, and the scissors with the broken blade. But in recent years, scientists have developed assays sensitive enough to isolate and quantify both bound and free forms of the PSA molecule. The goal is to characterize these forms of PSA in the blood, measure each part, and determine what these levels mean over time—so we can chart the course of normal and abnormal growth of the prostate. This separation of PSA into bound and free forms can help men in two important ways: It can make the PSA test more specific, for one thing. It can also help determine how aggressive a man's cancer is.

A more specific test: the free PSA test. As we'll discuss later in this chapter, an elevated PSA level does not automatically mean that you have prostate cancer. What it means is that you have prostate trouble—which could mean cancer, enlargement, infection, or even be a result of recent trauma—and you need to see a urologist to figure out exactly what's going on in there. The most common reason for a higher-than-normal PSA level is benign enlargement—BPH. It is common for a man's PSA to be as high as 10 percent of his prostate weight; for example, if a man has an enlarged prostate that weighs 60 grams, he may well have a PSA of 6—but not have cancer. Now: For reasons that are not entirely clear, when a man's PSA level rises because of BPH, more of the PSA is in the free form. (An easy way to remember this is: "The higher the free PSA, the more likely that you are *free of cancer.*") But men with prostate cancer are more likely to have low levels of free PSA (also known as "percent-free" PSA): Thus, if a man has an elevated PSA and most of it is free, then it's probably coming from BPH; if it's mostly bound, then the PSA elevation is probably coming from cancer. This is where free PSA is especially useful.

Can the free PSA test reduce your risk of an unnecessary biopsy? Probably. Can overreliance on free PSA mean that your prostate cancer might be missed? Possibly. In one study, researchers used a free PSA cutoff of 19 percent in men with total PSA levels between 3 and 4, and detected 90 percent of all cancers. Another study, of men with PSA levels between 2.6 and 4, had a higher cutoff—27 percent free PSA—but also detected 90 percent of cancers. This study found that 18 percent of unnecessary biopsies could be avoided by using this cutoff. Note: Again, because men with low free PSA levels are more likely to have aggressive cancers and more advanced disease found at the time of radical prostatectomy, even if the needle biopsy is inconclusive, or shows little cancer, if the percent-free PSA is lower than 15 percent, a man is likely to be harboring more tumor than a man with a higher level of free PSA.

Another study of men with higher PSA levels (between 4 and 10) found that using the free PSA test—and performing biopsies only on men with lower than 25 percent free PSA—could diagnose 95 percent of the cancers, but reduce unnecessary biopsies by 20 percent. However, some scientists, worried about diagnosing that remaining 5 percent of cancers, object to this cutoff number, because it means that some will be missed.

Should you get it? There are several points to consider: One drawback to the free PSA test is that it's twice as expensive, because two blood tests must be measured—the total amount and the free amount, from which the percent-free number is calculated. Although many doctors are overlooking the additional costs involved in this, free PSA testing has not yet become widespread. Some urologists, guided by free PSA measurements, recommend biopsy only when the percentage of free to total PSA is lower than 25 percent. This is good, in that it reduces the number of unnecessary biopsies, but it also means that about 5 to 10 percent of cancers may be missed. It may come down to what bothers you most—the thought of missing cancer at the earliest possible diagnosis, or having an unnecessary biopsy because of a false alarm.

However, there are two situations in which percent-free PSA can be particularly useful: Say a man has had multiple biopsies, because his total PSA is higher than normal. Every biopsy is negative—yet the worry remains. Here, if the free PSA is high, the man and his doctor can relax. If it's very low, it means he will need further biopsies. The second situation is the man with a strong family history of prostate cancer, who worries that he is headed down the same pathway as his father, brother, or other male relatives—even though his PSA is low for his age. Here again, knowing the free PSA percentage can be reassuring: If it's high, this man can relax. If it's very low, this is a good reason to have a biopsy.

How aggressive is the cancer? A doctor can't determine, from looking at the total PSA level in a man with prostate cancer, the source of the PSA elevation. For example, in many men with small amounts of early-stage cancer, most of the PSA is actually coming from non-cancerous tissue in the epithelium. However, *if the free PSA is less than 15 percent, it's more likely that all of that PSA is coming from cancer, that the cancer is significant in size, and that it will prove aggressive.* The differences in PSA illustrate once again that not all prostate cancers are created equal: Some are very slow-growing, and never need treatment. Others can be fatal within a matter of years after they are diagnosed. So for scientists, just as important as finding cancer early is knowing which kind of cancer—the "good" or the "bad"—we're dealing with. Research at Johns Hopkins has established the guidelines on which men can afford to "watch and wait" (see Chapters 6 and 7). We are also working to pinpoint the men at the other end of the spectrum, those with aggressive cancers that will almost certainly be lethal if not treated immediately. New evidence shows that free PSA can predict which tumors will be aggressive—and need to be treated as soon as possible—several years before total, or "regular" PSA tests can even spot cancer. In one Johns Hopkins study, researchers made use of the massive database of the Baltimore Longitudinal Study of Aging. The recent Johns Hopkins study, led by urologist H. Ballentine Carter, compared blood samples from men who developed prostate cancer to men who did not, and found that *fifteen years* before cancer was diagnosed, all of the men who turned out to have aggressive prostate tumors had levels of free PSA that were lower than 15 percent. Men with slower-growing, nonaggressive cancer all had free PSA levels greater than 15 percent.

This landmark study suggests that percent-free PSA may be an excellent predictor of aggressive tumors that will need to be treated.

Other Approaches under Study

The more we know about PSA and its subtleties, the more we're learning about the chemistry of the prostate, and the many biochemical signals it sends out all the time—if we can only figure out how to read them. Several sophisticated tests looking at other prostate cancer markers are currently being investigated. These include:

"Complexed" PSA: This is another way of looking at the separation of bound from free PSA. A new assay measures the amount of PSA bound to the particular protein that binds it—a protein called alpha-1-antichymotrypsin (ACT). Several investigators have suggested that this approach—it's like taking the same picture, but using a different lens—can be just as useful as percent-free PSA. Although this is still being evaluated, one advantage over free PSA analysis is that it involves only one blood test, and thus is more cost-efficient.

BPSA: This is a particular form of free PSA produced by the prostate's transition zone, a thin ring of tissue that surrounds the urethra, in BPH, benign enlargement of the prostate (refer back to Fig. 1.3). BPSA is not so much a marker for prostate cancer as a marker for BPH: Researchers at Baylor College of Medicine found that BPSA levels in men with prostate cancer and men with BPH were significantly different. One day, BPSA may be a helpful means of pinpointing the cause of an elevated PSA.

hK2: PSA is in a family of proteolytic (protein-cutting) enzymes called kallikreins. Another member of this extended family, one of PSA's cousins—like PSA, it's expressed by the prostate, can be measured in the blood, and responds to hormones—is called human kallikrein-2 (hK2). Laboratory studies suggest that cancerous cells make more hK2 than do normal prostate cells; also, hK2 appears to be higher in men with advanced cancer than in men with the more indolent form of the disease. Because of these promising studies, investigators hoped hK2 would prove to be a specific marker that could distinguish men with BPH from men with cancer. That hasn't happened yet, and it seems that hK2 alone is not enough of a crystal ball. It may be that measuring hK2 in combination with free PSA proves more helpful.

PMSA: Prostate-membrane-specific antigen, or PMSA, is a protein that is made on the surface of prostate cells. Several years ago, scientists hoped this test would be even more specific than the PSA test. However, it turns out that a number of other proteins in the body share a similar structure—particularly, a prominent one in the brain. For this and other reasons, the most recent studies indicate that PMSA won't live up to its original promise. PMSA is not higher in men with more advanced cancer than in men with localized disease; in fact, the levels of PMSA are exactly the same in men and women!

PSA density: This technique begins with a theory—that most men in the age group for prostate cancer also have at least some BPH, which can elevate the PSA concentration and make diagnosis more difficult. One way to distinguish between BPH and cancer, some doctors believe, is *PSA density*—the blood PSA score divided by the volume of the prostate, as determined by transrectal ultrasound. Basically, if you have benign disease, your PSA should be approximately 10 percent, and no higher than 15 percent, of the weight of your prostate (which translates to a PSA density of 0.1 to 0.15). For example, if you have a PSA of 8 and your prostate weighs 80 grams, most of the PSA is probably coming from BPH. But if your prostate weighs only 30 or 40 grams, your PSA level is too high to be explained by BPH alone.

The next question you might have is, "How do we weigh my prostate?" Well, there's the problem. It's impossible to estimate a man's prostate size without an invasive procedure such as transrectal ultrasound, and thus, PSA density has not proven to be of widespread value in screening for prostate cancer. For men who—because of an abnormal PSA or rectal exam—do undergo ultrasound-guided biopsy, PSA density can be helpful in determining how much cancer is in the prostate. It can also be useful in men who have had repeated negative biopsies, to determine whether they need to go further in searching for cancer.

In a study of sixty-one men, scientists found a difference in PSA density between prostate cancer and BPH; the average PSA density value for 41 men with clinically localized cancer (confined to the prostate) was 0.58; for the twenty men with BPH, it was 0.04. About 83 percent of the men with prostate cancer who had a normal PSA test had an elevated PSA density score; only two men with prostate cancer had a PSA density under 0.05. The highest PSA density reading for any of the men with BPH was 0.117; most men with BPH had a PSA density level under 0.1.

PSA velocity: Another promising approach to PSA is to look at *PSA velocity*—its rate of change from year to year. The supposition is this: If cells double at a much faster rate in prostate cancer than in BPH, and if prostate cancer produces more PSA than BPH does, it's likely that PSA's yearly rate of change will be much greater in a man with prostate cancer than in a man with BPH.

However, for this technique to be accurate, at least three PSA measurements should be obtained during a two-year period—or, the tests should be taken at least eighteen months apart. It is not helpful for a man to have two PSA tests in a short span of time—a couple of months apart, for example—because there is a natural fluctuation in PSA readings that may be as much as 15 to 30 percent. Say you have a PSA test result of 4.1; two months later, your next PSA test is 4.7. This could be a normal variation—yet it could well spark a panic if you believed you had cancer and it was growing fast.

In one study, using data from the Baltimore Longitudinal Study of Aging, investigators looked at three groups of men—those with BPH, those with prostate cancer, and a control group of men with no prostate disease. Studying twenty years' worth of stored blood samples, investigators found that PSA—for those who know how to read it properly—is a veritable crystal ball at predicting prostate cancer. The men who turned out to develop prostate cancer had "significantly greater rates of change in PSA levels than those without prostate cancer *up to ten years before diagnosis*." In other words, by tracking changes in PSA levels, they were able to detect prostate cancer *years before it could be diagnosed by other means.* For example, at five years before diagnosis—when PSA levels weren't appreciably different between men with BPH and men with prostate cancer—there was already a big difference in PSA velocity in men who turned out to have prostate cancer versus men who had BPH and the control group.

PSA velocity is highly valuable in detecting prostate cancer, and in distinguishing it from BPH early—particularly now, when an increasing number of men are returning to their doctor every year for a digital rectal examination and PSA test. But the whole idea here with PSA velocity is that it's a fluid continuum, not a cut-and-dried, one-shot reading. It's like having a prostate barometer—your doctor doesn't have to wait for the PSA score to reach a magic number (currently, it's 4 nanograms per milliliter). With PSA velocity, what matters is a significant change over time—an average *consistent* increase of more than 0.75 nanogram per milliliter a year, over the course of three tests. Say over eighteen months a man's PSA level went up from 1.2 to 2.3 to 3.6. Clearly, something's going on here. This obvious, steady rise could enable a doctor monitoring PSA velocity to detect clinically significant, curable prostate cancer in its earliest stages, instead of waiting for the PSA level to reach the magic 4, and then doing further tests. With PSA velocity, we can make a more accurate diagnosis of prostate cancer at even lower levels than the raw cutoff of 4, because it works at any level. (At present, it's unclear what rate of change is significant in men with PSA greater than 10.) Also, PSA velocity is more specific. If doctors use the PSA level of 4 as a cutoff point, about 40 percent of men who only have BPH undergo unnecessary biopsies. But with PSA velocity, this number is reduced; only 10 percent of these men with BPH undergo an unnecessary biopsy.

Although PSA velocity is a big improvement over looking at a bald PSA score and trying to figure out what it means, even this isn't a perfect system. It's important to note that 25 percent of men with prostate cancers that are growing do *not* have a big increase in their PSA. So, just because your PSA isn't high, and just because your PSA isn't going up, that doesn't mean you don't have cancer, and it doesn't mean that your cancer isn't growing.

PSA and a man's age: Which brings us to the idea of age-specific PSA. The theory here is this: As a man ages, his prostate gets bigger. Therefore, why should the PSA cutoff point be the same for a forty-year-old man as for an eighty-year-old man (who probably has a higher PSA level anyway, due to BPH)? It doesn't make sense: The younger man almost certainly has a much smaller prostate. Studies show that using a cutoff of 2.5 in men under age fifty will enable doctors to catch about 20 percent more cancers—but only require 5 percent more biopsies. Because detecting prostate cancer early is more important in these younger men whose lives are likely to be cut short by malignancy, this is a good rationale for using a lower cutoff for these men. Some scientists have suggested using a higher cutoff for men over age sixty, because so many older men have enlarged prostates. However, in doing this, some significant, curable cancers will be almost certainly missed. Therefore, *we do not recommend raising the PSA bar over 4 for anyone.* Because of this and other work, we now recommend a cutoff of 2.5 for men in their forties, a maximum of 3.5 for men in their fifties, and a cutoff of 4 for all other men.

PSA and race: There is no question that black men without cancer have higher PSA levels than their counterparts of other races; for example, in one retrospective study by Chicago researchers, the average PSA level of black men was slightly higher than in white men and Hispanic men; black men had higher PSA density levels as well. This might suggest that there should be a higher PSA cutoff for African-Americans. However, the other side of the coin is that black men also have a *greater risk of developing cancer* (see Chapter 3), and when they are tested with the same PSA cutoff level as white men, are more likely to be harboring a cancer. In one study, using a PSA cutoff of 4, 38 percent of white men were found to have cancer, but 52 percent of black men turned out to have cancer.

Should there be race-specific guidelines for PSA? Said one study, published in the *Journal of the National Cancer Institute:* "Criteria for normal PSA level and density have been derived primarily from white men, and may not be directly applicable to other populations. Race-specific data are needed to fully optimize PSA as a tumor marker in racial populations that are at high risk for prostate cancer death." African-American men are at a greater risk of developing prostate cancer, of being diagnosed at a later stage, and of dying from it than any other men. Thus, although they are more likely to have a higher PSA than other men with the same size prostate, African-Americans are also at highest risk of developing prostate cancer. In order to keep the test in these men as sensitive as possible, some scientists recommend making the PSA cutoff for African-American men in their forties lower than that for white men.

Why do black men have higher PSA levels than white men? This may simply reflect the higher activity of hormones in African-American men, due to a more active androgen receptor (discussed in Chapter 3). More research is needed to determine the guidelines for PSA testing in black men. However, it is quite clear that African-American men are more likely to develop the disease—and to have a more advanced, lethal form of it—and they need to be followed carefully. It may be that combining PSA with additional tests, such as free PSA, will prove to be most useful for these men.

CAN IGF PREDICT PROSTATE CANCER?

The Physician's Health Study, like the Baltimore Longitudinal Study of Aging (described in this chapter), has a bank of stored blood collected from participants. But instead of the BLSA's serial blood samples, this study took only a single blood sample from each participant. Scientists using data from the Physician's Health Study published some controversial results in the journal *Science:* They reported that a growth factor called IGF-1 (called insulin-like growth factor, because its molecular structure is similar to that of insulin), found in the blood, was a strong predictor—stronger, even, than PSA—of prostate cancer development. The fact that IGF-1—unlike PSA—is not prostate-specific was troubling to several scientists, including Johns Hopkins urologist H. Ballentine Carter and scientist Mitchell Harman at the Gerontology Research Center of the National Institute of Aging. They decided to ask this same question using the BLSA database, with its multiple blood samples from each participant. "In our study, it turned out that IGF-1 blood levels were associated with the risk of prostate cancer development," says Carter. "Men with the highest levels of IGF-1 had a threefold greater risk of developing prostate cancer compared to men with the lowest levels. However, unlike the study findings published in *Science,* PSA proved a much stronger predictor of future cancer development. Men with the hightest PSA levels were 12.5 times as likely to develop prostate cancer as men with the lowest levels." Thus, Carter adds, "Given the predictive power of PSA, it appears unlikely that knowing your serum IGF-1 level would be helpful."

ON THE HORIZON:
BRAINY COMPUTERS TO HELP PREDICT CANCER RISK

Johns Hopkins urologist Alan Partin loves statistics, facts, and figures: rearranging them, making sense out of them, and using what he's come up with to help patients. A prime example: The "Partin Tables" he developed, which filled a great need by correlating three facts about a man's disease—PSA level, Gleason score, and clinical stage—and accurately estimating the extent of a man's prostate cancer to help him make an educated decision about treatment (see Chapter 6)

Now, instead of just three pieces of information, he's taking more than a dozen, feeding them into a sophisticated neural network—a "thinking" computer program he has helped develop—and asking new questions, such as: What will the results of this man's biopsy be? What will be the pathologic stage of his tumor? Will he have positive lymph nodes?

"Neural networks are not new," says Partin, "but they're fairly new to medicine. The stock market uses them all the time: They watch trends; the network tells them what's going to happen in the next quarter, so they know which stock to buy. Factories use them to measure the temperature of water, steam coming out of the pipes, the noise level in the building—about fifteen or twenty variables that they continuously monitor—and they know two days before the machine's going to go down, because they've seen the pattern before. The neural network says, 'You're going to be in trouble, you'd better stop the line and fix something.'"

With a neural network program he and colleagues developed with funding from the National Cancer Institute, Partin says, "I can take a man's PSA, his age, his race, digital rectal examination, free PSA, and I can give him a very good estimate of his probability of having prostate cancer if he were to get a biopsy. Instead of saying 'That's a little high, maybe you should get a biopsy,' I can say, 'You've got a 48 percent chance of having cancer.'"

Neural networks recognize patterns, "just as you can recognize your child five hundred yards away by glancing." Their answers are educated guesses. The neural networks—so called because they function like artificial brains, and have the ability to learn from their mistakes—can see a bigger picture, says Partin: "For the last fifteen years, we have been looking at tumor markers, looking at pathologic information, trying to make predictions for prognosis. We look at slides, Gleason scores; we measure PSAs, we have new blood tests. We've been doing image analysis—looking at the shape and texture and organization of the DNA in the nuclei of prostate cancer cells. Some of these tests are good, some are great, and some are okay. No single one of them can tell us the answer, but maybe all of them together would give us more of an idea what the future holds for men."

But no human, Partin adds, can comprehend so many variables at one time. Enter the neural network, which uses complex mathematical-statistical analysis "to compare variables that aren't inherently coordinated with each other." The network doesn't even try to figure them out. "It simply doesn't care whether the variables make sense together; it's just looking for a pattern."

How, then, does this brainy computer work? Partin gives the example of a kid trying to learn Spanish with flash cards. Hold up a card, the kid looks at the symbols and takes a guess. "If he's right, we put that card aside, and pick up the next card. If he's wrong, we tell him the correct answer, put the card back in the stack, and ask him again in a few minutes. Keep going through the flash cards, and eventually he'll learn Spanish," Partin says. "Then you can give him words he's never seen before, and because he's learned all the prefixes, suffixes, and conjugations he can make a guess, and often he'll get it right." The neural network is simply a matter of training a computer to look at a complex series of results and determine a pattern—the possibility of cure, perhaps, or the likelihood that cancer will be aggressive. "The computer does this thousands of times until, like a brain, it gets pretty good at guessing which horse is going to win the race."

Compared to standard statistical patterns, the neural network's conclusions, based on retrospective data from prostate cancer patients—five hundred so far—are "far superior," says Partin, who is on a committee with the World Health Organization and the International Union of Cancer Control to investigate neural network technology worldwide. He believes the network has the potential to save millions of men from unnecessary biopsies. "Last year, 25 million men in the U.S. had PSA tests; 20 million of them have had a negative prostate biopsy and don't know what to do next year. We just can't afford to biopsy 20 million men every year. If the neural network can say, 'You don't need that biopsy,' if all the knowledge that we can grasp is saying that a man is probably okay, then that's where this technology is going to help."

Who Needs Screening?

When to start? If you're an American man, you should begin testing for prostate cancer at age fifty, unless your risk is higher than average—that is, if you're an African-American man, or if you have a strong family history of the disease (especially if more than one man in your family has had prostate cancer, or developed it before the age of fifty-five). In this case, you should begin at age forty. Another way to look at it is, every man who can expect to live at least ten to twenty more years, and *who does not want to die from prostate cancer*, should be screened.

Now, what does that mean? Simply that if a man's age or health suggests that he won't live longer than ten years, there is no reason to make an early diagnosis of prostate cancer. If a man who is very old, or very ill, has early, localized prostate cancer now, it is unlikely that he will live long enough for the cancer to become a problem. If the cancer progresses, there are many ways to control the disease and keep symptoms at bay for years. Creating anxiety about what to do—what treatment decisions to make—is not helpful for these men. One of the major missing pieces here—especially as the average life span lengthens—is, how does a man *know* how long he's going to live? One urologist has said that he would not perform a PSA test on a man older than eighty unless he was brought to the office by both of his parents. But we desperately need an accurate way to distinguish the eighty-year-old man who will live to be one hundred from his counterpart, who may die the next year.

But what about the phrase, "who does not want to die from prostate cancer"? Obviously, nobody wants to die from prostate cancer—or heart disease, or any ailment, for that matter. For many men, however, this is much more than an abstract concept: It is a great fear. These men have seen death from prostate cancer, watched the suffering of their father, brother, or a friend, and prayed it wouldn't happen to them, too. But other men don't understand this. They only know what they read in the newspapers and hear on television—that treatment of prostate cancer is associated with a lot of side effects, a thing to be avoided at all costs. As we've discussed, it took a few years of better treatment and earlier detection before scientists could show a drop in the number of men dying from prostate cancer. This is why, for years, so many skeptics stated that "there is no evidence that the treatment of localized prostate cancer reduces deaths." That was a half-truth even then; there was also no evidence that it did *not* reduce deaths. That's because a study testing this statement was never done. It couldn't have been. To know whether early diagnosis and treatment would reduce deaths from prostate cancer, doctors needed to be able to identify patients with curable cancers, treat them, and then follow them for fifteen or twenty years, and then compare those results to patients who were not screened. We can't know the results of such a study, because it's only been in the last ten years that we've been able to diagnose men at an early, curable stage, and the results of a study that is ongoing will not be known for another fifteen to twenty years. (Actually, the way this study, called the PLCO study, is set up, we may never know the answer; see Chapter 7.) The good news is that we may not have to wait that long: The recent figures are so dramatic that they have silenced many of these critics: In 1995, 40,400 men died of prostate cancer; in 2001, the number of deaths from prostate cancer is estimated to be only 31,500.

Why not take prostate cancer screening a step further, then? Why not begin testing *all* men at age forty? One obvious reason is that the disease is less common in men under age fifty. On the other hand, prostate cancer discovered in younger men is more likely to be curable. Thus, Johns Hopkins urologist H. Ballentine Carter and colleagues began looking for a way to improve prostate cancer screening.

They used an approach that has worked well to answer such questions (such as when to start and how often to screen) in cervical and breast cancer programs: a highly sophisticated computer model, called a Markov model, which mathematically simulates the progression of a disease in a group. "Basically, it takes a hypothetical population of individuals and walks them through life," Carter explains, with some men developing prostate cancer, some dying of prostate cancer, and some never getting the disease, and eventually dying of other causes—just like in real life. Setting up the model was the hard part. But then, the researchers used it to test various screening strategies to see how they affected the death rate from prostate cancer, and how many PSA tests and biopsies were needed to detect each cancer.

The results, published in the *Journal of the American Medical Association*, were unexpected: For men who are *not* at higher risk of developing prostate cancer, the current approach (beginning screening at age fifty) was not the best strategy. Instead, they found, a more effective strategy was to give PSA tests at age forty and at age forty-five, and then at age fifty (or earlier, if PSA is 2 or above), start testing every *other* year, instead of every year. "That was the only strategy that did three things: It reduced the death rate of prostate cancer, reduced the overall number of PSA tests, and reduced the overall number of prostate biopsies for each cancer detected," says Carter.

Interestingly, the study also found that lowering the PSA threshold for biopsy below 4 did not save more lives, but did dramatically increase the number of prostate biopsies. So what about the recommendations to use lower PSA thresholds in younger men, and test yearly beginning at age fifty? "The model assumes that everybody is perfect and every man returns for PSA testing when he should," says Carter. In this ideal setting, when testing starts at age forty, "it may not make much difference in terms of curability whether the cancer is detected at a PSA of 2.5 or 4." Thus, Carter doesn't advocate changing the standard policy based on these preliminary findings alone. However, he hopes that they will stimulate further research, and that scientists will begin asking "whether the current approach to screening is the best."

In the meantime, it may be possible to use PSA to identify men who are more likely to develop prostate cancer—and also, those who are more likely not to develop it. Scientists at the Physicians Health Study noted that men with PSA levels above 2 had more than twelve times the likelihood of being diagnosed with prostate cancer within the next decade than men with PSA levels below 1. This means that if a man's PSA remains low, he may be unlikely to develop prostate cancer, and may need less frequent PSA testing.

But what about younger men—in their forties and fifties—with low PSA levels? Can their lifetime risk of developing (or evading) prostate cancer be predicted, as well? Carter and colleagues used data from the Baltimore Longitudinal Study of Aging to investigate the relationship between a PSA level and the later risk of developing prostate cancer in men in their forties, fifties, and sixties. They found that men in their forties and fifties with a PSA *above 0.6–0.7* had a fourfold greater risk of developing prostate cancer over the next two to three decades than men with lower PSA levels—and furthermore, were able to use PSA as a crystal ball, to target a man's risk of developing prostate cancer. For example: Two decades after a PSA measurement taken in their forties, 91 percent of men with PSA levels above 0.7 were free of prostate cancer, compared to 99 percent of men with lower PSA. For men in their fifties, 73 percent with PSA levels over 0.7 were free of prostate cancer two decades later, compared to 95 percent of men with lower levels. For men aged sixty-five and above, the researchers found, when PSA levels are below 0.5–1.0, it is very unlikely that prostate cancer will be diagnosed by age seventy-five.

PROSTATE CANCER RUNS IN MY FAMILY: SHOULD I THINK ABOUT GENETIC TESTING?

At the moment, that's all you can do—think about genetic testing, because it isn't available yet. But it soon will be. This means, theoretically, that the 9 percent of men who inherit a defective gene involved in prostate cancer can have their blood drawn, and find out whether they're at extra risk for prostate cancer.

Right? Well, the answer is, maybe. Today, we have identified and characterized two genes that have been linked to hereditary prostate cancer: HPC-1, located on Chromosome 1, and HPC-X, on the X chromosome. Several other genes have been identified, too, although we don't know as much about them, and there will almost certainly be more such discoveries to come. The next steps are to pinpoint the actual genes—because, although we know the general neighborhood, we haven't yet found the exact street address on the chromosome. This is necessary before a blood test can be developed.

Then, once a blood test is developed, what will happen? Once we have a test, men with prostate cancer who have a strong family history can be tested to see whether they harbor one of the mutated genes. (There will probably turn out to be several genes involved.) If the man tests positive, after a lot of counseling about the consequences of testing, other family members can be tested to determine whether they, too, carry the gene and are at high risk.

In Chapter 3 (where it's discussed in much more detail), we talked about how cancer starts—the "domino effect," or chain reaction caused when a single gene goes bad, then causes another to mutate, until finally the result is cancer. Some men are born with the deck stacked against them; they're born with a bum gene. In HPC-X, this means they're more susceptible to prostate cancer. In HPC-1, research at Johns Hopkins suggests that every man who inherits this mutated gene will eventually develop cancer. Now, this doesn't mean a man with this sword hanging over him can't *delay* cancer—for example, by changing his diet: Although we don't know for certain yet, a lot of research suggests that this may be so. And it definitely doesn't mean that a man with an inherited gene linked to prostate cancer should start making out his will, or take up hang gliding or bungee jumping. Actually, the more we can learn about how these genes go astray, the better the news is for everybody. For one thing, if we can figure out which proteins or nutrients are deficient in these men, we may be able to restore the genetic balance through diet or medication and *prevent* cancer. (In fact, a whole new science is developing, in which nutrients can be added to food in this way—a process known as creating "nutraceuticals.") For another, you now have a "heads-up"—a warning that your father and grandfather never received.

Thankfully, *we are talking about a disease that can be cured if it's caught early enough*. Many families with inherited illnesses—Huntington's disease, for instance—would give their eyeteeth to face an enemy that can be beaten. And this brings us to one of the great ethical issues of genetic testing. For some families, the counseling and preparation process in genetic testing is extensive. This is because, sadly, some diseases are so horrible, and so dreaded, that diagnosis is sometimes accompanied by suicide.

But prostate cancer is not such a disease. Not only is it curable if caught early, there are many good treatments that can prolong life, and the next decade will see a virtual explosion—not only of new drugs, but of new approaches aimed at turning incurable prostate cancer into a chronic illness, like diabetes, which might not be eradicated, but which can be stopped. The bottom line: *There is much hope here, more than ever before.*

And yet, many men who are reading this book have watched their forebears die of prostate cancer, in agonizing pain and suffering, and these men with a strong family history of prostate cancer are haunted by the possibility that they, too, may have inherited the disease, and may have passed it on to their sons. Indeed, for some men, the family history is so frightening that, as have some women with a family history of breast cancer, they may ask for prophylactic treatment of prostate cancer—they may want to have their prostate removed before cancer develops. Genetic testing is a medical Pandora's box of ethical dilemmas that we will all wrestle with—because this is new territory for everybody, and we're feeling our way as we go.

Finally, if you have a strong family history of prostate cancer, and you turn out not to have one of the identified genes, this doesn't mean you won't just develop it anyway, over time, like so many American men.

Is genetic testing for you? It's not available yet. Which means you have plenty of time to decide. In the meantime, if you are at increased risk, do everything you can to stay ahead of the game—start screening at age forty, change your diet (for more on food, see Chapter 4), and keep learning as much as you can about this disease.

MY PSA IS ELEVATED: WHAT ELSE COULD IT BE?

Just as having a low PSA doesn't mean that you don't have prostate cancer, having a high PSA doesn't automatically mean that you do. If your PSA is high, you have some form of prostate disease—trauma, enlargement, infection, or cancer—and you need to see a urologist to figure out which one it is.

For example: Trauma—even a particularly vigorous rectal exam—can make a man's PSA levels shoot up temporarily. (To illustrate how complicated PSA is: In one study, French scientists found that the rise in PSA after a rectal exam is mainly in *free* PSA—still, the number went up, and the result could be misleading.) This means that, ideally, your blood should be drawn *before* you have a rectal exam or any other procedure, such as cystoscopy, a prostate biopsy, or transurethral resection of the prostate (TURP), which could affect the prostate, and falsely elevate PSA. For this reason, it makes sense to wait six or eight weeks after you have a needle biopsy before having your PSA taken if you are planning to use the results for treatment decisions. And even then, it can still be higher than it was before your biopsy—so if this happens, don't panic, thinking your PSA is shooting up uncontrollably. BPH itself can elevate PSA. Conversely, taking the drug finasteride (Proscar) to treat BPH can artificially *lower* the PSA reading by as much as half. (Also, the drug Propecia, used to deter hair loss, is a low-dose form of finasteride and can lower PSA as well.) To account for this, the PSA number of men taking finasteride should be multiplied by two. (Fortunately, finasteride does not appear to affect percent-free PSA.)

A mild case of prostatitis can raise PSA, and an acute infection, such as bacterial prostatitis, can cause it to skyrocket. Because of this, many physicians treat an abrupt rise in a patient's yearly PSA test with antibiotics for several weeks, followed by another PSA test, just to rule out infection as a possible cause (and avoid an unnecessary biopsy). If the trouble is indeed prostatitis, and the episode is severe enough, it may take four to six weeks of antibiotics for PSA to return to its normal, or baseline, levels—although in some men, the baseline level moves up to a new plateau, and falls no further.

Sexual activity can elevate PSA as well: PSA levels can increase by as much as 41 percent in less than an hour after ejaculation. (Thus, it is wise to abstain from having sex for two days before you are due to have your PSA tested.)

An episode of urinary retention (from BPH, or urinary tract infection) can also cause an abrupt elevation in PSA, and take as long as a week to return to normal. In rare cases, BPH can block blood supply to areas of the prostate. This is called a prostate infarction, and the cutoff of blood is much like that in a myocardial infarction, or heart attack. An episode of prostate infarction can trigger urinary retention, and also cause a temporary jump in PSA, sometimes to startling levels—as high as 100 or 200. One study by Michigan scientists found that infarcts can elevate not only levels of PSA, but of acid phosphatase (another enzyme made by the prostate; see Chapter 6), and that "infarcts may be responsible for some otherwise unexplained levels" of both of these enzymes in the blood.

Finally, a mistake in the medical laboratory can cause a wrong PSA reading—and create needless anxiety in the process. For all of these reasons, no treatment decision should be made on a lone PSA reading. (For more on confirming the diagnosis of prostate cancer, see Chapter 6.)

Note: One activity that does not raise PSA levels (and create a false warning of cancer) is bicycling. In one study, published in the *Archives of Family Medicine*, scientists studied twenty men, aged twenty-seven to fifty-four, who were members of a cycling club. They found that even long-distance cycling (although it did seem to cause numbness in the perineum, the area between the scrotum and rectum) did not raise blood levels of PSA. A larger study, of 260 men who competed in a four-day race, found no significant change in PSA levels. (However, four of these men already had PSA levels higher than 4, and these levels did increase slightly after the race.)

Prostate Cancer Screening: What Should I Do?

Have a *digital rectal exam* and

PSA test at age forty, forty-five, and every year starting at age fifty, until old age or ill health suggest that your life span is less than ten to fifteen years. (If you are African American, or if you have a family history of prostate cancer, you should begin yearly testing at age forty.)

If the rectal exam is positive: Have a *biopsy, even if your PSA is low.*

If the rectal exam is negative, the next step depends on your PSA: You should have a biopsy if your PSA is:

- Greater than 2.5 and you are age forty to forty-nine
- Greater than 3.5 and you are age fifty to fifty-nine
- Greater than 4.0 and you are sixty or older
- Lower than the above ranges, but has increased by more than 1.5 over the last two years

These recommendations do not include free PSA. Should you have your free PSA tested? It may come down to what bothers you most—the thought of missing cancer at the earliest possible diagnosis, or having an unnecessary biopsy because of a false alarm.

You can relax until the next rectal exam and PSA test if your PSA is:

- Less than 2.5 and you are age forty to forty-nine
- Less than 3.5 and you are age fifty to fifty-nine
- Less than 4.0 and you are age sixty or older

Again, these recommendations use total PSA alone, and not free PSA. If you are worried about having cancer, and your free PSA is less than 25 percent, then you should undergo a biopsy even if your total PSA is within the above ranges.

6

DIAGNOSIS AND STAGING

Read This First

Do you have prostate cancer? Maybe your PSA was abnormal, or it's higher than it was last year, and the year before that. Maybe your doctor felt something suspicious during the rectal exam. What happens now? The next step is to determine whether you have cancer, and the only way to do that is with a biopsy.

But before we go on, we should note that if it is cancer, there is no need to panic and make any hasty decisions. If you have cancer, it didn't start today, this month, or even this year; it's been in there a long time—most likely, at least ten years, growing very slowly. A few more weeks, for you to be absolutely certain of the diagnosis, to determine the extent of the disease, to decide on the right treatment, and find the best doctor to administer that treatment, won't mean that you miss your window of opportunity to be cured. Instead, taking a few weeks to be sure you have enough information to make the right decision may be the best investment in your health, and your life, that you'll ever make.

Once you have all of this information, it's time for some hard decision-making. It's time to ask yourself: *What are my options? And what should I do?* For most men, the diagnosis of prostate cancer is unexpected—like a sudden punch in the stomach. As with any other unexpected calamity in your life, you've got to face it square on, and collect all the facts. At your fingertips are three facts you will probably come to know as well as your Social Security number—your PSA, Gleason score, and clinical stage. With just these three facts, almost immediately you have a good idea where you stand. The cancer either appears to be clinically localized to the prostate—the most common scenario in the United States today, because of improved diagnostic testing—or the cancer has spread locally, but does not appear to be present at distant sites; or rarely, less than 10 percent of the time, the cancer has been caught later, and it has spread to either the lymph nodes or bone. Once you have reached this point, of knowing where you stand, your next move is to examine the options for treatment, and find the one that you feel is best for you.

Diagnosis and Staging

Do you have prostate cancer? Maybe your PSA was abnormal, or it's higher than it was last year, and the year before that. Maybe your doctor felt something suspicious during the rectal exam. What happens now? The next step is to determine whether you have cancer, and the only way to do that is with a biopsy.

But before we go on, we should note several things: First of all, the chances are good that the biopsy will be negative—only 25 percent of men with a PSA between 4 and 10 will turn out to have cancer. And

even if it is cancer, there is no need to panic and make any hasty decisions. *Nothing has to happen today.* If you have cancer, it didn't start
today, this month, or even this year; it's been in there a long time—
most likely, at least ten years, growing very slowly. A few more weeks,

---

TRANSRECTAL ULTRASOUND: BEAUTIFUL PICTURES, LIMITED VALUE BY ITSELF

Like sonar on a submarine, ultrasound creates pictures using sound
waves. Transrectal ultrasound can sometimes detect differences between cancerous and normal tissue in the prostate by means of a probe,
inserted in the rectum (that's what transrectal means—literally, "through
the rectum"). This probe—in effect, a big microphone—is a dramatic improvement over what we had years ago—a lower-frequency, lower-resolu-
tion technique, in which sound waves had to travel all the way through
the abdomen to reach the prostate.

Several years ago, many doctors believed transrectal ultrasound could
be a "male mammogram," another means of screening for and detecting
prostate cancer early. That hasn't happened. Transrectal ultrasound is neither quick nor cheap, and the results often depend on the skill of the doctor using the ultrasound equipment. But the biggest drawback is that even
though ultrasound can produce spectacular images of the prostate, they
are often misleading.

Hit or miss: Originally, imaging specialists believed cancers could be
distinguished from surrounding tissue because they lacked internal
echoes—thus, the sound waves would "bounce" differently, in distinct
patterns. Unfortunately, however, this has not turned out to be a depend-
able system: Just as prostate cancer can *feel* different to a doctor's finger,
based on many factors (see Chapter 5), it can also *sound* different from
man to man. Transrectal ultrasound misses about half of prostate cancers
greater than a centimeter in size because they sound just like regular
prostate tissue. And, because some normal tissue sounds just like cancer,
ultrasound also mistakes many benign lesions for cancer. Thus, most cancers are not seen on ultrasound, and most lesions that *are* seen on ultrasound are not cancer. The main role for transrectal ultrasound is in guiding
the needle biopsy, to make sure that the prostate is systematically sam-
pled. Ultrasound can also be useful in determine the weight of a man's
prostate, which can, in turn, determine PSA density.

The bottom line on ultrasound: It can neither diagnose cancer, nor rule
it out. Beware of the doctor who wants to do an ultrasound "just to see if
there's cancer there"—because, again, ultrasound is not a diagnostic
study. Its only purpose is in helping the urologist aim the biopsy needle.

for you to be absolutely certain of the diagnosis, to determine the extent of the disease, to decide on the right treatment, and find the best doctor to administer that treatment, won't mean that you miss your window of opportunity to be cured. Instead, taking a few weeks to be sure you make the right decisions may be the best investment in your health, and your life, that you'll ever make.

Now, how do you make any wise investment? By learning as much as you can before you commit to a plan of action. So let's move ahead, with this crash course on biopsy:

Biopsy

Until the early 1990s, biopsy of the prostate was done "blind"—doctors couldn't see what they were doing—and often, the biopsy wasn't actually in the part of the prostate doctors thought they were reaching. Today, using transrectal ultrasound as a guide, urologists can see what they're doing in "real time," as they're doing it. So a biopsy of the prostate is more accurate—and, because the needle is smaller than ever, it's less painful, and complications are minimal.

Imagine the prostate as a large strawberry—except this strawberry has just a few seeds, maybe seven little black dots in all. These seeds are tumors (because prostate cancer is "multifocal," there are usually several cancerous spots, not just one; see Chapter 5), and they can be millimeters in size. This is the challenge facing urologists, for whom the prostate biopsy is a critical scouting mission. Our tactical weapon in this search for cancer is a spring-loaded biopsy gun, a tiny device attached to the ultrasound machine. It's a sophisticated needle, hollow in the center, designed to capture tiny cores, or glands, of tissue—each about a millimeter thick—which pathologists will then analyze under the microscope.

Before the biopsy, you will be asked to have an enema, and take some antibiotics to minimize the risk of infection. (For more, see "Before and After the Biopsy," below.) The biopsy is done with you wide awake, lying on your side. The urologist inserts the ultrasound probe through the rectum, and uses the ultrasound image to direct the needle to strategic sites in the prostate.

Although needle biopsies are much better than they used to be, they still aren't perfect, and don't always provide definitive answers. Sometimes what's under the microscope is almost impossible to label definitively as cancer. Just as often, the needle misses the cancer—because it's just plain tricky to hit a tiny seed inside a strawberry, especially one you can't see.

Thus, we hedge our bets. It used to be that urologists took four measly samples of tissue, one from each quadrant of the prostate. Then the number increased to six (one from the top, middle, and bottom of the gland on the right and left sides). Now it's clear that taking ten or twelve samples is better still. We have also become much more strategic in where we fish for cancer: We know, for instance, where the cancer is most likely to be hiding—in the prostate's peripheral zone, extending along its sides like a shallow horseshoe (see Fig. 6.1). We also know that it's likely to spread laterally—like a thin sheet—and that it's easy to stick the needle in too deep, and overshoot the target area. Urologists are learning to guide the needle so it catches the edge of the prostate, rather than sampling tissue from the center, for a "higher yield" of cancer cells. In a Johns Hopkins study, urologist H. Ballentine Carter found that if only six biopsies are taken in the usual way (from the top, bottom, left, and right sides), 25 percent of prostate cancers are missed. However, if six samples are taken from the area where the cancer most probably is—right along the edges of the peripheral zone—only 12 percent of cancers are missed. But the odds of finding cancer are even better if more samples—ten to fourteen—are taken. And men with very large prostates (especially men with benign enlargement) should have even more samples taken: If, say, instead of a large strawberry, you were trying to pinpoint tiny cancers in an orange, it just makes sense that you're in for a tougher job, unless you sample a greater portion of tissue.

"Breast or lung cancer makes a solid nodule, just like a fist, that you usually can detect by palpation or imaging," says Johns Hopkins pathologist Jonathan Epstein. (See "Biopsy: Why You Should Get a Second Opinion," below.) But prostate cancer tends to infiltrate normal tissue, meandering around normal cells. Or, as Johns Hopkins scientist Don Coffey explains, it spreads out like a hand, whose fingers flow into nearby tissue "like a river flooding a valley." This means that there can be a significant amount of cancer—even if it's not in the form of an obvious lump that's easy to feel or see on ultrasound.

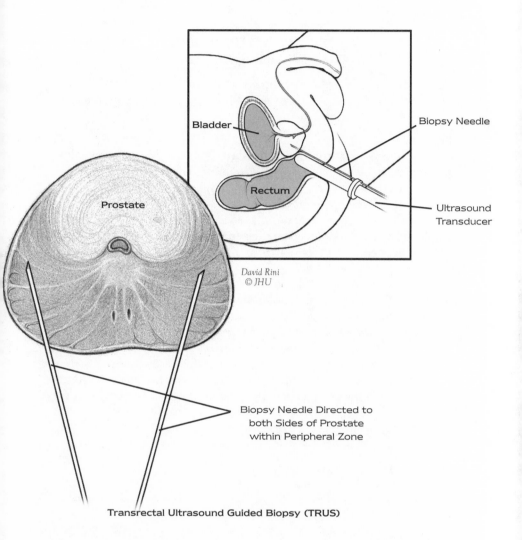

Bladder

Biopsy Needle

Rectum

Prostate

Ultrasound
Transducer

David Rini
© JHU

Biopsy Needle Directed to
both Sides of Prostate
within Peripheral Zone

Transrectal Ultrasound Guided Biopsy (TRUS)

FIG. 6.1 Fishing for Cancer

Cancer is most likely to be hiding in the prostate's peripheral zone, extending along its sides like a shallow horseshoe. Because prostate cancer tends to spread laterally—like a thin sheet—it's easy to stick the needle in too deep and overshoot the target area. Urologists are learning to guide the needle so it catches the edge of the prostate, rather than sampling tissue from the center, for a higher yield of cancer cells.

BEFORE AND AFTER THE BIOPSY: WHAT TO DO, AND WHAT TO EXPECT

The specifics (such as, how long before the procedure you should stop taking aspirin) vary from hospital to hospital, but here are some basic guidelines:

BEFORE:

• No dietary restrictions. Eat breakfast or lunch before you go to the hospital. Drink plenty of fluids—juice, coffee, or water.

• Give yourself an enema (such as Fleet's) the morning of the biopsy.

• Continue taking your regularly scheduled medications, but *DO NOT TAKE* aspirin, arthritic medication, vitamin E, Motrin, or any blood-thinning medications (such as Coumadin or heparin). If you have pain, take Tylenol (acetaminophen). *Your biopsy will likely be canceled if you take any pain medication other than Tylenol.*

• If you are taking a daily dose of aspirin, stop taking it one week before the biopsy. If you have taken any aspirin within one week of the biopsy, it is safest to reschedule the procedure.

• Do not urinate or empty your bladder just before the procedure. Your bladder should be partially full (this makes it easier for the ultrasound to get a good image).

• Take antibiotics ahead of time: You should receive antibiotic tablets to minimize the risk of infection. (The most common antibiotic used here is a fluoroquinolone, such as levofloxacin or ciprofloxacin.) They should be taken the day before the biopsy, on the day of the biopsy, and for two days afterward.

DURING:

• The biopsy will take about thirty minutes.

• You will be asked to lie on your side. The procedure itself is uncomfortable, but usually not painful. (See below.)

AFTERWARD:

• Your urine will probably be tinged with blood; you may even pass a few blood clots during urination, and see blood when you have a bowel movement. This is normal; do not be alarmed. The bleeding should stop the same day, or the next morning.

• "Force fluids"—basically, this means drink a lot—the rest of the day. The reason for this is to dilute your urine, to prevent the formation of blood clots in the bladder.

• Do not drink any alcoholic beverages for twenty-four hours after the biopsy.

• Resume any prescription medications *except* blood-thinning agents such as Coumadin or heparin. (Don't start taking these again until your urologist gives you the go-ahead.)

• No heavy lifting or straining for five days after the biopsy.

> • You may see blood in your ejaculate for several months after the biopsy; this is normal.
>
> **CALL YOUR DOCTOR IMMEDIATELY IF:**
> • You have fever or chills.
> • Your bladder feels very full and you are unable to urinate (this is serious; if necessary, go directly to the emergency room).
> • Rectal bleeding (usually with a bowel movement) lasts for more than two to three days, or is significant.
> • Blood in the urine persists for more than five days.

What Complications Can I Expect from My Biopsy?

Prostate biopsy is an invasive procedure—a minor one, but invasive all the same, and there is a minor risk of complications. These include:

Pain: Although nobody would describe a biopsy as fun, for most men the experience is more in the category of "discomfort" than significant pain. However in some men—particularly those who have ten, twelve, or more tissue samples taken—the biopsy can really hurt. What's hurting is not, as you may think, the rectum (there are no pain fibers in the tissue lining the rectum); the pain is from the needle traveling through the prostate itself. How can you make the biopsy less painful? Explore the options with your urologist. One choice is what's called "conscious sedation." This is what doctors use in procedures such as colonoscopy, and patients feel no pain, and remain conscious throughout the procedure—but don't remember anything that happened during it. (So be aware that even though you may carry on a full conversation with your urologist during the biopsy, afterward you will almost certainly ask the same questions all over again, because you won't remember asking them the first time.) Note: Sedation of any kind increases the cost of a procedure, and also introduces the rare but serious risk that there will be complications from the sedation itself. A safer, cheaper solution is the use of a prostatic block—a local anesthetic, similar to the kind your dentist uses to numb your gums before you have a cavity filled. This block is injected into the tissues surrounding the seminal vesicles on both sides of the prostate (this area is called the pelvic plexus). The same nerves that are responsible for erections (these are the neurovascular bundles, and are discussed in detail in Chapter 8) also carry pain fibers that run to the prostate. Simply blocking these fibers can reduce pain markedly. Alternatively, some urologists believe that the procedure is less painful if an anesthetic jelly is used to lubricate the probe.

Infection: Despite the fact that the biopsy is taken through the rectum, infection is hardly ever a problem, if its risk is kept to a minimum—if a cleansing enema is given beforehand, and antibiotics are given both before and after the biopsy. In most patients, this means getting an oral dose of an antibiotic (in the category of fluoroquinolones) an hour or so before the biopsy, and then taking it two to three days afterward. In some men, however, this may not be enough: If you have a chronic illness such as diabetes, for instance, you may be more susceptible to infection, and may need a longer course of antibiotics. Also, if for some reason the trauma to the rectum is greater than usual, infection can develop. This is terribly important: *If you have any fever after the biopsy, contact your urologist immediately.* In very rare cases, infection can be fatal. In the vast majority of men, however, infection never happens, and complications are minimal.

Bleeding: The urethra, the tube that carries urine from the bladder out of the body, runs right through the prostate (see Fig. 1.2). It is very common, therefore, for a man who has had his prostate biopsied to notice a little bit of blood in his urine immediately after the procedure. You also may notice traces of blood in the ejaculate, sometimes for weeks afterward. This is because the prostate is like a sponge, riddled with tiny ducts, and any bleeding caused by the biopsy can seep into its many nooks and crannies. This blood turns brown with age, and although it's unpleasant, it is no cause for concern, and it absolutely does not signal some turn for the worse in your cancer. It's just old, dried-up blood.

Now, there's a different type of bleeding that can occur during the biopsy, and although this, too, is rare, this can also be serious and require immediate attention: If a man has large hemorrhoids, and the biopsy needle inadvertently punctures one of these veins, this can cause significant rectal bleeding, and may result in another procedure on the spot—sewing up or tying off the broken vein to stop the bleeding.

Impotence: A much rarer complication after biopsy is erectile dysfunction. Some men have reported that their erections after their biopsy are not as strong as they were before the procedure; rarely, a man will even experience impotence. If this happens, it is most likely because the biopsy needle hit too close to one of the neurovascular bundles (for more on these, see Chapter 8), and this is a temporary problem. It's temporary because the nerves are still there, and still intact, and there should be a full recovery of sexual function once the bruised nerve heals. *Again, this is extremely rare—and most important, you should never let the fear of temporary impotence keep you away from a biopsy.* Urologists don't schedule biopsies lightly, and you wouldn't be getting one if your doctor didn't think you needed it.

If I Have Cancer, Will the Biopsy Spread It?

This is an excellent question, and a very common fear. It just makes sense, doesn't it, that if you poke a hole in a wall that's holding back cancer, the cancer might escape. Doctors have worried about this, too, in many forms of cancer. *But the good news is that there is no evidence that this has ever happened, or that it could happen.* Think about it: Almost every cancer you can think of—breast, colon, lung, prostate—is diagnosed by biopsy. If the biopsy itself could spread cancer, then the whole concept of early diagnosis and treatment wouldn't work. But many thousands of people—all of whom had initial biopsies to confirm what they had—have been cured of cancer.

But what if some cancer cells escape into my bloodstream? Well, they may. In fact, the more we learn about cancer in the prostate and elsewhere, the more we understand that the circulation of cancer cells in the blood is probably a fairly common event—even in cancers that are curable. And it's not unreasonable to assume that a few more cancer cells may find their way to the bloodstream when the tumor is manipulated, as it is during a biopsy. *The key is the stage of your cancer.* When cancer is confined to the prostate, even if a few cells escape into the blood, they won't survive. This is because they haven't yet gotten the hang of living outside the area where they developed. But over time, cancer cells change with age. They get more aggressive, and they become, in many ways, "smarter." They not only move to distant sites, but have the wherewithal to thrive in these new locations as well. So there are two different issues: One is the *presence* of cancer cells in the blood; the other is the *survival* of these cells in distant locations. Prostate cancer cells are simply unable to live outside their normal environment until they develop this ability, called metastatic capability.

They Didn't Find Cancer: Am I Off the Hook?

Perhaps the most troublesome thing about prostate biopsies—already a troublesome subject—is figuring out what to do if the cells aren't cancer. Does that mean there's no cancer there—and if so, then why did your PSA go up, or what was that hard lump your urologist felt during the rectal exam? If something suspicious prompted the biopsy in the first place, that something is still there. If that something was palpable during the rectal exam, then you should probably get a repeat biopsy immediately. One explanation for a no-show of cancer is that if a doctor can feel a tumor, that means it's hard—and sometimes, when a needle hits this hard tissue head-on, it just glances off the edge of it, without actually penetrating the tumor and taking a sample of it. Similarly, if your PSA is significantly higher than it should be for your age, or if it's been going up more rapidly than it should, or if your free PSA is low (see Chapter 5 for PSA guidelines), it's possible that the needle biopsy simply missed the cancer. In this case, you should have another biopsy. It's not uncommon for a needle biopsy to be negative—*even though cancer is present.* This is called a "false negative," and it can give both the urologist and the patient "a false optimism that the cancer isn't there," says Johns Hopkins pathologist Jonathan Epstein. Imagine the difficulty of trying to capture this elusive tissue in a biopsy, using only a tiny needle. In some cases, it's like looking *with* a needle in a haystack.

Recently, pathologists at Johns Hopkins looked at seventy-four men who needed more than one biopsy and were eventually found to have cancer. What was the problem here? Why did these men need several biopsies? Was it just that they had very little cancer? For most of the men, no—they had significant cancer, but it was hard to find it: Many of the men had large prostates (greater than 75 grams) or cancer in an out-of-the-way place, up at the top of the prostate, near the pubis (in the anterior or lateral part of the prostate; see Fig. 1.3)—not where a needle would normally go.

Interpretating the Biopsy Findings

Is a biopsy ever just negative? Yes, often the pathologist will state that no cancer is seen, that everything that was biopsied was benign. That is what's called a "negative biopsy" (although you should still seek a second opinion; see below). However, there are two other diagnoses that sound like cancer is not present, but which can be misleading. The first is a word that pathologists love, "atypical." "Atypical" means that the cells can't definitely be called cancerous, but then again, cancer can't be ruled out with certainty. In other words, "atypical" means "maybe." It also means two other things: It means you should have your slides reviewed by a pathologist who is an expert in prostate cancer, to be sure that cancer isn't present. And if the pathologist concurs that it is atypical, you need a repeat biopsy. Another common result is PIN, for "prostatic intraepithelial neoplasia." PIN cells aren't cancerous, exactly, but they are good indicators that cancer is either nearby, or that it's coming soon. If PIN is found, especially if it is high-grade (grade 2 or 3), then you're at an increased risk of harboring a cancer, and you, too, should have a repeat biopsy immediately. (For more on PIN, see below.)

Making Sense of the Gleason Score

Under the microscope, prostate cancer is a mess. Imagine some work of modern art, a painting with countless shades of gray—some nearly white, some nearly black, most subtle variations of shades in the middle. This is prostate cancer—a hodgepodge, a mixed-up batch of cells that range all the way from the almost normal-looking, to cells that are so poorly differentiated and obviously diseased that they could never be considered normal.

The concept here is known as *heterogeneity*, and it's one of the most frustrating aspects in determining how serious a man's prostate cancer is. A pathologist looks at cores of tissue taken in a needle biopsy, and cells from one part of the prostate may look one way, and those from another part may look completely different. So vexing is this, in fact, that for years, pathologists felt that it was impossible to classify, or grade, prostate cancer cells at all.

Then Donald F. Gleason did what nobody else was able to do: He made sense out of these cells. For years, Gleason, the reference pathologist for the Veterans Administration Cooperative Group, studied thousands of prostate cancer biopsies. Gradually, he was able to identify five specific patterns of cancer cell architecture that could be seen under a low-powered microscope. These patterns are called "grades." He then found that if he added the number of the most common pattern to the second most common pattern, he came up with a score—such as, 3 + 3 = 6, or 3 + 4 = 7—and this combination, the score, proved more accurate than just picking one pattern alone. Now the

Gleason scoring system is accepted universally as the best way to assess the aggressiveness of prostate cancer cells.

The lowest possible Gleason score is 1 +1 = 2; the highest is 5 + 5 = 10. However, although in theory this creates nine distinct risk groups, in practice it works a little differently. Today, hardly any men with Gleason 2, 3, and 4 cancers—the least aggressive, and least likely to metastasize—are diagnosed by biopsy. These tumors are most often found in the transition zone—the home of BPH, benign prostatic enlargement. They're usually found when tissue samples from a transurethral resection of the prostate (TURP) are sent to a pathologist for routine testing; they're generally considered "harmless," and usually are managed with watchful waiting. These are the slow-growing "incidental" cancers (discussed in Chapters 3 and 5) that show up in as many as half of all men by age eighty (even Asian men, who hardly ever need treatment for prostate cancer). These, too, are the cancers that critics of PSA testing worried would be found by regular screening for prostate cancer, leading to unnecessary treatment in men with cancer that would never become a threat.

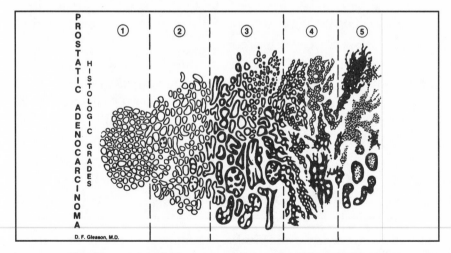

FIG. 6.2   The Many Faces of Prostate Cancer: The Gleason Scoring System

This is prostate cancer—a hodgepodge, a mixed-up batch of cells that range all the way from the almost normal-looking (pattern 1), to cells that are so poorly differentiated and obviously diseased that they could never be considered normal (pattern 5). The Gleason system of evaluating prostate cancer is based on these five specific patterns of cancer-cell architecture, called *grades*. Pathologists add the number of the most common pattern to the second most common pattern and use this *score*—such as (3 + 3 = 6), or (3 + 4 = 7)— to assess the aggressiveness of prostate cancer cells.

But again, these very low-grade tumors are also the ones we hardly ever see on needle biopsy: Fewer than 2 percent of men who have a needle biopsy turn out to have a Gleason score of 2, 3, or 4 cancer. Fortunately, there is good news on the other side of the Gleason scale—we only see high-grade Gleason tumors—Gleason 8, 9, and 10—in about 8 percent of all biopsies. The vast majority of men diagnosed with prostate cancer fall right in the middle of the Gleason scoring system—Gleason 5, 6, and 7. Gleason 5 and 6 tumors are much alike; they behave similarly, and are both relatively slow-growing—the kind of cancers that can be cured. To get a Gleason 7, it means that one part of the equation is a 3 and the other is a 4, which means it's more aggressive. However, Gleason 7 is still different from Gleason 8; more on this later. Furthermore, there is a difference between Gleason 3 + 4, where most of the tumor is Gleason grade 3, and Gleason 4 + 3, where more of the tumor is Gleason 4. It is now known that tumors with more Gleason 4 behave more aggressively. (Thus, when talking about Gleason 7, it's important to know which tumor grade is predominant.)

The Gleason grade ranks *cell differentiation* (Fig. 6.2). Basically, the pathologist asks, how clear-cut are the cancer cells' structure and edges? The architecture of normal, well-differentiated cells involves distinct, clearly defined borders. Well-differentiated cells have clear centers. "They're like little round doughnuts," says Johns Hopkins pathologist Jonathan Epstein. When cancer cells become poorly differentiated, they seem to melt together into malignant clumps. These cancers are the most aggressive. They run rampant, sweeping through nearby tissue and launching missiles to distant sites in the body, no longer respecting boundaries—their own, or those of other cells. The results are often devastating: Without treatment, the fastest, most out-of-control cancer cells can kill a man within several years of their initial clinical presentation. Well-differentiated cancers, in contrast, tend to progress very slowly. Poorly differentiated cancers tend to spread like wildfire.

Cancers with a high Gleason score are more likely to be "margin-positive" (to have cancer that has penetrated the prostate wall to a point where it can't all be removed in surgery; more on this in Chapter 7), more likely to have spread to the seminal vesicles, and more likely to defy treatment than cancers with a lower score. With a high Gleason score, there's also a higher likelihood of cancer spreading to the lymph nodes. Therefore, if a man has a high Gleason score, there is a greater probability that his cancer has spread beyond the prostate wall and maybe to nearby organs.

This is how prostate cancer spreads: First, of course, it grows inside the prostate. (Most—about 72 percent of cancers—begin in the peripheral zone, 20 percent start in the transition zone, and 8 percent originate in the central zone. For more on the prostate's zones, see Chapter 1.) It reaches, and then penetrates, the prostate wall, also called the capsule. Then it starts to creep along the wall of the prostate, heading north, toward the seminal vesicles, ultimately extending in advanced cases into the bladder, the urethra, and the pelvic side walls. (However, it hardly ever reaches directly into the rectum.) Biologically, for whatever reason—certain growth factors, perhaps, or supporting structures—prostate cancer cells seem to need the particular environment that spawned them. However, once the tumor has matured enough to live on its own outside the prostate—that is, once it can grow around the seminal vesicles—it is also more likely to have spread to distant sites. That's why the finding of cancer cells around the seminal vesicles is so important. It is a sign that this cancer can survive outside the environment of the prostate. When doctors speak of "distant metastases" of prostate cancer, they generally mean it has hitched a ride via the bloodstream to the lymph nodes (channels that run throughout the body), bone—the spine, ribs, or pelvic bones—or the lungs.

What if It's PIN?

As any pathologist will tell you, diagnosing prostate cancer is like trying not to fail a particularly tough multiple-choice test—the kind with bewildering answer options like "All of the above" and "Other." Which brings us to another wrinkle in the ambiguous world of needle biopsies—PIN, or prostatic intraepithelial neoplasia. For lack of a better description, PIN cells (which, when present, are found in the tissue lining the prostate) are "funny-looking." They're not cancerous, but they're not benign, either. They're "other." *They're abnormal, and they're strongly linked to prostate cancer.*

Pathologists refer to PIN as a form of "atypical hyperplasia," or an abnormal hyperactivity of growth. Like cancer itself, PIN has its own distinct patterns—mild (PIN1), moderate (PIN2), and severe (PIN3). It's generally believed that mild PIN is insignificant, and that it doesn't require further evaluation.

But most pathologists now believe that moderate and severe PIN (PIN2 and 3) should be grouped together as "high-grade" PIN, and that these cells should be taken very seriously. Some even call these "premalignant" cells (although technically, it's not clear that the cells themselves actually go on to become cancerous). "We'll often find high-grade PIN next to cancer," explains Johns Hopkins pathologist Jonathan Epstein. If high-grade PIN is found but cancer is not, he says, instead of indicating that a man's prostate is cancer-free, the more likely scenario is that cancer may have been missed. High-grade PIN, he believes, "is a marker for prostate cancer," a harbinger that means— if PIN is found in your prostate—you need another biopsy to rule out cancer. (In the largest studies of men with high-grade PIN, the repeat biopsy was positive for cancer 25 to 40 percent of the time.) Moreover, you need this biopsy right away, not six months or so down the road.

What About Perineural Invasion?

As cancers grow, they compress normal tissue, looking for "elbow room"—spaces with less resistance, where they can spread. Nerves are usually surrounded by some empty space; for cancer, this is the real estate equivalent of a nice suburban lot with a big backyard—plenty of elbow room. Thus, it's not uncommon to find prostate cancer in the spaces around the nerves; this is called "perineural invasion." Because the nerves are most common close to the surface of the prostate, the finding of perineural invasion on a biopsy suggests that the cancer is close to the edge of the prostate, and may well have penetrated the capsule. However—this is important to keep in mind— *cancer that has penetrated the capsule can still be cured.* Which makes this a paradoxical finding—because, although men with perineural invasion are more likely to have capsular penetration than men without it, *perineural invasion has no long-term impact on whether or not a man can be cured.* For this reason, some noted pathologists have suggested that it should not even be commented on when found in a biopsy, because it's not worth worrying about.

Rare Forms of Prostate Cancer

Almost all—95 percent—cancers of the prostate are of a type called adenocarcinomas. These are cancers that form in the tiny glands within the prostate. (For an illustration of the prostate, see Chapter 1.)

But there are some rare exceptions: One of these is *small cell carcinoma.* This form of cancer develops in different cells, called neuroendocrine cells, in the prostate. Small cell carcinoma of the prostate is very similar to small cell carcinoma of the lung. It grows rapidly, and is very difficult to cure. The main treatment is chemotherapy. It is rare for small cell carcinoma to be diagnosed initially; usually, it's found in patients who were initially diagnosed with "regular" prostate cancer, an adenocarcinoma, that was not controlled by surgery, radiation, or chemotherapy. In these men, cancer typically comes back as a large pelvic mass, or as metastases to organs such as the liver. The tip-off to this diagnosis is that small cell carcinoma does not make PSA. Thus, if a man has a large, local cancer, and a low PSA, he should be evaluated for small cell carcinoma.

Another rare form of prostate cancer is *transitional cell carcinoma.* (Note: This is different from cancer that is found in the prostate's transition zone.) This cancer arises from the prostatic ducts and the prostatic urethra, the stretch of urethra that runs through the prostate. It is the same kind of cancer seen in men with bladder cancer—so if this diagnosis is made, a man should be checked for bladder cancer as well—and the treatment is often directed at removing both the prostate and bladder.

Finally, *sarcoma of the prostate* is very rare. These tumors arise from the stroma, the smooth muscle and connective tissue within the prostate, and they can be very large at the time of diagnosis. Treatment, as with "regular" prostate cancer, is based on the extent of the tumor.

BIOPSY: WHY YOU SHOULD GET A SECOND OPINION

You're a pathologist staring at cancer cells under a microscope. Just a few tiny cores of tissue, and a man's life may depend on what you have to say about it. You make the call: Your word is a huge part of the treatment decision-making. So think, think—what about those funny-looking cells over there? Is it cancer?

The prostate biopsy can be a pathologist's worst nightmare. "Of all biopsies, prostate biopsies are probably the hardest" explains Johns Hopkins pathologist Jonathan Epstein, who is world-renowned for his expertise and accuracy in judging prostate cells, and who has probably examined more prostate tissue than any other pathologist. "You're dealing with such a limited amount of tissue, and cancers tend to creep around the benign gland," rather than forming as a solid mass. Imagine a Tootsie Roll, wrapped in paper. The cancer is like the paper, a veneer over an expanse of healthy tissue. And the veneer is often maddeningly ambiguous. So not only can the hollow-core biopsy needle overshoot and miss the cancer, the cancer cells it *does* get don't always match the pictures in the textbook.

One result of this is the biopsy labeled "atypical"—a diagnosis that appears in about 5 percent of biopsies at most institutions, says Epstein. "Basically, what that means is that a pathologist will see something that he thinks could be cancer, but is not comfortable calling it cancer." For many patients, the next step is having a repeat biopsy—and the value of this is often questionable, he says. "The problem is, in about 20 percent of cases, the biopsy can miss cancer—so even if it's negative, it doesn't mean the patient doesn't have cancer; in fact, the cancer can be extensive. We've seen some missed entirely. They were called totally benign, yet they were cancer." So instead of having a repeat biopsy, the next step should be getting a second opinion on the "atypical" diagnosis.

Another problem Epstein has found is that many pathologists seem just as likely to overdiagnose cancer: "There are many mimickers of prostate cancer under the microscope, and people not as familiar with prostate biopsies can diagnose cancer when it's not." About one and a half percent—six to eight men—of the patients who come to the Brady Urological Institute each year with a diagnosis of prostate cancer are found to have been misdiagnosed. "We switch the diagnosis. We say, 'This is not cancer, this is benign.'"

Perhaps the best option in the case of tricky diagnoses, says Epstein, is to have the slides sent to an expert. "About 70 to 80 percent of the time, it can be resolved as being definitively benign, or definitely cancer." But even biopsies that seem straightforward deserve another look. "We recommend getting a second opinion before anybody undergoes any form of treatment," says Epstein. "*It's just as important as getting a second opinion for surgery or radiation. You could have the best surgeon in the world, but if you don't have the right pathology, you could have the wrong thing done for you.*"

On this point, Epstein is blunt: "We have done numerous studies showing the reproducibility of Gleason scores" at academic medical centers and in the general pathology community, looking at the Gleason grade based on a biopsy and then comparing it to the actual specimen removed during surgery. Although the "before" and "after" Gleason grades are usually in excellent agreement at academic medical centers, "by and large, the Gleason grading that's performed in the community is disappointing. All across the map, it doesn't correlate with what you see in a radical prostatectomy. People are having decisions made—surgery or radiation, or watchful waiting—based in part on a Gleason grade, when it's not accurate." In an effort to improve prostate cancer diagnosis, Epstein has designed an online tutorial for pathologists. (Pathologists interested in learning more can find the Web site at www.pathology.jhu.edu. The Gleason's grading tutorial is under the "Divisional Web Sites" heading.)

Beware the low-grade Gleason score: Particularly erroneous, Epstein has found, are biopsies given low Gleason scores. "From the standpoint of patient care, the low-grade Gleason (a score of 2, 3, or 4) doesn't exist, and it gives a false sense of optimism. Even if I call something a 2 + 2 = 4 in a biopsy, when the prostate is removed in a radical prostatectomy, it will turn out to be Gleason 5, 6 or higher." Low-grade Gleason tumors do exist, Epstein says, "but where they exist is in the central transition zone of the prostate, not in the peripheral zone where you do biopsies. A low Gleason score is the kind of thing that shows up more in a transurethral resection of the prostate" (TURP), a procedure used to treat benign prostate enlargement, in which tiny bits of tissue from the center of the prostate are chipped away and removed through the urethra. "If a tiny focus of low-grade cancer shows up on a TURP, it's not as worrisome as a tiny bit of intermediate tumor found on a biopsy. A low-grade Gleason score is valid on a TURP, but not on a needle biopsy."

The Diagnosis Is Cancer: What Next?

Do you need further tests? Probably not, if you have localized prostate cancer. At this point, you and your doctor have the major information you need to determine the extent of your cancer, and to decide on a course of treatment. The Gleason score tells you the *kind* of cancer cells you have; the next step is to estimate the extent—*how far* these cells may have spread. This is called determining the *clinical stage* of the cancer. (Or "staging" the cancer—doctors often use it as a verb.) Is cancer confined to the prostate? Or has it spread, and if it has, how far?

Until recently, staging of prostate cancer was based on the Whitmore-Jewett system, which had four basic categories, ranging from cancer too small to be felt, to cancer that had metastasized to the lymph nodes and bone. However, it became clear that more refinements were needed for localized cancer categories, and for this reason, the International Union Against Cancer and the American Joint Committee on Cancer have promoted the use of the TNM system. Here, T represents the local extent of the tumor, N indicates the presence of metastases to the lymph nodes, and M is for distant metastases. The T stage is divided into eight categories, depending on whether the cancer can be felt during a rectal examination—and, if so, how extensive it is. If your prostate feels normal on examination, you have T1 disease; the T2 category describes whether the cancer can be felt in half of one lobe, one entire lobe, or both lobes. Note: Many men, and even some

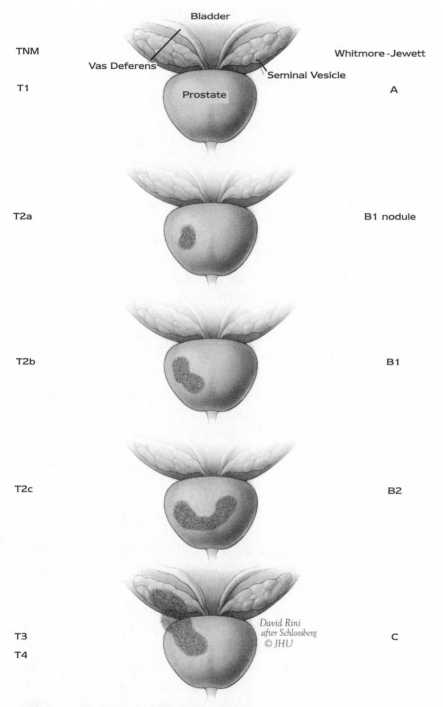

TNM

T1

T2a

T2b

T2c

T3
T4

Bladder

Vas Deferens

Prostate

Seminal Vesicle

Whitmore-Jewett

A

B1 nodule

B1

B2

C

David Rini
after Schlossberg
© JHU

FIG. 6.3 The Stages of Prostate Cancer

This illustration, using both the 1992 TNM and the Whitmore-Jewett systems, shows prostate cancer in all its stages, ranging from cancer that's too small to be felt, to cancer that has spread to the seminal vesicles.

doctors, confuse *bilateral biopsies* with *bilateral palpable disease*. If your cancer is present on biopsy in both lobes of the prostate, but nothing can be felt on examination, you have T1 disease.

The first TNM classification for prostate cancer was developed in 1992; it's a good system, and the one we use in this book (see Table 6.1). However, in 1997, it was meddled with by the American Joint Commission on Cancer. For mystifying reasons, the 1997 modification streamlined three distinct stages of localized cancer—T2a, T2b, and T2c—into two. We feel strongly that this is a mistake. In the 1997 definition, stages T2a and T2b of the 1992 system were combined—see Table 6.1. It may seem nitpicky, but the distinctions are important. Here's why: Men diagnosed with stage T2a according to the 1992 definition (palpable cancer, involving less than half of one lobe of the prostate) have a better prognosis than men with stage T2b disease, as defined by the 1992 definition (palpable cancer, involving more than half of one lobe). (Actually, under the 1992 definition, stage T2b disease has much in common with, and behaves similarly to, stage T2c cancer, which is "bilateral," involving both lobes of the prostate.) Thus, if you are told that you have stage T2a or T2b disease, you need to know exactly what your doctor is talking about. There is at least one proposal to return to the 1992 TNM system, and this may happen. In the meantime, we will only use the 1992 system in this book. Because it is more specific, this is the optimal system to use with the Partin Tables as well (discussed below).

Where Do I Stand? The 2001 Partin Tables

Is the cancer so small that it may not need to be treated? Is it bigger than that, but still localized within the prostate, and curable? Or has it spread to a distant site, and the best hope is to control the cancer? By themselves, the various tests you've had aren't enough to paint the whole picture. For example, the digital rectal exam is not able to pick up microscopic cancer spread to the prostate wall and beyond. Because of this, the digital rectal exam tends to underestimate the stage of cancer. Studies have found that a significant number of cancers initially staged as T2b end up being classified as higher because the cancer has invaded the capsule of the prostate or the seminal vesicles. For cancer with an initial clinical evaluation of T2c, this degree of "understaging" ranges from 39 to 66 percent. One reason for this is that the digital rectal exam is subjective; it depends on the expe-

TABLE 6.1

TNM STAGING SYSTEM

The 1992 and 1997 systems are almost the same, except for one major change: Stages T2a and T2b of the 1992 system were merged into one category in the 1997 system. We believe this is a mistake, because these are distinct stages, and behave in different ways. Thus, we use only the 1992 system in this book.

1992 Stage	1997 Stage	Description
T1a	Same	Not palpable in a rectal exam; found incidentally, when benign tissue is removed by a TURP; 5 percent or less of the removed tissue is cancerous.
T1b	Same	Not palpable; found incidentally; but greater than 5 percent of the tissue removed by the TURP is cancerous.
T1c	Same	Not palpable; identified by needle biopsy because of elevated PSA.
T2a	Same	Palpable; involves less than half of one lobe of the prostate.
T2b	T2a	Palpable; involves more than half of one lobe, but not both lobes.
T2c	T2b	Palpable; involves both lobes.
T3, T4	Same	Palpable; penetrates the wall of the prostate and/or involves the seminal vesicles.
N+	Same	Has spread to the lymph nodes.
M+	Same	Has spread to bone.

rience and perceptiveness of the doctor performing it. Another is that the digital rectal exam can only give information about the prostate gland itself—and not even all of it, at that. And it certainly can't tell anything about the nearby pelvic lymph nodes or bones. Also, if a man has had other surgery on the prostate—a TURP, for instance, for BPH—this can cause the prostate to feel different on an exam, and it can throw off the digital rectal exam.

What about PSA? We know PSA can signal the presence of cancer. But can PSA be more specific—can it tell the stage of a man's tumor? Yes, it can. As always, though, PSA is tricky. As a tumor gets bigger, the

PSA level generally goes up. However, as the tumor grows, it tends to be overrun by more malignant, poorly differentiated cancer cells that have a higher Gleason score. These poorly differentiated cancer cells are different from normal prostate cells, and as a consequence, they make less PSA. In fact, these cancer cells elevate PSA less per gram of tissue than well-differentiated cancer cells—which means that as cancers grow, the PSA level doesn't go up in a directly corresponding way. That's why PSA can be normal even when cancer has spread to the seminal vesicles or pelvic lymph nodes, or it can be higher than expected in men with cancer that's confined to the prostate. *PSA does not accurately estimate the growth of cancer. Thus, the true meaning of PSA can't be interpreted without knowing the Gleason score.*

By itself, the tests you have had are pieces to a puzzle. Scientists at Johns Hopkins have found a more accurate way to estimate the exact extent of prostate cancer, using a special table that puts these pieces together—correlating clinical stage, Gleason score, and PSA, based on information from thousands of men. The result is called an *estimated pathologic stage.*

The best way to predict a cancer's curability is to remove it, and have a pathologist examine every bit of it; this is called the *pathologic stage.* The information you're working with before treatment—the *clinical stage*—is an estimate, what a doctor *believes* a man's prostate cancer to be, based on the rectal exam, PSA, transrectal ultrasound, and needle biopsy. However, pathologic stage is much more certain for predicting the likelihood of cure, because a pathologist has been able to examine actual prostate tissue and, often, tissue from the lymph nodes—not just make guesses about it based on a few cells and test results.

The Partin Tables were developed at Johns Hopkins by urologists Alan Partin and Patrick Walsh, after Partin studied the course of prostate cancer in hundreds of Walsh's radical prostatectomy patients. They're designed to help men and their doctors predict the definitive pathological stage before treatment and then determine the best course of action. The 2001 Partin Tables, which appear at the end of this chapter, are based on the results of 5,079 men who underwent surgery at the Johns Hopkins Hospital between 1994 and 2000. It is important to use these updated tables (as opposed to older ones you can find on the Internet or those your doctor may have) because they reflect the improvement in cancer control that has come with increasingly earlier diagnosis. There are five tables, and they can predict the likelihood of a man's having organ-confined disease, capsular penetration (cancer that has reached the prostate wall), cancer in the seminal vesicles, and cancer in the lymph nodes with 95 percent accuracy. (These are the numbers in parentheses in the table; they indicate that only 5 percent of the patients will fall on either side of those limits.)

These tables are the next best thing to "virtual surgery"—they help predict what would be found if the prostate were removed surgically, and examined by a pathologist. This provides an excellent way to predict the chances of cure—the chances that treatment will eliminate the disease forever, and that no cancer cells have escaped the prostate. If the tumor is found to be confined to the prostate, or even if the tumor has penetrated the capsule of the prostate, but the surgeon can obtain a clear margin (the margin is the edge of the removed tumor; a clear margin means there aren't any cancer cells on the edges—an excellent sign the surgeon got it all), then the chances for cure are very good. To determine the chances for cure with each pathologic stage, see pages 296–297. If the cancer has invaded the nearby seminal vesicles, it is likely that some cancer cells have escaped the "local area," the prostate and its immediate vicinity. However, about 40 percent of men who have seminal vesicle involvement will have an undetectable PSA (in surgeons' terms, an undetectable PSA equals cure) ten years after radical prostatectomy. Finally, if cancer has spread to the lymph nodes, it is very unlikely that the PSA will be low ten years later. But there still may be a role for radical prostatectomy in some men (see below).

Whatever the finding, don't get discouraged. Even cancer in the highest stages can be controlled and kept at bay indefinitely, sometimes for many years. There is always hope. Even men with cancer in their lymph nodes can live for many years clinically disease-free (without any symptoms). There will be much more about this in later chapters.

How to use the tables: To figure out where you fit into these tables (at the end of the chapter), start by plugging in your PSA score. For example, if a man has a PSA less than 4, and a small tumor involving less than half of one lobe of his prostate (T2a disease), with a Gleason score of 6, there is almost a 98 percent probability that the cancer will be confined to the "surgical specimen"—what would be removed in a radical prostatectomy, if the man chooses this avenue of treatment—and a very low probability (1 or 2 percent) that the cancer has escaped to the seminal vesicles or lymph nodes. This is clearly a curable cancer. Conversely, the higher the PSA, more poorly differentiated the cancer, the more advanced the clinical stage, the lower the likelihood of cure. For example, if a man has a PSA of 14, palpable cancer involving both lobes of the prostate (T2c), and Gleason 8 disease, the probability that the cancer will be confined to the surgical specimen is 47 percent, and the likelihood that it will involve the lymph nodes or seminal vesicles is 53 percent. In this scenario, it is likely that micrometastasis to distant sites has occurred.

Now, having said all this: We also have to point out that, although these figures are as accurate as we can make them, *they are just statistics.* There are no absolutes; every man's situation is different. Thus, other factors, beyond cold, hard numbers, can be terribly important in determining the best course of action. For example, in situations where cure is unlikely *but possible:* For a man in good health who otherwise could expect to live at least ten to fifteen more years, the side effects of radical prostatectomy are low enough that it's worth it to attempt a cure. For older men, or men with other health problems (because radical prostatectomy, a major operation, does take a certain physical toll), who are more likely to have severe side effects from surgery and less likely to receive the same benefit, radiation is probably a better choice.

So take this information as your starting point. Consider carefully your overall health and potential longevity. Then you and your doctor can decide whether or not it's reasonable to select curative forms of therapy, or simply to adopt a policy of watchful waiting, in which the tumor is treated only after it produces symptoms.

Caveats That May Affect Your Outlook

Age: Age is one of the most important factors in making a decision about treatment, and it's also one of the hardest. For most of us, on the scale of unpleasant things to do, the idea of estimating how many more years we have left to live would rank somewhere below having a root canal. But now is the time for you to make an honest appraisal of your general health. If you appear to have localized cancer, but you've got some other medical problems—say you've had a heart attack, or you have trouble breathing—then it may only be necessary to keep an eye on the tumor initially, a treatment that's called watchful waiting. Or, you should opt for one of the less strenuous forms of treatment. On the other hand, if your family has a history of longevity (if your parents lived to their eighties or nineties), if your blood pressure is low, if you don't have diabetes, you don't smoke, and have no history of heart disease, then you may live long enough to need to be cured, and your cancer may be aggressive enough that it requires aggressive therapy.

We used to believe that prostate cancer was an "old man's disease"—rather doddering, slow to progress, and more harmless than cancer in younger men. We don't believe that anymore. Research has shown that in older men, prostate cancer is often more aggressive than it is in younger men, and it's often diagnosed at a later stage. A recent Johns Hopkins study, led by urologist H. Ballentine Carter, has shown that older men have larger volumes of tumor, and they're more likely to have Gleason 7 tumors.

Why is this? Simply because the cancer has been there longer. As prostate tumors grow, they become more heterogeneous, and poorly differentiated. They accumulate more mutations, and become more aggressive. Prostate cancer generally is a slow grower. In its early stages, it can take months or even years for a tumor to double in size. Before a tumor ever gets big enough for a doctor to feel—about 1 cubic centimeter in volume—it has to double at least thirty times. But after this, it only takes about ten more doublings for prostate cancer to become fatal—when it reaches 1 kilogram in volume. Each time the tumor doubles, there are more mutations. The cancer begins to grow faster; it becomes more aggressive, and the cells learn how to live outside the comfortable environment of the prostate. So in some older men, it may be wise to undertake aggressive therapy, if it is likely that they will be living for many more years.

Race: For reasons we do not understand, African-American men are not only more likely to develop prostate cancer (as discussed in Chapter 3), but to die from it. Is it due to inadequate medical care—making it more likely that cancer will be diagnosed later, rather than sooner? One editorial in the journal *Urology* cited evidence that black American men are "significantly less likely than white men to have a regular doctor, and to have had a digital rectal examination and PSA testing performed." Clearly, the editorial states, "socioeconomic factors, differences in attitudes towards health care and differences in access to health care need to be urgently addressed." Or is it because of some genetic factor that makes tumors in these men more aggressive? Unclear, although there are genetic factors that suggest black men are more susceptible to prostate cancer (discussed in Chapter 3). What is clear, however, is that African-American men with prostate cancer have a serious condition that needs to be approached with the intent to cure. Some studies have suggested that African-American men who undergo radical prostatectomy are more likely to have cancer that has already spread; however, other studies disagree. Regardless, if you are a black man diagnosed with prostate cancer, you and your doctor need to go after it now, aggressively.

Stage T1c cancer: Of all the categories of prostate cancer, this is probably the one that's hardest to make precise predictions about, because it contains a broad spectrum of tumors—from the tiniest, to some that are quite extensive. Because of this, the averages on the Partin Tables give only a rough index as to extent of disease. If you have T1c cancer, the main thing you should know is that you probably have significant cancer, and that it's curable. Cancer that can be cured, and that probably should be. What we can't give you, because nobody knows it yet, is a more precise estimate for your particular cancer. However, there are two distinct subcategories of stage T1c diseases that we do know something about:

Low-volume T1c cancer: The advantage of any screening program for cancer is that it's designed to detect cancer early. The disadvantage to such programs, including the ones for breast cancer, is that some cancers may be found at such an early stage that they don't need to be treated. This can be the case in men with T1c cancer: About 10 to 20 percent of these men have "low-volume" cancers—tumors smaller than 0.2 cubic centimeter. Do you? And does this mean you're one of those lucky men whose cancer won't ever grow enough to cause trouble? The findings reported by the pathologist on the needle biopsy (see above), your PSA density, and free PSA percentage can help here. If the pathologic findings suggest that you may have a small tumor, your PSA density should not be more than 10 or 15 percent of the weight of your prostate. If it's higher, this suggests that something more than benign disease is responsible for your elevated PSA, and that the needle biopsy just didn't sample it adequately. Similarly, if the PSA is coming from BPH, your free PSA should be high—above 15 percent. If it's less than 15 percent, then it is likely that cancer, not benign disease, is causing your PSA to rise—in which case, the cancer is probably more significant than it seems.

If you're a healthy man under the age of sixty with many years still ahead of you, you should strongly consider curative treatment. Expert pathologist Jonathan Epstein of Johns Hopkins says he does not know which cancer is so small in a young man that it won't grow to the point of threatening his life over time. But if, for reasons of age or health, your projected life span is less than ten years, your cancer may never become significant, and may never need to be treated. This is a form of treatment, too—it's called watchful waiting. We discuss it more thoroughly in the next chapter, but here are some factors that can help predict which cancer is significant and which is not. *Note: These factors apply only if the cancer is not palpable, and if the biopsies have included at least six cores:*

Stage T1c cancer is significant if . . .
It's found in three needle cores, OR
It's present in greater than half of any one needle core, OR
If the Gleason score is 7 or higher, OR
If the PSA density is greater than 0.1–0.15, OR
If the free PSA is less than 15 percent.

Stage T1c cancer is probably NOT significant if . . .
It's found in only one or two needle cores, AND
It makes up less than half of each needle core, AND
The Gleason score is 6 or lower, AND
The PSA density is less than 0.1–0.15, AND
The free PSA is greater than 15 percent.

The key word here is "predictive." (Remember, *any* clinical stage is a prediction. The only certainty is pathologic stage.) This prediction is the best we have, based on all we know, and it's only about 75 percent accurate. This means that about 75 percent of the men who are predicted to have low-volume cancer actually are found to have it when they undergo radical prostatectomy. There's a caveat here, too: *It all depends on your pathology.* It is possible that the doctor's needle did not adequately sample the prostate, for all the difficulties with needle biopsy that we discussed earlier in this chapter.

What about the remaining 25 percent? The news is good: Although there's more cancer, it is almost always confined to the prostate, and curable. However, 25 percent is a large number of men with significant prostate cancer. That's why we feel that if you're a younger man who may have low-volume disease, you should be very cautious about embracing a watchful waiting philosophy. Prostate cancer is not always forgiving. There are not many second chances with this disease. You need to understand the seriousness here before you take this step. What if the cancer, which is curable now, spreads from one PSA test to the next?

If your health is otherwise good, and you can expect to live at least ten years, and you decide to select watchful waiting, you will need to watch this cancer like the proverbial hawk. For starters, if you did not have *twelve samples taken* during your biopsy, you should have this done now. This will help you be more certain that there isn't more cancer than the original biopsy suggested. If these samples do not reveal more cancer, you should have a rectal exam and PSA every six months, and have intermittent biopsies to make sure the primary tumor has not changed. Unfortunately, as we discussed above, PSA is not perfect in estimating the growth of a tumor: In one Johns Hopkins study, 25 percent of men with progressively growing cancers showed no increase in their PSA. What do we know about watchful waiting in men who appear to have these small tumors? So far, most studies of this have been short-term, because this condition has been recognized for less than a decade. But several studies suggest that 25 to 50 percent of these men who are followed closely will develop progression of cancer within three to five years. At that point, if they choose to undergo surgery, many—but not all—of them will have curable disease.

Very high PSA: You have T1c disease, but your PSA is through the roof. It is possible that you may have curable disease. There is an unusual form of prostate cancer, in which men with *curable disease* can have very high PSAs—as high as 300, for example. How can this be? The cancer is in the transition zone—the site usually reserved for BPH, benign enlargement of the prostate. This is a thin ring of tissue surrounding the urethra, and if cancer is here, it may be trapped in the center of the prostate by a thick band of smooth muscle. In this location, tumors can grow to be quite large *without escaping the prostate.* This is the site, too, of the low-grade Gleason tumors, as discussed above, that probably wouldn't be diagnosed if it weren't for a TURP procedure. For reasons we don't understand, tumors here are usually well differentiated—and men with transition zone cancer are usually curable. How do you know if you have it? First, cancers in the transition zone are hardly ever felt during a rectal exam, because they're smack in the middle of the prostate. Second, they're hard to diagnose, and a typical patient will have undergone two or three negative biopsies before the cancer is found. And finally, the tumors are usually less than Gleason 7. If these criteria apply to you, you may well have curable cancer.

Acid Phosphatase

Acid phosphatase is an enzyme that, just like PSA, is secreted by the prostate gland. When a prostate becomes cancerous, the ductal system stops working properly. So, like PSA, acid phosphatase builds up in the prostate, leaks out, and is reabsorbed by the bloodstream. That's why elevated acid phosphatase levels can signal that something's wrong with the prostate. However, unlike PSA, acid phosphatase is made by many organs other than the prostate. For example, after radical prostatectomy, PSA falls to zero, but acid phosphatase still remains in the normal range; thus, acid phosphatase is not as specific as PSA.

There are two ways of looking at acid phosphatase: Radioimmunoassay, and enzymatic assay. The radioimmunoassay test is *not* helpful. It is often elevated in men with BPH, and therefore it gives little useful information. The enzymatic test, however, can be helpful, because, if it is elevated, it usually signifies advanced disease. But, like PSA, acid phosphatase can be tricky. There are many men with advanced disease in whom acid phosphatase is not elevated.

The PSA test is much more sensitive, and its increasingly widespread use has led some doctors to question the value of acid phosphatase. For instance: In one study of 460 men with prostate cancer, twenty-one men had elevated Pap scores. But for seventeen out of these twenty-one men, advanced cancer had been detected either by an abnormal digital rectal exam or PSA score—so the Pap test provided helpful information for only four men out of the whole group! (This is what scientists call a "low yield" of unique information.) And sometimes when Pap is elevated, it's wrong—a false positive, creating needless anxiety and confusion. Therefore, acid phosphatase is no longer considered a must-have test before a doctor can determine the best therapy. It is most helpful in determining the extent of an advanced tumor.

Transrectal Ultrasound and Staging

Most studies have found transrectal ultrasound to be a rather mediocre predictor of the presence of cancer that has penetrated the prostate wall, and to be downright poor in finding cancer that has reached the seminal vesicles. In two studies, only 30 percent of tumors that had spread to the seminal vesicles could be found by ultrasound. One investigation, of thirty men undergoing radical prostatectomy, found ultrasound's sensitivity in spotting cancer that had worked its way beyond the prostate wall was a measly 5 percent. Another study, comparing ultrasound and pathological staging in 121 men, found ultrasound's overall accuracy in staging was only 66 percent—better, but still not reliable enough. And a multicenter study of 230 men found that ultrasound correctly staged 66 percent of locally advanced cancer and only 46 percent of the cancers confined to the prostate.

Ultrasound's main difficulty is its inability to "see" microscopic cancer spread. So, to sum up: *No definitive decision about a man's course of treatment should be made on the basis of ultrasound alone, and ultrasound readings shouldn't be the cause of a man's exclusion from surgery that potentially could cure his disease.*

Bone Scan (Radionuclide Scintigraphy)

In a bone scan, doctors inject into the bloodstream a radioactive tracer, a chemical that's attracted, like a magnet, specifically to bone. (This substance is harmless and soon passes out of the body.) Then, using a device called a gamma camera, doctors take pictures of the bones. Normal bone absorbs the radioactive tracer at a lower level. But in areas of new growth—of bone regeneration, as in a healing fracture, or cancer—the tracer accumulates; more is absorbed, and this surplus shows up as a "hot spot" on the image.

Bone scans are not perfect. Many men feel that if their bone scan is negative, they're home free. Unfortunately, that's not always true. Microscopic prostatic cancer cells, as we've discussed earlier in this chapter, can sneak out of the prostate and move into bone. But these cells are called micrometastases for a reason—they're tiny. It could take five, ten, or even fifteen years for them even to show up on a bone scan. Thus, a negative bone scan doesn't mean you don't have micrometastases—so it's not very sensitive. Worse, it's not terribly specific. Any form of bone disease will show up as a hot spot mimicking cancer: a new or old fracture, infection, arthritis, anything that's got to do with the bone in question. For example, one man went through a terrible scare because a hot spot suggested the prostate cancer had spread to his skull. It turned out to be an old football injury, the man's cancer was removed, and his PSA remains undetectable. But he and his family experienced needless stress, at an already stressful time. Thus, routine bone scans are not useful in men with localized prostate cancer. The likelihood of metastases is extremely low, and most of the lesions the scan does pick up aren't cancer anyway. Today, bone scans are rarely performed on patients with PSA levels less than 10, unless they are experiencing bone pain. For men diagnosed with more advanced disease (PSA greater than 10, Gleason score greater than 7, clinical stage T3 or greater), a bone scan can be very helpful. If it demonstrates that cancer has spread to bone, then the treatment at this point is clear—immediate hormonal therapy. If the bone scan is inconclusive, more tests will be necessary to find out what form of bone disease is present. Plain X-rays can rule out the presence of benign conditions, such as an old fracture, arthritis, or Paget's disease (in which there is an overgrowth of bone). If these X-rays are clear, it is possible that there is a small bit of underlying cancer—in which case, the next step is usually an MRI of bone. If the answer is still not clear, rarely, some men undergo biopsies of bone to exclude metastases.

Optional Imaging Tests for Staging Prostate Cancer

MRI (magnetic resonance imaging): MRI is painless and noninvasive; it gives a three-dimensional scan of the body, producing images that are like slices of anatomy. It creates better pictures than CT scans (see below), but it's expensive and time-consuming (an average scan lasts about forty-five minutes). Also, being inside an MRI machine, according to one typical patient, is "like being a sardine in a can." Some patients (5 percent or fewer) actually become claustrophobic while they lie in the machine's tubelike embrace. To help prevent this, some hospitals play soothing music while patients are being imaged. (One bit of advice for men about to undergo an MRI scan, although it's easier said than done: It really helps to relax, close your eyes, and, if you can, try to go to sleep.) The newest generations of MRI machines are moving away from the torpedo-tube design, and are more open.

The appeal of MRI is that it produces beautiful images of the prostate. The problem is, we can't rely on these gorgeous images to stage a man's prostate cancer accurately. Several years ago, we hoped a new transrectal coil would fine-tune the accuracy. (Like the probe in transrectal ultrasound, this allowed pictures to be taken through the rectum, instead of through the abdomen.) It didn't—at least not enough to let us determine whether a man had capsular penetration, involvement of the seminal vesicles, or cancer in the lymph nodes. A variation of this approach is magnetic resonance spectroscopy (MRS)—but again, although the high-tech images are beautiful, they just aren't accurate enough to show the true stage of a man's prostate cancer. The problem in both approaches is the nature of prostate cancer itself: In its early stages, it does not make a large mass. Even when cancer penetrates the capsule of the prostate, it usually juts out by just a millimeter or two from the surface of the prostate before the cells begin to meander upward, toward the seminal vesicles. At most, this "extracapsular extension" never reaches more than 5 millimeters. To catch this tiny bit of cancer poking out of the prostate requires microscopic precision—which the images of MRI, although beautiful, are unable to achieve. Further, many of the lesions MRI does pick up are not cancer, and cancers greater than 1 centimeter often don't show up. We believe that MRI has little value in staging prostate cancer, and should only be used to check for pelvic lymph node metastases in men who are at very high risk.

CT (computed tomography) scan: Getting a CT scan basically means having a circular series of X-ray pictures taken by a machine that goes around the body. Then a computer puts the pictures together, generating images that, as in MRI, are like slices of anatomy. The CT tube where a patient lies is bigger than an MRI machine, so claustrophobia is not such a problem, and this technology is faster than MRI. However, the pictures aren't terribly good either. (One way doctors can enhance CT images is to give patients an intravenous dye; however, this can cause an allergic reaction in some people.)

When it comes to imaging the prostate, CT has turned out to be something of a dud. It can't visualize cancer in the prostate, and it's not very good at showing cancer that has spread beyond the prostate. This is mainly because CT looks for sizable masses. It can't spot tiny invasions; and sadly, this is how most prostate cancers spread to new territories. (For example, the overwhelming majority of metastases to the lymph nodes start out on a microscopic level.)

In detecting localized spread of prostate cancer (beyond the prostate wall, or into the seminal vesicles), CT has been found to have a sensitivity of 50 percent at best. It also has an unfortunate false-positive rate in diagnosing prostate cancer in the seminal vesicles. We do not recommend routine CT scans for men who appear to have localized disease. In men with advanced disease, where we are concerned that cancer may be in the lymph nodes, MRI is the preferred means of imaging.

Chest X-ray: The presence or absence of cancer in a man's lungs can help doctors stage prostate cancer. But metastases to the lungs in men with localized prostate cancer are very rare. A chest X-ray is definitely optional—but not necessary. The greatest value of this test is in detecting heart and lung disease, rather than the spread of prostate cancer.

Molecular Staging of Prostate Cancer

Scientists are exploring several promising new means of hunting for prostate cancer cells in the blood. This kind of testing is called molecular staging, because the techniques it uses come from the high-tech field of molecular biology.

RT-PCR: There are several ideas at work here. One is that PSA is only made by prostate cells. (This is not entirely true; PSA is also manufactured in tiny amounts at other body sites such as the urethral glands and submandibular gland.) Another is that PSA-secreting cells can be identified in the blood using a state-of-the-art technique called reverse transcriptase polymerase chain reaction, or RT-PCR.

You may have read about PCR, an extremely powerful way for scientists to amplify DNA; it works like a tiny, molecular Xerox machine, churning out countless copies of bits of genetic material. Well, RT-PCR is just as powerful, but it's more cell-specific. (While DNA, the genetic code, can be extracted from every cell in the body, RNA, like a genetic "fingerprint," can be traced to particular cells—in this case, to prostate cancer cells.)

Note: This technique should not be confused with simpler PSA measurements—it's a different kettle of fish altogether. Other PSA tests (discussed earlier), determine how much PSA is circulating in the plasma, the liquid part of blood. In the RT-PCR technique, scientists extract cells from the blood to determine whether those cells *can make PSA*. The assumption is that if there are circulating cells that can make PSA, then these must be future micrometastases—cells that have escaped the prostate, that will inevitably spread the cancer elsewhere. Initial reports of RT-PCR suggested that men who were found to have advanced cancer at the time of radical prostatectomy were more likely to be RT-PCR-positive. One center even reported that men who had a positive RT-PCR before radical prostatectomy were more likely to have an elevated PSA after surgery than men who were RT-PCR negative. These early reports, as one University of Pittsburgh urologist puts it in a scientific review article, "electrified many prostate cancer investigators who scrambled to duplicate these results." The problem was, he continues, "the assay was as temperamental as it was sensitive . . . reproducible results were extremely dependent on the technique." Most of the researchers who tried to use the RT-PCR technique found that the results had little to do with stage, grade, or a man's eventual prognosis.

But what about these cancer cells floating around in the bloodstream? Isn't this a scary thing? The answer is, sometimes. For years, it has been known that cancer cells can be present in the blood of patients with many different types of cancer *that can still be cured.* (The cancer is curable because, as we discussed earlier, these cells have not yet developed the ability to survive at distant sites.) In fact, in one study, 25 percent of men *with curable cancer* had a positive RT-PCR test; their results were false positives. And this tells us something we already knew, that just because a man has cancer cells circulating in his blood, this doesn't mean his cancer can't still be cured. For these cells to set up a new home in bone, they must develop aggressive techniques to help them survive in a new, hostile environment outside the prostate. Thus, the fact that cancer cells happen to be floating around in the bloodstream is not evidence of metastases—it's like a criminal case based only on circumstantial evidence; it wouldn't hold up in court. A final matter that needs to be explored here is the possibility that this RT-PCR test may not even be a true measure of PSA. It may actually be measuring a molecule that bears a striking resemblance to PSA, but isn't.

A promising new approach: magnetic beads: A remarkable new technique, developed at Johns Hopkins, allows scientists to isolate a single cell from a milliliter of blood—a feat indeed, considering that in this dollop (about one fifth of a teaspoon) of blood are some six million cells.

"The whole technology of being able to isolate single cells out of the bloodstream is a major breakthrough," says urologist Alan Partin, who helped develop this technique. This research, published in *Journal of Urology*, used the technique to answer a question—one we discussed earlier in this chapter—that has long worried doctors and patients: Is it possible that the act of removing the prostate, or even removing some of its tissue in a biopsy, might somehow allow prostate cancer cells to escape into the bloodstream? The answer was reassuring—most likely, no, "and if some cells do break free, it's not significant."

But the technique can also answer questions in men after surgery: Are there still prostate cells floating around, and if so, are they cancer cells? With this test, says Partin, "we can tell if it's a prostate cell, we can tell if it's cancerous." The test accomplishes what RT-PCR has not consistently been able to deliver. RT-PCR, explains Partin, was designed to zero in on a "piece of DNA that looked like it might have come from a prostate cell."

The new test, in contrast, uses tiny magnetic beads, coated with antibodies, that act as flypaper: "They attach to the white blood cells and remove them," says Partin. "Whatever's left is stained for PSA, which lights up in a fluorescent field. Everything else is black, and there's that big prostate cell beacon shining at you."

Someday, this test may be used as a follow-up monitoring test, perhaps as part of routine PSA tests after surgery, to detect any stray prostate cells as soon as possible. The advantage here is that, ultimately, once we know the genetic characteristics of a metastatic cell, these circulating cells could be tested to see whether they—like criminals on the FBI's Most Wanted list—"match the profile." This might become one of several crystal balls we've been seeking—a valuable way to predict the biological behavior of these perplexing cells in the bloodstream.

ProstaScint scan: This test uses an antibody stuck to a radioactive isotope called indium. This antibody, injected in the bloodstream, is designed to zoom in on prostate-membrane-specific antigen, or PMSA, a protein that's made on the surface of prostate cells, and is highly expressed in advanced cancers. The idea is that this test—a nuclear medicine scan of the abdomen and pelvis—could show the extent of disease, highlighting cancer in the prostate, in the area immediately around it, and even spotting pockets of cancer elsewhere, such as the lymph nodes. The test has much promise. For now, however, ProstaScint scans are difficult to read, and there seems to be a great deal of subjectivity in interpreting them. Because the results are often inscrutable, many physicians are reluctant to rely on this test—which leads to the question, why perform a test if you're not confident in the result? Also, for technical reasons, the antibody that is currently used can identify only those cells that are dead; a new antibody is being developed. Until these scans can be improved, it is unlikely that they will or should be widely used.

Lymphadenectomy

Just as the best way to stage cancer is to look at it after the fact (after it's been removed during surgery), the best way to check the lymph nodes in the pelvis for cancer is to go in there and get them—to remove them surgically, and let a pathologist examine them. If a large, suspicious-looking lymph node is seen on an imaging study, it is possible to do a needle biopsy (similar to a needle biopsy on the prostate) without surgery. However, when prostate cancer metastasizes to the lymph nodes, they rarely become enlarged; thus, if it's essential to know the status of the lymph nodes, surgical removal is necessary.

The lymph nodes can be tested during a prostatectomy operation (see Chapter 8), but this technique, called *frozen section analysis,* often misses small amounts of tumor. So again, if it's absolutely essential to know whether cancer is in a man's lymph nodes, the best approach is surgery.

The least invasive approach is called a *laparoscopic pelvic lymphadenectomy.* Picture someone ice-fishing—cutting a tiny, inconspicuous hole, dropping a line, and bringing out a big fish. That's the idea here; laparoscopic surgery is much less invasive than traditional surgery that involves an incision, and the benefits to patients include shorter hospitalization, quicker recovery time, less postoperative pain, and a better cosmetic result—a few tiny holes, for example, instead of a scar several inches long. Alternatively, a procedure called a *mini-lap* (mini-laparotomy staging pelvic lymphadenectomy) can be performed. This requires a slightly longer incision, but the recovery period is about the same. (This is more familiar to most urologists than the laparoscopic technique.)

Who should get it? The only man who should be subjected to one of these procedures is someone to whom it will make a dramatic difference in the decision-making process. For example, say a man has a large, palpable cancer that invades the muscles in the pelvic side wall (stage T3), a Gleason score of 8, and a PSA of 30. There is no reason for this man to go ahead with a lymph node dissection. His disease is already extensive, and treatment for him should be aimed at controlling the cancer, and relieving symptoms and pain. To put this man through the rigors of a procedure that ultimately won't help him is neither helpful nor kind. Instead, this technique is most helpful in men who appear to have clinically localized prostate cancer, but a grade of Gleason 8 or greater. If a man with Gleason 8 disease has any cancer in the lymph nodes, he has an 85 percent chance of having metastatic disease within five years. On the other hand, if the lymph nodes are negative, he has a good chance of being cured at five years. Here, the status of the lymph nodes can provide critically important information. But in men with Gleason 7 or less, the information from the lymph nodes is not as important. As we will discuss in Chapter 7, men with Gleason 7 disease and positive lymph nodes have only a 15 percent chance of having metastatic disease at five years. And there is some evidence suggesting that even men with positive lymph nodes may live longer if their prostate is removed. Thus, we only perform staging pelvic lymphadenectomies in men with Gleason 8 disease who are candidates for surgery, and who are potentially curable.

On the Horizon: New Markers for Staging Prostate Cancer

In Chapter 5, we mentioned some new tests being designed to monitor prostate cancer—including hK2, PMSA, and BPSA. Here are a few more ideas that may prove helpful in staging cancer:

Microvessel density: The idea here is also the idea behind one of the most exciting new approaches for treating advanced cancer, a series of drugs called *angiogenesis inhibitors.* When prostate cancers advance, they pave the way ahead, laying down a track of new blood vessels. This process is called *angiogenesis.* Some scientists believe that measuring the extent of these blood vessels (along with other cancer-nourishing substances made by tumors, called *endothelial growth factors*) can give insight into how aggressive the cancer is.

Immunohistochemistry/laser capture microscopy with microarray analysis. There's a mouthful! The idea here is also to help scientists figure out which cancers are most aggressive by tracking the many genetic changes a cell goes through in its transformation from normal to cancerous, and beyond that to aggressive, advanced cancer. Immunohistochemistry (using antibodies to label and target certain proteins in cells), and its more sophisticated research partners, laser capture (in which a laser picks out a particular cell from under a microscope), and a technique called microarray analysis, are means by which scientists can look through thousands of genes for certain changes that have been linked to aggressive cancer. The big drawback here is the confounded heterogeneity of prostate cancer. When we examine a cancerous prostate removed during radical prostatectomy, we can see, on average, seven separate cancers. And as you might expect, these cancers may all be different in terms of DNA content, the characteristics of the various tumors, and even their aggressiveness. (This is why a needle biopsy tells so little of the story of a man's prostate cancer.) Because of the tremendous variability of prostate cancer, it will be difficult—even with the most sophisticated techniques—to say, "we need to find X, Y, and Z," because those may be just a few of many genetic "bad guys" that determine whether, and how, a cancer will spread.

For most men, the diagnosis of prostate cancer is unexpected—like a sudden punch in the stomach. As with any other unexpected calamity in your life, you've got to face it square-on, and collect all the facts. At your fingertips are three facts you will probably come to know as well as your Social Security number—your PSA, Gleason score, and clinical stage. With just these three facts, almost immediately you have a good idea where you stand. The cancer either appears to be clinically localized to the prostate—the most common scenario in the United States today, because of improved diagnostic testing—or the cancer has spread locally, but does not appear to be present at distant sites; or rarely, less than 10 percent of the time, the cancer has been caught later, and it has spread to either the lymph nodes or bone. Once you have reached this point, of knowing where you stand, your next move is to examine the options for treatment, and find the one that you feel is best for you.

THE 2001 PARTIN TABLES

Scientists at Johns Hopkins have found a more accurate way to estimate the exact extent of prostate cancer, using a special table that puts these pieces together—correlating clinical stage, Gleason score, and PSA, based on information from thousands of men. The Partin Tables are designed to help men and their doctors predict the definitive pathological stage before treatment, and then—based on this more accurate information—determine the best course of action. There are five tables. They can predict a man's likelihood of having organ-confined disease, capsular penetration (cancer that has reached the prostate wall), cancer in the seminal vesicles, and cancer in the lymph nodes with 95 percent accuracy. (These are the numbers in parentheses in the table; they indicate that only 5 percent of the patients will fall on either side of those limits.) To determine the chances for cure with each pathologic stage, see pages 296–297.

PSA 0–2.5 ng/ml

Gleason Score	Path Stage	Clinical Stage T1c		T2a		T2b		T2c	
2–4	Organ-Confined	95	(89–99)	91	(79–98)	88	(73–97)	86	(71–97)
	Capsular Penetration	5	(1–11)	9	(2–21)	12	(3–27)	14	(3–29)
	Seminal Vesicles Involved	0	(0–0)	0	(0–0)	0	(0–0)	0	(0–0)
	Lymph Nodes Involved	0	(0–0)	0	(0–0)	0	(0–0)	0	(0–0)
5–6	Organ-Confined	90	(88–93)	81	(77–85)	75	(69–81)	73	(63–81)
	Capsular Penetration	9	(7–12)	17	(13–21)	22	(17–28)	24	(17–33)
	Seminal Vesicles Involved	0	(0–1)	1	(0–2)	2	(0–3)	1	(0–4)
	Lymph Nodes Involved	0	(0–0)	0	(0–1)	1	(0–2)	1	(0–4)
3+4=7	Organ-Confined	79	(74–85)	64	(56–71)	54	(46–63)	51	(38–63)
	Capsular Penetration	17	(13–23)	29	(23–36)	35	(28–43)	36	(26–48)
	Seminal Vesicles Involved	2	(1–5)	5	(1–9)	6	(2–12)	5	(1–13)
	Lymph Nodes Involved	1	(0–2)	2	(0–5)	4	(0–10)	6	(0–18)
4+3=7	Organ-Confined	71	(62–79)	53	(43–63)	43	(33–54)	39	(26–54)
	Capsular Penetration	25	(18–34)	40	(30–49)	45	(35–56)	45	(32–59)
	Seminal Vesicles Involved	2	(1–5)	4	(1–9)	5	(1–11)	5	(1–12)
	Lymph Nodes Involved	1	(0–4)	3	(0–8)	6	(0–14)	9	(0–26)
8–10	Organ-Confined	66	(54–76)	47	(35–59)	37	(26–49)	34	(21–48)
	Capsular Penetration	28	(20–38)	42	(32–53)	46	(35–58)	47	(33–61)
	Seminal Vesicles Involved	4	(1–10)	7	(2–16)	9	(2–20)	8	(2–19)
	Lymph Nodes Involved	1	(0–4)	3	(0–9)	6	(0–16)	10	(0–27)

PSA 2.6–4.0 ng/ml

Gleason Score	Path Stage	Clinical Stage T1c		T2a		T2b		T2c	
2–4	Organ-Confined	92	(82–98)	85	(69–96)	80	(61–95)	78	(58–94)
	Capsular Penetration	8	(2–18)	15	(4–31)	20	(5–39)	22	(6–42)
	Seminal Vesicles Involved	0	(0–0)	0	(0–0)	0	(0–0)	0	(0–0)
	Lymph Nodes Involved	0	(0–0)	0	(0–0)	0	(0–0)	0	(0–0)
5–6	Organ-Confined	84	(81–86)	71	(66–75)	63	(57–59)	61	(50–70)
	Capsular Penetration	15	(13–18)	27	(23–31)	34	(28–40)	36	(27–45)
	Seminal Vesicles Involved	1	(0–1)	2	(1–3)	2	(1–4)	2	(1–5)
	Lymph Nodes Involved	0	(0–0)	0	(0–1)	1	(0–2)	1	(0–4)
3+4=7	Organ-Confined	68	(62–74)	50	(43–57)	41	(33–48)	38	(27–50)
	Capsular Penetration	27	(22–33)	41	(35–48)	47	(40–55)	48	(37–59)
	Seminal Vesicles Involved	4	(2–7)	7	(3–12)	9	(4–15)	8	(2–17)
	Lymph Nodes Involved	1	(0–2)	2	(0–4)	3	(0–8)	5	(0–15)
4+3=7	Organ-Confined	58	(48–67)	39	(30–48)	30	(22–39)	27	(18–40)
	Capsular Penetration	37	(29–46)	52	(43–61)	57	(47–67)	57	(44–70)
	Seminal Vesicles Involved	4	(1–7)	6	(2–12)	7	(3–14)	6	(2–16)
	Lymph Nodes Involved	1	(0–3)	2	(0–6)	4	(0–12)	7	(0–21)
8–10	Organ-Confined	52	(41–63)	33	(24–44)	25	(17–34)	23	(14–34)
	Capsular Penetration	40	(31–50)	53	(44–63)	57	(46–68)	57	(44–70)
	Seminal Vesicles Involved	6	(3–12)	10	(4–18)	12	(5–22)	10	(3–22)
	Lymph Nodes Involved	1	(0–4)	3	(0–8)	5	(0–14)	8	(0–22)

PSA 4.1–6.0 ng/ml

Gleason Score	Path Stage	T1c		T2a		T2b		T2c	
2–4	Organ-Confined	90	(78–98)	81	(63–95)	75	(55–93)	73	(52–93)
	Capsular Penetration	10	(2–22)	19	(5–37)	25	(7–45)	27	(7–48)
	Seminal Vesicles Involved	0	(0–0)	0	(0–0)	0	(0–0)	0	(0–0)
	Lymph Nodes Involved	0	(0–0)	0	(0–0)	0	(0–0)	0	(0–0)
5–6	Organ-Confined	80	(78–83)	66	(62–70)	57	(52–63)	55	(44–64)
	Capsular Penetration	19	(16–21)	32	(28–36)	39	(33–44)	40	(32–50)
	Seminal Vesicles Involved	1	(0–1)	1	(1–2)	2	(1–3)	2	(1–4)
	Lymph Nodes Involved	0	(0–1)	1	(0–2)	2	(1–3)	3	(1–7)
3+4=7	Organ-Confined	63	(58–68)	44	(39–50)	35	(29–40)	31	(23–41)
	Capsular Penetration	32	(27–36)	46	(40–52)	51	(44–57)	50	(40–60)
	Seminal Vesicles Involved	3	(2–5)	5	(3–8)	7	(4–11)	6	(2–11)
	Lymph Nodes Involved	2	(1–3)	4	(2–7)	7	(4–13)	12	(5–23)
4+3=7	Organ-Confined	52	(43–60)	33	(25–41)	25	(18–32)	21	(14–31)
	Capsular Penetration	42	(35–50)	56	(48–64)	60	(50–68)	57	(43–68)
	Seminal Vesicles Involved	3	(1–6)	5	(2–8)	5	(3–9)	4	(1–10)
	Lymph Nodes Involved	3	(1–5)	6	(3–11)	10	(5–18)	16	(6–32)
8–10	Organ-Confined	46	(36–56)	28	(20–37)	21	(14–29)	18	(11–28)
	Capsular Penetration	45	(36–54)	58	(49–66)	59	(49–69)	57	(43–70)
	Seminal Vesicles Involved	5	(3–9)	8	(4–13)	9	(4–16)	7	(2–15)
	Lymph Nodes Involved	3	(1–6)	6	(2–12)	10	(4–20)	16	(6–33)

PSA 6.1–10.0 ng/ml

Gleason Score	Path Stage	T1c		T2a		T2b		T2c	
2–4	Organ-Confined	87	(73–97)	76	(56–94)	69	(47–91)	67	(45–91)
	Capsular Penetration	13	(3–27)	24	(6–44)	31	(9–53)	33	(9–55)
	Seminal Vesicles Involved	0	(0–0)	0	(0–0)	0	(0–0)	0	(0–0)
	Lymph Nodes Involved	0	(0–0)	0	(0–0)	0	(0–0)	0	(0–0)
5–6	Organ-Confined	75	(72–77)	58	(54–61)	49	(43–54)	46	(36–56)
	Capsular Penetration	23	(21–25)	37	(34–41)	44	(39–49)	46	(37–55)
	Seminal Vesicles Involved	2	(2–3)	4	(3–5)	5	(3–8)	5	(2–9)
	Lymph Nodes Involved	0	(0–1)	1	(0–2)	2	(1–3)	3	(1–6)
3+4=7	Organ-Confined	54	(49–59)	35	(30–40)	26	(22–31)	24	(17–32)
	Capsular Penetration	36	(32–40)	49	(43–54)	52	(46–58)	52	(42–61)
	Seminal Vesicles Involved	8	(6–11)	13	(9–18)	16	(10–22)	13	(6–23)
	Lymph Nodes Involved	2	(1–3)	3	(2–6)	6	(4–10)	10	(5–18)
4+3=7	Organ-Confined	43	(35–51)	25	(19–32)	19	(14–25)	16	(10–24)
	Capsular Penetration	47	(40–54)	58	(51–66)	60	(52–68)	58	(46–69)
	Seminal Vesicles Involved	8	(4–12)	11	(6–17)	13	(7–20)	11	(4–21)
	Lymph Nodes Involved	2	(1–4)	5	(2–8)	8	(5–14)	13	(6–25)
8–10	Organ-Confined	37	(28–46)	21	(15–28)	15	(10–21)	13	(8–20)
	Capsular Penetration	48	(39–57)	57	(48–65)	57	(48–67)	56	(43–69)
	Seminal Vesicles Involved	13	(8–19)	17	(11–26)	19	(11–29)	16	(6–29)
	Lymph Nodes Involved	3	(1–5)	5	(2–10)	8	(4–16)	13	(5–26)

PSA > 10.0 ng/ml

Gleason Score	Path Stage	Clinical Stage							
		T1c		T2a		T2b		T2c	
2–4	Organ-Confined	80	(61–95)	65	(43–89)	57	(35–86)	54	(32–85)
	Capsular Penetration	20	(5–39)	35	(11–57)	43	(14–65)	46	(15–68)
	Seminal Vesicles Involved	0	(0–0)	0	(0–0)	0	(0–0)	0	(0–0)
	Lymph Nodes Involved	0	(0–0)	0	(0–0)	0	(0–0)	0	(0–0)
5–6	Organ-Confined	62	(58–64)	42	(38–46)	33	(28–38)	30	(21–38)
	Capsular Penetration	33	(30–36)	47	(43–52)	52	(46–56)	51	(42–60)
	Seminal Vesicles Involved	4	(3–5)	6	(4–8)	8	(5–11)	6	(2–12)
	Lymph Nodes Involved	2	(1–3)	4	(3–7)	8	(5–12)	13	(6–22)
3+4=7	Organ-Confined	37	(32–42)	20	(17–24)	14	(11–17)	11	(7–17)
	Capsular Penetration	43	(38–48)	49	(43–55)	47	(40–53)	42	(30–55)
	Seminal Vesicles Involved	12	(9–17)	16	(11–22)	17	(12–24)	13	(6–24)
	Lymph Nodes Involved	8	(5–11)	14	(9–21)	22	(15–30)	33	(18–49)
4+3=7	Organ-Confined	27	(21–34)	14	(10–18)	9	(6–13)	7	(4–12)
	Capsular Penetration	51	(44–59)	55	(46–64)	50	(40–60)	43	(29–59)
	Seminal Vesicles Involved	11	(6–17)	13	(7–20)	13	(8–21)	10	(3–20)
	Lymph Nodes Involved	10	(5–17)	18	(10–27)	27	(16–39)	38	(20–58)
8–10	Organ-Confined	22	(16–30)	11	(7–15)	7	(4–10)	6	(3–10)
	Capsular Penetration	50	(42–59)	52	(41–62)	46	(36–59)	41	(27–57)
	Seminal Vesicles Involved	17	(10–25)	19	(12–29)	19	(12–29)	15	(5–28)
	Lymph Nodes Involved	11	(5–18)	17	(9–29)	27	(14–40)	38	(20–59)

*Numbers represent percent predictive probability (95 percent confidence interval). Ciphers indicate lack of sufficient data to calculate probability.

Source: Partin, A. W., P. C. Walsh, J. I. Epstein, and J. D. Pearson, "Contemporary Update of Prostate Cancer Staging Nomograms (Partin Tables) for the New Millennium," *Urology* vol. 58, 2001.

7

WHAT ARE MY OPTIONS?

Read This First

What's the best treatment for prostate cancer? This is a trick question. There is no single best treatment, because prostate cancer isn't a "one-size-fits-all" disease. It's different in every man. There are many factors—not only the clinical stage of your cancer, but your own age and general health—involved in choosing the treatment that's right for you.

Fifteen years ago, most men who had prostate cancer were diagnosed at an older age, and with more advanced disease. Most efforts were palliative, aimed at relieving symptoms (as opposed to curative, aimed at eradicating the cancer), and men often died within a few years. Today, thankfully, the tables have been turned: Now, most

American men are diagnosed with localized prostate cancer, and are curable. It is possible today to prevent a man from dying a painful death of prostate cancer fifteen or twenty years in the future. Now, the goal is to achieve this *and* leave the patient with an excellent quality of life—cured of cancer, continent, potent, as if nothing had ever happened, and the diagnosis and treatment of cancer were just a rough patch on the road. If you have localized disease (this includes locally advanced disease), you have three main choices: watchful waiting, surgery, or radiation therapy.

The best thing you can do now is educate yourself—not just about prostate cancer, but about the doctors who treat it. You're building a bridge here, and you can only go so far by yourself. Ultimately, you are going to have to find a physician you trust to help you find your way through this very complicated disease.

What Are My Options?

Prostate cancer is a complicated disease—so complicated, in fact, that it's unique in every man. Your brother-in-law had prostate cancer? Your neighbor, too? And now you—three men with three distinct cancers. There is so much variability here. Because the disease is completely different from man to man, you may find that the treatment that's best for your neighbor is not the one that's best for you. You can't go by anybody else's experience with prostate cancer, because you've each got your own custom-made case. And yet, you're all part of the same club, a group nobody wants to join—the "reluctant brotherhood" of men with prostate cancer.

What's the best treatment? This is a trick question. There is no single best treatment, because, again, prostate cancer isn't a "one-size-fits-all" disease. There are many factors—not only the clinical stage of your particular cancer, but your own age and general health—involved in choosing the treatment that's right for you. Even personal preferences enter into this decision: Some men, for example, would rather take action—even if their cancer is incidental—than drive themselves crazy with worry, living from one PSA test to the next in watchful waiting. To other men, the idea of surgery is so disturbing that they would rather take their chances with diet, meditation, and other lifestyle changes than go "under the knife." For some men—such as an eighty-one-year-old man with diabetes and congestive heart failure—any form of aggressive treatment, with side effects and recovery time, would not only be unhelpful, but could produce complications that can make the "golden years" needlessly unpleasant. For others—a seventy-six-year-old man who swims two miles a day, who has two teenage children and parents who died in their nineties—not going after this disease aggressively would be uncharacteristic, and unthinkable.

Fifteen years ago, most men who had prostate cancer were diagnosed at an older age, and with more advanced disease. Most efforts were palliative, aimed at relieving symptoms (as opposed to curative, aimed at eradicating the cancer), and men often died within a few years. Today, thankfully, the tables have been turned: Now, most American men are diagnosed with localized prostate cancer, and are curable. The use of PSA testing has given us a five-year lead time in diagnosis. It is possible today to prevent a man from dying a painful death of prostate cancer fifteen or twenty years in the future. Now, the goal is to achieve this *and* leave the patient with an excellent quality of life—cured of cancer, continent, potent, as if nothing had ever happened, and the diagnosis and treatment of cancer were just a rough patch on the road. If you have localized disease (this includes locally advanced disease), you have three main choices: watchful waiting, surgery, or radiation therapy. As you work through your decision about treatment, ask yourself questions like these: What's more important? Knowing that you're cured of cancer, but realizing that there's a trade-off—in other words, you might have some side effects from treatment? Or, would it be better for you to get the treatment with the fewest side effects, hoping that you may die of something else before cancer catches up?

If You Have Localized or Locally Advanced Disease

As we discussed in Chapter 6, prostate cancer grows relatively slowly for many years. When it's localized—confined within the prostate—it can take years for a tumor to double in size. And here is the confounding thing: *Cancer can stay in the prostate indefinitely.* It takes a long time and many steps involving subtle genetic changes before a normal cell, which is designed to live and die, becomes a cancer cell—before some switch is activated that makes the cell think it's immortal—and before such cells start dividing endlessly. (As we've discussed earlier, in high-risk men, some of these steps are short-ened.) But—although we're working to improve our means of prediction—as yet, nobody can "mind-read" localized prostate cancer. There is no crystal ball to tell us what it's going to do.

If localized prostate cancer is found in a sixty-five-year-old man, for example, it could stay in the prostate for years and he may die *with* prostate cancer, not *of* it. This is what happens to hundreds of thousands of men, and it's one of the factors that can make treatment decisions so cloudy. But—and this is the crux of the issue— once it escapes the prostate to distant sites, the lymph nodes and bones, today there is no way to stop it. It can rarely be cured, although it can often be controlled. (And with an explosion of new treatment strategies for advanced disease, our ability to control cancer will keep getting better.) Just a few years ago, once cancer had spread to bone, the average life expectancy was three years. (Again, as new treatment strategies are tested and made available, this can be expected to change—see Chapter 12.)

So: If you have localized disease, the big, blunt question you need to ask yourself is, *how long are you probably going to live?* Nobody wants to think about this question, but there it is. In men over sixty-five who don't have heart disease or another form of cancer, life expectancy can vary from two years to thirty-seven years. The factors, in order of importance, that can shorten your life expectancy are: hypertension, smoking, diabetes, consuming more than four drinks of alcohol a day, and not exercising. In contrast, factors that can help you live longer are getting regular exercise, eating a diet low in fat and high in fruits and vegetables, and having a high HDL (the "good" kind) of cholesterol.

The next question is, *is your cancer curable?* What is the chance that the cancer has not extended to the seminal vesicles or the lymph nodes? Remember, even if the cancer has penetrated the capsule, it can still be cured in most cases. But it's harder to cure the cancer if it's involved the seminal vesicles, and prostate cancer is rarely curable if it involves the lymph nodes. You probably have a pretty good estimate of this from the Partin Tables in the last chapter. And next, how old are you? This is different from the question about your life expectancy. If you are in your fifties or younger, even if the odds of cure don't appear to be in your favor, you will tolerate surgery better than an older man, and you should probably consider it. If you are older, the situation gets a bit more complicated. Men over seventy who undergo radical prostatectomy are more likely to have problems with impotence and incontinence. (Note: Both of these can be treated, and the rates of complications vary significantly, depending on the expertise of the surgeon who performs the operation.) Men over seventy are also more likely to have more cancer than younger men. For example, in men with stage T2 cancer, the tumor is more often organ-confined in men in their fifties than in men in their seventies. Why? This is because the cancer has been there longer, and had a chance to grow, and possibly become more malignant. Recently, Johns Hopkins urologist H. Ballentine Carter studied five hundred men with T1c disease who underwent radical prostatectomy. He found that older men were more likely to have Gleason 7 tumors (in the mid-range, moderately well differentiated) than men in their fifties, and that age was a statistically significant factor in the prediction of curable disease.

Let's go back to our sixty-five-year-old man. He's in otherwise good health, and he can reasonably expect to live at least fifteen or twenty more years. *His cancer is curable now.* If he does nothing about it, if he opts for watchful waiting, he may miss his golden opportunity for cure. Remember, right now we have no way of estimating the biological potential of prostate cancer. We can't determine if it's harmless or deadly; we don't know *if* or *when* it will make that leap beyond the prostate. Even in its earliest stages, prostate cancer doesn't always spread considerately, in logical, creeping, easy-to-predict steps.

At the other end of the spectrum is the man in his eighties. Even if his cancer is organ-confined and curable, it's not likely that he will live long enough for major treatment to be worthwhile. Older men are less resilient; as we mentioned before, aggressive treatment is much harder on them. What's the point of risking incontinence, a result of surgery, or rectal bleeding, a result of radiation, in an eighty-five-year-old man? If his disease progresses to the point where he has difficulty with urination, there are many ways to treat such symptoms, ranging from a TURP (transurethral resection of the prostate, to relieve urinary obstruction) to hormonal treatment. For most older men, the *number of years of life*—the long-term survival—is not nearly as important as the *life in those years*—the quality of life.

Why Do I Need to Be Treated? Making Sense of Some Controversial Studies

Remember the doctors we talked about in Chapter 5, who hate PSA and don't believe it does any good to detect prostate cancer early? We see a similar strain of fatalism here, in delaying treatment or selecting watchful waiting (also called "conservative management," "expectant following," or "deferred treatment") as the main strategy for men with localized disease that is considered curable.

There are a lot of doctors out there who steer their patients with curable disease toward watchful waiting. Their main basis for this: Studies that suggest the death rate for men who don't get treatment is low, about the same as for men who don't have prostate cancer. For a number of years, doctors who saw no value to treating prostate cancer quoted a study from Sweden, where the main treatment option is watchful waiting. This study suggested that men with localized prostate cancer rarely died from it. It's pretty clear now that this study had many flaws, one of which was in the interpretation. In that study, at ten years only 13 percent of men had died from prostate cancer. But the disease had progressed in another 50 percent of the men, and most of these men eventually needed castration or hormonal therapy to treat urinary obstruction, bleeding, or pain.

However, some other data have come out of Sweden to challenge the questionable conclusions in that study. One recent study was a retrospective analysis of 536 men known to have prostate cancer who died in Göteborg, Sweden, between 1988 and 1990. In some cases, the time between diagnosis and death was as long as twenty-five years. This study made two important points: First, if you're going to find out whether localized prostate cancer can go on to kill a man, you need to follow him—however long it takes—until he dies. Ten years is simply not long enough to give us all the answers. And in this study, 63 percent of men who were diagnosed with localized disease and survived more than ten years eventually died of prostate cancer. This study also emphasizes the importance of age at diagnosis: In men who were diagnosed with prostate cancer before age fifty-five, *100 percent eventually died from the disease.* In yet another recent study from Sweden, the age at diagnosis was also shown to be an important prognostic factor: For example, in men with low-grade tumors, the years of life lost to prostate cancer ranged from eleven years in men aged forty-five to fifty-five, to 1.2 years in men aged seventy-five to eighty. These studies may explain the low estimates of death from prostate cancer in that first Swedish study: There, the men had an average age of seventy-two, and follow-up evaluation did not extend beyond ten years. What that first study—the one quoted by so many doctors—did, in effect, was to close the book before the last few chapters and assume the story had a nice ending, because everything was all right at that point.

Sweden has the third highest death rate for prostate cancer in the world. Now, if localized prostate cancer doesn't kill, why are there so many deaths from prostate cancer in Sweden? And why do 50 percent more men in Sweden die of prostate cancer than women die of breast cancer—when, in the United States, where we actually treat and cure prostate cancer, fewer men die of prostate cancer than women die of breast cancer?

In Sweden, watchful waiting means ignoring early prostate cancer, sending the patient home and telling him to come back when he has some symptoms—when the cancer has spread—so that he can be treated with hormonal therapy. This is not what watchful waiting means in the United States (more on this below). But it's the most cost-effective solution in a socialized system of medical care. It doesn't require expensive therapy or skilled therapists. The only drawback is that men die, and men suffer—needlessly. These statistics are particularly distressing when we consider this: Today, when localized prostate cancer is diagnosed in men who have a life span longer than fifteen years, *the decision not to offer these men potentially curable therapy may be a death sentence.* Because in most patients, the disease is going to progress.

Now, what about studies from the United States? A review article published in the *New England Journal of Medicine* summarized a number of other studies involving watchful waiting. In these studies, the authors reported, the men treated with watchful waiting were carefully selected from a large group of patients because they were felt to have slow-growing cancers that were unlikely to spread. These patients were not representative of the usual patient who walks into a doctor's office—in other words, they were almost all "best-case scenarios." Even so, ten years later, 40 percent of the men in these elite groups who had Gleason scores from 5 to 7 had metastases to bone, and by fifteen years, that number had increased to 70 percent. Again, what we see here is that prostate cancer marches on; it continues to progress in most men—even those with the mildest-looking disease. And if a man with localized prostate cancer does not get effective treatment, and if he lives long enough, he will very likely die of prostate cancer.

One of the most recent investigations of watchful waiting was a large study conducted by doctors in Connecticut and published in the *Journal of the American Medical Association.* Here, the researchers looked at men who were treated with watchful waiting, and the number of men who died of prostate cancer five, ten, and fifteen years later. It concluded that men with low-grade cancers faced a minimal risk of dying from prostate cancer. (Remember, those Gleason 2–4 tumors are rarely diagnosed today, and only make up about 2 percent of men with localized prostate cancer.) For men with Gleason 5–7 scores, the investigators concluded, the risk of death from prostate cancer is a "modest" one, that increases slowly over at least fifteen years of follow-up. "These men face a risk of dying from prostate cancer," the researchers conceded, "but it is unclear from a population perspective what percentage of these men will actually benefit from treatment" and from aggressive screening to detect their cancer.

There is a huge problem with this story, one that goes to the heart of prostate cancer treatment itself: Why were these men treated with conservative therapy in the first place? Mainly because they were in the group of men we'll talk about later in this chapter, men who were considered too old or too ill to live longer than ten years. Most of these men beat prostate cancer on a technicality—they died of other causes before they lived fifteen years. In other words, they didn't die of prostate cancer because some other disease killed them first. Thus, this study grossly underestimates the risk of dying from prostate cancer in men who actually lived fifteen years. And in doing so, the study fails to tell a young, otherwise healthy man—who could live for twenty or thirty more years—the true probability that his cancer will progress and kill him.

Results of still another study show something different: In men with clinically localized prostate cancer, radical prostatectomy reduced the development of metastases and death from prostate cancer by 50 percent when compared with men who were followed with watchful waiting.

The PLCO Study

This is another salvo in the argument whether treatment for prostate cancer has any effect on long-term survival. Critics have stated, loudly, that "there is no evidence that definitive treatment of localized prostate cancer increases survival." However, there has been no large, well-designed study to evaluate the effectiveness of early prostate cancer treatment in prolonging lives. Sadly, there still isn't. (Thus, to be truthful, these critics should also admit that there is no evidence that treatment *doesn't* prolong life.)

The PLCO study is an attempt to answer the question. This is a massive, multimillion-dollar study, sponsored by the National Cancer Institute, involving prostate, lung, colon, and ovarian cancers. For prostate cancer, the point is to determine whether or not screening makes a difference in life expectancy. (This also has a lot to do with the controversy surrounding the PSA test's effectiveness—see Chapter 5.) Men will be screened once a year for four years, and then followed for twelve years. This is similar to the screening intervals used in a study to determine mammography's effectiveness in spotting breast cancer. However, prostate cancer is much slower-growing than breast cancer, and some doctors worry that four years isn't going to be long enough for PSA's yearly rate of change to be as meaningful as it has the potential to be.

Another worry is that the screening isn't being done in the best possible way up front, and thus the follow-up, which will be expensive, will be worthless. The study was planned a long time ago, using the then-state-of-the-art PSA cutoff of 4. But as we learn more about PSA testing, we realize that there are going to be better ways to do it—in fact, PSA testing's already improved, and keeps getting better. What's the best way to use PSA? Is PSA density the way to go? Free PSA? PSA velocity or age-specific ranges? Scientists just don't know. So initiating a long-term study without using the best techniques appeared, to some investigators, to be premature.

The investigators heading this study have had great concern that their control group might be "contaminated" by PSA screening outside of the study—that a man might have a PSA test on recommendation of his family physician, or because he read about it in the newspapers. This "contamination" could markedly affect the ability of this study in the long run to compare men who have been screened and men who have not been. For this reason, these NIH investigators have made a concerted effort to discourage PSA testing through scientific presentations and the use of the media. They are also active in getting this message out to potential patients. These efforts may have helped to protect the integrity of their study, but at what cost? Several of these patients, men who avoided screening based on these doctors' advice, have come to Johns Hopkins and been diagnosed with more advanced disease that was difficult to cure.

Also, in this study, treatment is up in the air—once a diagnosis is made, the choice of treatment (or no treatment) is left up to the patient and his physician, with no mandate to pick the most effective treatment to cure the man's cancer. (This is in contrast to the studies that demonstrated the efficacy of mammography—in which women diagnosed with breast cancer underwent radical mastectomy.) Remember that the end point here is death from prostate cancer. *So how can we know if PSA makes a difference in life expectancy if men pick ineffective therapy?* And finally, the age range for the study is not meaningful; it includes men up to age seventy-four. The unfortunate fact is that many of these men probably won't be alive to see the end of the twelve-year follow-up period. It is unlikely, then, that they will live long enough to provide any new insights into the long-term effectiveness of treatment.

So it seems a shame that this massive study, which taxpayers are funding, is proceeding without a more thoughtful design.

The PIVOT Study

Another attempt to shed light on prostate cancer treatment is the national PIVOT (Prostate Cancer Intervention versus Observation Trial) study, led by a Minnesota internist and a Seattle urologist and funded by the Department of Veterans Affairs and the National Cancer Institute. Its aim is to find out which works better for clinically localized prostate cancer—radical prostatectomy with early intervention (such as radiation therapy) in case the cancer comes back, or watchful waiting, with treatment for symptoms if the cancer spreads.

"We're not looking at radiation as a primary treatment," comments the internist who's heading the study, "because studies indicate that radiation is at least not better than radical prostatectomy." Instead, the PIVOT study will "compare watchful waiting with the most frequently recommended, and probably the best, of the early intervention approaches—radical prostatectomy."

Like the PLCO study, the PIVOT study is long; it has a three-year enrollment period, and a twelve-year follow-up; two thousand men will be able to participate. Men up to age seventy-five are eligible—but these older men, like the rest of the men in the study, must be healthy enough to be considered fit for surgery. Only men with prostate cancer who are considered candidates for surgery may take part in the study; they will be assigned to one of two groups—either they'll undergo a radical prostatectomy, or they will be followed closely with watchful waiting and treated as needed for specific symptoms or metastases. Many cancer centers and Veterans Administration hospitals throughout the country are participating in this study.

What's the measure of success here? It's what you might call the ultimate end point—death or survival. "Really, that's what the patient cares about," says the internist. "Will my disease be cured? Is my life better without the surgery? We don't know the answer to either of those questions. Those in favor of radical prostatectomy say, 'How can doctors dare not treat? They're killing people with watchful waiting!' And the watchful waiting people say that surgery doesn't prolong survival. These are two groups of intelligent, caring people, and there is information to support either of these two views."

Men in the study will be examined at least every three months the first year and every six months afterward, and periodically they will answer questionnaires about their quality of life. Their doctors will check for any evidence that prostate cancer has progressed, and they will document any changes in the patients' condition. If the patient dies—for any reason—all of this information will go to an independent review committee, which will study all the accumulated data and determine whether the man's death was definitely, probably, possibly, or definitely not due to prostate cancer.

The PIVOT study is interesting for several reasons; despite the age limit of its patients—it's hard to know how many seventy-five-year-old men will be around for the study's conclusion—the selection criteria seem fairly strict. Men who obviously are not good candidates for surgery, the study's directors say, will not be included. Also, because of its size, the study promises highly specific results.

Final thoughts on these two studies: The results of these studies will not be known for many years, and the outcome will not be helpful to patients who have to make a decision about treatment today. It may be that these studies will have to be terminated if the death rates from prostate cancer in the United States (see Chapter 3) continue to fall. This would be the best sign that the transformation in the treatment of prostate cancer from a know-nothing, do-nothing philosophy, which lasted until the mid-1980s, to an approach of early diagnosis combined with more effective therapy has proven to be a winning strategy.

Watchful Waiting

Watchful waiting is certainly not a new approach. It's long been a mainstay of prostate cancer treatment; in fact, for years, one third of men with prostate cancer have been treated with watchful waiting. Note: Watchful waiting in the United States is not the same as watchful waiting in Sweden. In this country, it means to be followed carefully, to delay definitive treatment until it becomes clear that the tumor is growing. This has the immediate advantage of avoiding unpleasant treatment and its side effects. For men with curable disease, it has the major disadvantage of missing the "golden window" of curability. When cancer escapes from the prostate, it doesn't send out a press release announcing the event; it just goes, as silently as it appeared in your body in the first place. Then it's too late to close the proverbial barn doors. We can't put cancer back in the prostate. We can do our best to cure it if it's still locally advanced. If it spreads to the lymph nodes or bone, however, the best we can do for now is control it.

Who should opt for watchful waiting? To put it bluntly, at the top of this list should be men who are too old or too ill either to undergo the rigors of treatment or to live another ten years—long enough for such treatment to be worthwhile. These men are very unlikely to die of prostate cancer, and if the cancer progresses, their symptoms can usu-ally be managed well with hormonal therapy. (Frankly, these men should not have had a PSA test and biopsy in the first place.)

Also in this group should be men who don't want to experience the side effects associated with surgery or radiation, men who are diagnosed with stage T3, T4, or N+ disease who don't yet have symp-toms (although for some men with cancer in the lymph nodes, there may be a role for radical prostatectomy; see below); some men whose prostate cancer is truly incidental and not yet something to worry about (some men with stage T1a cancer, see Chapter 6); and older men with stage T1c disease who have favorable pathology, low PSA densities, and high free PSA (see Chapter 6).

Besides its initial freedom from side effects, watchful waiting has another advantage at first—it's the cheapest option, because there's no expensive treatment to pay for. If you have no symptoms, you simply live your life, and return to the doctor every six months or so for a checkup

Remember, in the United States watchful waiting doesn't mean "do nothing," and it doesn't mean your doctor has written you off—it means you get treatment for specific symptoms when you need it. It can mean active treatment as soon as there are signs that the tumor is progressing, such as hormone therapy or spot radiation to ease bone pain; it can mean a TURP or other procedures to bring relief when the prostate cancer becomes large enough to obstruct the urinary tract; it can mean a host of options aimed at tackling specific problems, prolonging life, and easing pain.

Watchful waiting and curable prostate cancer: The benefits of watchful waiting aren't terribly clear for younger men with localized disease—men who probably could be cured if they act in time. The biggest disadvantage, again, is that the "window of curability" may silently close from the time of one checkup to the next.

If you have curable disease and opt for watchful waiting, you will have to live with uncertainty about the future. At present, there is no reliable way to tell when the disease is just beginning to progress, even if it hasn't yet escaped the prostate. In about 25 percent of men with growing prostate cancer, there is never a significant, telltale rise in PSA.

Some scientists have dubbed watchful waiting for men with curable disease "watchful progression." In a study from British Columbia of 113 men, about 40 percent of the men with T1 disease and 51 percent of the men with T2 disease had growth of the cancer found on rectal examination within two years, and this increased to 60 percent at three years. Using digital rectal examination as the guide, the findings demonstrated high rates of clinical progression within the watchful waiting population.

So if you're a man under age seventy with a life expectancy greater than ten years and localized, curable prostate cancer who decides to watch and wait—with the hope that if the cancer grows, it will be caught in time—think hard about this risk. You should return to your doctor at regular intervals—every six months—for repeat digital rectal examinations, PSA tests (even though, as discussed above and in Chapter 6, PSA doesn't always go up correspondingly when cancer advances), and periodic prostate biopsies to help doctors find out if the cancer that's in your prostate is staying put or if it's on the move. PSA tests alone aren't sufficient to monitor the growth of the cancer because—as Johns Hopkins urologist H. Ballentine Carter reported— in 25 percent of men with cancers that were progressing, PSA levels did not change. You also need to understand the risks you could be facing down the road if cancer spreads—the long-term symptoms, and the side effects and costs of treatment for advanced disease.

Now, what about quality of life in men with curable disease who choose watchful waiting? In a study from Denmark, of fifty-two men with localized cancer who were treated with watchful waiting (the men reported their own symptoms on questionnaires for an average of about three years), 31 percent had undergone a TURP to relieve urinary symptoms, 8 percent underwent radiation therapy, and 44 percent received hormonal treatment. When asked about incontinence, 21 percent of the men said they were using pads, and 37 percent said that they leaked daily; 21 percent of the men said urine dripping or leaking was a substantial problem. Impotence was another problem; 81 percent of the men said they were able to have an erection before their cancer was diagnosed. At the time of the questionnaire, 77 percent said that their ability to have an erection was reduced, and only 29 percent had an erection after the prostate cancer was diagnosed. For 12 percent, impotence was a problem.

When watchful waiting may be a safe gamble: Having said all this, it is difficult to extrapolate this information from Denmark to the American man with small, nonpalpable T1c cancer. But it does show that prostate cancer progresses; as it progresses, it spreads beyond the prostate, and eventually it's no longer curable. It produces symptoms, and men need further treatment just for basic quality-of-life issues like being able to urinate voluntarily, without dribbling throughout the day (fortunately, a TURP can bring significant relief to this problem). Thus, for most men with curable prostate cancer, watchful waiting is *not a way to make the problem go away so you'll never have to think about it again.*

But what if you're in your sixties or younger, and you have small T1c or T1a cancer? You're young and healthy enough to have surgery, and your disease is certainly considered curable—in fact, it's microscopic, possibly incidental prostate cancer. Why seek treatment now?

There used to be two polarized schools of thought about this: One was that everybody with this small cancer needed treatment as soon as possible. "We can definitely cure it now. Time's wasting—let's get going!" some doctors said. They urged patients to have their cancer "nipped in the bud," treated when the chances of curing it were at their peak. The other group was not nearly so optimistic; these doctors believed that treatment didn't really prolong life by that many years anyway, so what was the point? (Amazingly, a number of doctors still feel this way, as discussed above.)

Beware of extremes. One of the first lessons a doctor learns in medical school is that "There are always two things you never say—always and never." The truth is probably somewhere in the middle.

Before the 1970s at Johns Hopkins, the approach was that if a man had cancer found at a TURP (for treatment of benign enlargement of the prostate) but not a tumor large enough to be felt in a rectal exam (men with stage T2 cancer), then his cancer was the incidental kind, with "low malignant potential" and not much clinical significance— the kind of cancer men die "with," not "of." And so they weren't treated.

In 1976, Johns Hopkins investigators embarked on a pioneering study using tumor volume to predict cancer patients' prognosis. They analyzed the medical histories of more than one hundred of these men who were not treated, and they followed their progress for an average of seven years. Their findings: One group of these men did reasonably well; their cancer rarely progressed. But another group did not fare so well; their cancer continued to grow.

What was the difference between these two groups? The clue, investigators found, was in the percentage of cancer removed during the TURP. This work provided the now standard classifications for stage T1 disease. (TURPs are not performed as commonly as they used to be; there are many other treatments for BPH. And when a TURP is performed, the tissue is often vaporized, instead of removed in little chips, so there is nothing to send to a pathologist.)

When *5 percent or less* of the tissue was cancerous, only 17 percent of the men went on to develop more advanced cancer within seven years; this is now the classification for stage T1a disease. But when *more than 5 percent* of the resected tissue was cancerous, 68 percent of these men went on to develop cancer progression within seven years; this now is the classification of stage T2a disease. "It is felt that the amount of cancer in almost all of these patients is significant enough to warrant therapy," says one of the investigators.

Further analysis has shown that when men with stage T1a disease undergo radical prostatectomy, about 25 percent of them turn out to have a significant amount of cancer in the prostate—the kind of cancer that's found in men with palpable tumors. This is because, as we discussed in Chapter 6, the biopsy is not perfect. It's a glimpse at what is probably within the prostate, and from that, pathologists make their most educated guess.

So: Some men with stage T1a cancer require treatment. Some don't. How to tell the difference? Our old friend PSA comes back to help us again. As it turns out, the level of PSA three months after TURP can be helpful in identifying the men at highest risk of cancer progression. If the PSA is less than 1.0, virtually all of the men with stage T1a disease have an insignificant amount of cancer. "And we feel that these men can probably be followed with careful digital rectal examinations and PSA tests every six months or a year," says one of the study's chief investigators.

If the PSA is greater than 10, all of these men are likely to have significant cancer remaining, and all should have definitive therapy before it's too late.

What about the patients in the middle, with PSA levels between 1.0 and 10—the range for about half the men with T1 disease? Currently, there's just no way to predict exactly how much cancer remains in the prostate—and, therefore, who will need treatment and who won't. Some doctors have advised these men to undergo a repeat TURP; but there's no real evidence to suggest that this will provide any helpful information. It's hard on the patient, too. Also, a repeat TURP may make it more difficult for a surgeon to perform a subsequent radical prostatectomy, if the man then has to undergo yet another procedure.

Other investigators are enthusiastic about the use of ultrasound and random needle biopsies as follow-up measures for these men, but the long-term success rate for these procedures has yet to be determined; cancer could still slip outside the prostate and not be caught in time. The safest guideline here may be the patient's age: If he's younger than sixty, aggressive, curative therapy should be strongly considered.

Another group who could have insignificant cancer are men with stage T1c disease (found by needle biopsy, after an elevated PSA score). Ten percent of these men with a PSA greater than 4 have insignificant cancer. If you have T1c disease, can you afford to wait? This is discussed in more detail in Chapter 6, but here are some factors that can help predict which cancers are truly incidental, and which need to be treated. If your cancer is incidental, your pathology should suggest low-volume disease (cancer in one or two needle cores, involving less than half of any core and a Gleason score of 6 or less), *and* your PSA should not be more than 10 or 15 percent of the weight of your prostate. If it's higher, this suggests that something more than benign disease is responsible for your elevated PSA. Similarly, if the PSA is coming from BPH (benign enlargement), your *free PSA* should be high—above 15 percent. If it's less than 15 percent, then it is likely that cancer, not benign disease, is causing your PSA to rise—in which case, the cancer is probably more significant than it seems. The key words here are "likely" and "probably." Even expert pathologist Jonathan Epstein of Johns Hopkins says that he does not know which cancer is so small in a young man that it won't grow to the point of threatening his life over time, and that using these estimates, 25 percent of men with T1c cancer still have a significant amount of cancer.

What happens to cancer cells over time: Some men who opt for watchful waiting take solace in the fact that their cancer cells are well differentiated. But unfortunately, just because you have well-differentiated cancer cells today does not mean they'll stay that way forever. There are two concepts here; one is *genetic drift.* As a cancer progresses—as its cells double again and again—the DNA becomes less stable. The cancer develops new mutations; it becomes more aggressive. As the tumor progresses, well-differentiated cells deteriorate into poorly differentiated cells. The other concept is *heterogeneity,* or clonal selection. By the time a prostate cancer is large enough to be diagnosed clinically, its cell population is mixed—a diverse group of cells, all jockeying for position in one location. In this varied group are both well- and poorly differentiated cells, cells driven by hormones and cells untouched by hormones. And although an initial biopsy may find well-differentiated cancer cells, almost certainly some poorly differentiated ones have mingled in there as well. With time and further growth, these poorly differentiated cells grow at a faster rate than their more sedate, better-differentiated counterparts. Eventually, they will outpace the stately progression of the well-differentiated cells and dominate the tumor. So a well-differentiated cancer, one that's localized to the prostate, may be only a temporary condition. And unfortunately, we can't tell which well-differentiated cancers are going to stay that way.

What about lifestyle changes? There is a new subgroup of men who are choosing watchful waiting with a different strategy in mind: They do not have small tumors, or the lowest Gleason scores; some of them are very young—in their forties and fifties, with tumors that their doctors have described as "slow-growing." These men are deciding to avoid treatment now and "heal themselves," with lifestyle changes— dietary changes, antioxidants, herbal compounds, meditation, and complementary medicine. (Complementary medicine is discussed in Chapter 12.) They have a lot of support—on the Internet, especially, and also from diet specialists who claim to have the answers for beating prostate cancer, as well as heart disease, and various other illnesses.

Why diet? The rationale for diet and lifestyle changes goes back to the men we have heard so much about in this book—those remarkable Asian men, whose risk of getting prostate cancer is so much lower than ours, until they move to the United States. Then, their risk starts to climb. This is why so many scientists worldwide believe there is something in the Asian diet that prevents prostate cancer.

The men in this group who are shunning traditional curative treatment are doing it with the belief that if they start eating these same foods, and taking high-powered dietary supplements, their cancer will go away. Nobody knows where this approach will lead; it's too new. One day, diet may very well help American men *prevent* cancer from forming. But the idea that starting a diet *after cancer develops* can make the disease go away, to be blunt, is just not sound. Look at it this way: Smoking causes lung cancer. Men who don't smoke hardly ever get lung cancer (issues of secondary smoke aside), and if you stop smoking now, your risk of *developing* lung cancer begins to plummet. But what if you stop smoking *after* you find out you have lung cancer? Does the cancer go away? No, sadly, it doesn't. The reasons for this go back to the complicated chain of reactions we discussed in Chapter 3—the "domino effect" of damaged DNA, causing other genes to mutate, eventually resulting in cancer. Mutated genes cause the cancer to grow; these genetic errors are repeated, and get worse, every time the cells divide. Once the DNA has been damaged, there is no turning back. *You can't, as they say, "unring the bell."* Even if you stop the original "inciting agent," the factor that caused cancer in the first place, you will not cure that cancer by this means alone. You may prevent new cancers from forming, but that first cancer is there to stay, unless it is stamped out by treatment: Those genetic errors are irreversible.

To the best of our knowledge, prostate cancer arises from oxidative damage (discussed in Chapter 3). A normal prostate cell is transformed into a cancerous cell because of mutations to DNA caused by oxidative damage. But is it possible that fat itself can make the cancer grow more? We don't know for sure. It is possible that changes in diet and lifestyle could slow down cancer, but again, there's no evidence that they will make the cancer go away. (Breast cancer, lung cancer, and colon cancer are caused by similar oxidative damage. But here, too, there is no evidence that dietary therapy can make these cancers disappear.)

Cost is a factor, too: In the long term, it's unclear whether watchful waiting will actually result in a decrease in health care dollars, as some studies have claimed. The Swedish study mentioned above suggests that even under the best circumstances, about half of men with localized disease will live to see their cancer spread beyond the prostate, requiring further treatment for advanced disease. If these men decide to have hormonal treatment, the cost of this over two years, at hundreds of dollars a month, may be more than the expense of a radical prostatectomy or radiation therapy (which is about $12,000). Also, the symptoms from advanced cancer and the side effects of hormonal treatment and chemotherapy can be much worse than the side effects that can accompany treatment for early disease.

A recent study from Norway looked at the financial cost of watchful waiting. Prostate cancer is the most common cancer in Norwegian men, and at least half of the men with prostate cancer die of it. This was a study of 174 men who had cancer that was not considered curable; 95 percent of these men were symptomatic at diagnosis (which means they had advanced cancer, and urinary problems or bone pain). Sixty-two percent of the men died from prostate cancer; all but two were hospitalized for an average of one month; 36 percent needed round-the-clock nursing or a nursing home; 50 percent had complications that required hospitalization or long-term catheterization; 66 percent needed a TURP; 76 percent had hormone therapy; 16 percent underwent palliative radiation (to ease bone pain); and 50 percent received analgesics regularly, including opiates. These statistics paint a grim picture, one nobody wants to read, and one we would rather not write about. However, the point here is that most doctors and enthusiastic patients who talk about watchful waiting usually focus on the beginning of it —the good part about avoiding the up-front complications, the side effects from surgery or radiation. They don't talk about the rest of it—what happens when cancer spreads, and you're constantly playing catch-up, trying to stop specific symptoms and maintain some quality of life and dignity.

TREATMENT PROS AND CONS

Ideal candidate	Radical Prostatectomy	Radiation Therapy
Age	Under age 70	Over age 60
Stage	T1b, T1c, T2 (and some men with T1a disease)	T1, T2, T3, T4
Main advantages	If cancer is confined to the prostate, this is the best way to cure	Less invasive
Main disadvantages*	Side effects: Impotence 10–75% Incontinence 2–20% Death 0.2%	May not cure localized cancer; Side effects: Rectal injury 1–2% Impotence 20–70% Death 0.2%

*Note: Side effects vary greatly, depending on the skill of the surgeon or radiation oncologist.

If I Decide to Get Treatment, What Are My Choices?

For tumors that are confined to the prostate—stages T1 and T2—there are two main choices: Surgery (radical prostatectomy) and radiation therapy. Radiation also is used when the cancer has spread just outside the gland, to kill cancer cells and shrink the prostate. High-energy X-ray beams are aimed at the prostate and sometimes at nearby lymph nodes; sometimes this is combined with implanted "radiation seeds."

WHO SHOULD CONSIDER SURGERY?

T1a:	Most men with T1a disease have truly incidental cancer that rarely progresses. However, studies of radical prostatectomy patients show that about 25 percent of men with T1a cancer have significant disease. If a man has had a "simple" prostatectomy for treatment of BPH, and if, three months after that procedure, his PSA is less than 1, he probably has insignificant cancer, and is an ideal candidate for watchful waiting. If he is younger than 60, or has a PSA greater than 1 at three months after this procedure, he should consider surgery.
T1b, T1c, T2:	Decision should be made based on the Partin Tables, a man's age, and overall health. For older men with T1c disease, the presence of low-volume disease should be considered/excluded.
T3a:	Men with T3a disease are usually not good candidates for a radical prostatectomy. However, some patients with minimal spread of cancer, and Gleason scores lower than 8, may benefit from surgery, especially if they are in their fifties or younger. About 25 percent of these men turn out to have organ-confined disease.

Which Treatment Is Better for Localized Disease?

A better question might be, "Which treatment is right for me?" There are several important considerations here: your age, overall health and stage of cancer, the side effects associated with different treatments, and finally—most importantly—your own wishes.

When prostate cancer is localized *in men with a life expectancy of fifteen years or more,* the goal for treatment is cure. This sounds obvious, until we remember that when prostate cancer is advanced, the cancer can be controlled, but—for now—not eradicated.

The big advantage of radical prostatectomy is that *there is no better way to completely eliminate cancer that is curable* (see above). The disadvantages are the side effects, namely the risks of impotence and incontinence. And radical prostatectomy is no "walk in the park." It is major surgery, and the body must be in strong enough shape to handle it. (For more on complications of radical prostatectomy, see Chapter 8.) In men under sixty-five who undergo treatment by a surgeon who is an expert, the side effects of surgery and radiation therapy are similar. In men over seventy, incontinence and impotence are more common. *Note:* The side effects of surgery are highly variable, depending on the skill and experience of the surgeon.

Radiation therapy's great advantage is that it isn't surgery. But its major disadvantage, especially for the younger patient, is that *its ability to control the cancer may not last forever.* Remember (as we discussed in Chapter 6), prostate cancers are "multifocal," and the average prostate removed during radical prostatectomy turns out to have *at least seven separate tumors* in it. Thus, to cure prostate cancer with radiation, the entire prostate must be eliminated. There is always some uncertainty, especially for younger men, as to whether radiation's effect will last a lifetime. Also, radiation has some side effects (see Chapter 9). However, the chances of side effects with external-beam radiation are less "operator-dependent" than with surgery or seed implantation.

In choosing the treatment that's best for you, it's important to try for a balance between effectiveness and side effects. More information on each of these choices follows in this chapter, and the next chapters cover these treatments in significantly greater detail.

Radical Prostatectomy Is a Better Option for . . .

The ideal candidates for radical prostatectomy are the men most likely to benefit from it: men who are curable and who are going to live *long enough to need to be cured.* Men who are curable have organ-confined cancer, or even cancer that has penetrated the prostate wall *if* the cancer is well to moderately well differentiated and it's possible for doctors to get what's called a "clear surgical margin"—that is, if they can cut out all the tumor.

Men with stage T3 disease generally are not considered candidates for radical prostatectomy. However, sometimes the digital rectal examination can be wrong. Sometimes, doctors overestimate the tumor's actual extent—when indeed it may not have spread beyond the prostate. Twenty-five percent of these men who undergo surgery turn out to have organ-confined cancer. Younger men with Gleason scores of 7 or less should consider surgery for several reasons—for one thing, they tolerate the procedure much better than older men; for another, their quality of life will be better (see below).

The ideal candidates for surgery, then, are men in their forties, fifties, and sixties, in otherwise good health, with curable cancer. (Some otherwise healthy, fit men in their seventies may be individually selected for treatment as well.) This includes men with stage T1b, T2a, T2b, and T2c cancer. It also includes some men with stage T1a disease (discussed above), and most patients with stage T1c disease.

RADICAL PROSTATECTOMY IN MEN WITH POSITIVE LYMPH NODES

Conventional wisdom: Once cancer has escaped the prostate to distant sites, it can't be cured. Therefore, putting a man with advanced disease through the rigors of surgery is cruel and, more importantly, not helpful.

This belief is why, for years, many physicians have gone to such painstaking lengths to make sure a man has curable disease before performing "curative" treatment—radical prostatectomy.

Unfortunately, sometimes—even when cancer seems entirely curable—it has already spread invisibly, microscopically into the lymph nodes, and this isn't discovered until well after the operation is over. This is the whole purpose of frozen section analysis of the lymph nodes, the procedure-before-the-procedure (now performed much less frequently than it used to be; see Chapter 6) in which a man's pelvic lymph nodes are checked for the presence of cancer while he lies anesthetized on the operating table. If cancer is found, many—but not all—surgeons simply sew up the incision they just made, genuinely believing it's kinder to spare the patient the rigors of a tough operation. And the poor patient? Having prepared himself for surgery and its complications, hoping for a cure, he wakes up to a terrible psychological blow: He's got an abdominal incision to recover from—but his prostate, and his cancer, are still there. Nothing's changed, except perhaps the hopeful part of the picture for him.

Maybe the conventional wisdom is wrong. Results of a Johns Hopkins study suggest that in men with cancer in the lymph nodes, radical prostatectomy not only averts many complications—a finding Hopkins surgeons have previously published—but it may *prolong life* as well.

The investigators looked at 168 men diagnosed between 1983 and 1995 who were thought to have localized disease but were found at the time of surgery to have cancer in their lymph nodes. Of these, 127 had a lymph node dissection and a radical prostatectomy (most of these men turned out to have microscopic lymph node metastases); forty-one underwent the lymph node dissection alone (the situation described above). Reviewing the patients in each group, the surgeons found nineteen perfectly matched pairs of men—men with the exact same age, PSA score, Gleason grade, clinical stage, follow-up, and amount of cancer in the lymph nodes. The only difference was that, in each pair, one man had the surgery, one man didn't.

Many complications in advanced prostate cancer arise from the physical presence of the prostate: As the cancer grows, men often develop such problems as urinary retention and obstruction, blood in the urine, kidney and bowel trouble. Men with advanced cancer who have undergone a radical prostatectomy rarely have these problems. From this standpoint, their quality of life is better.

But do they live longer? This study suggests that they may. Ten years later, only 34 percent of the men who had the lymph node dissection alone were still alive. But 56 percent of the men who had the radical prostatectomy were still alive—a big difference in survival.

More research—specifically, a much larger study—is needed, because there are too few patients here to make a generalization for all men with lymph-node-positive prostate cancer. But this evidence suggests that there *may* be a role for radical prosatectomy, even in advanced disease.

Radical Prostatectomy Is Not a Good Option for . . .

Radical prostatectomy is not helpful for men with disease that has spread widely beyond the prostate. It also is not ideal for older patients (men over age seventy).

Once prostate cancer escapes the wall of the prostate to the point where it widely invades the seminal vesicles, pelvic lymph nodes, or bone, it can rarely be cured. The principal goal here is to control the tumor locally; this can be done with radiation, hormone therapy, or a combination of both. With late-stage cancer, the goal is simply to do everything possible to fight the cancer and buy more time, with the hope that one of the new treatment strategies currently being tested will be shown to work, and will be available in the near future. The focus changes to ensuring good quality of life, rather than a cancer-free life. The main line of treatment for late-stage prostate cancer is hormone therapy, chemotherapy, and spot radiation to treat painful metastases. Some promising new therapies are being tested as well. (See Chapter 9.)

Why is age a factor? Several reasons. One is that men over age seventy, as we discussed above, often have more advanced cancer than the clinical findings might lead a doctor to suspect, and are therefore less likely to be cured because the cancer has been there longer. As men age, the prostate enlarges from BPH—so by the time a doctor can feel a cancerous lump in these men with their larger prostates, it's probably bigger than the cancer that can be felt in a younger man with a smaller prostate. Studies have shown that for men with T2a disease, the likelihood that the cancer is confined to the prostate is less for men over seventy than for men in their fifties. Similar findings have been shown for men with nonpalpable T1c cancer.

Also, older men are more likely to suffer side effects from surgery than younger men; they're more likely to have incontinence because, as men get older, their muscles get weaker—all the muscles, including the ones responsible for urinary control. The problem is that the sphincter muscles involved are the ones men don't normally need to use (because the prostate and bladder neck bear the main burden of holding back urine and keeping urination a voluntary experience). Also, because most older men have BPH, their bladder has thickened from the extra work needed to overcome the obstruction caused by the enlarged tissue. For these men—instead of three gatekeepers—the lone stalwart holding back an overmuscled bladder is a weaker, untested sphincter that's never been asked to work this hard before, and may have some trouble adjusting to the job.

Sexual dysfunction is also more common, for a couple of reasons: First, as men age—in addition to losing muscle strength—they lose nerves, too. By age sixty, men have lost about 40 percent of all the nerves in their body. And during radical prostatectomy, nerves are often injured—some permanently, some temporarily. So if you have fewer nerves to begin with, and some of these are damaged, the critical number of nerves necessary for erection may be lost. Yet another aspect of aging is that the nerves don't heal as well—again, making recovery of sexual function less likely. And finally, because men over age seventy aren't likely to live as long as men twenty years younger, it's difficult to show that radical prostatectomy actually does more than radiation therapy to lengthen life expectancy in these men.

Radiation Is a Better Option for . . .

The ideal candidates for radiation treatment are patients who are older, or who are less likely to be cured by surgery.

Men who undergo radiation treatment are said to be "negatively selected"—they get radiation therapy because radical prostatectomy has been ruled out as the best option for them. They are generally older men, over seventy; men in poor health who aren't considered strong enough for surgery; or men who have disease that has extended beyond the prostate to the point where it can't be removed surgically (stage T3 or T4).

However, others who opt for radiation treatment are men with organ-confined disease who just don't want to have surgery. Most recently, younger men have been encouraged to have radiation, especially implanted seeds (a procedure called *brachytherapy*), because the treatment is easier to take, and because they've been told it works just as well as surgery, and with fewer side effects. All of this will be discussed in greater detail in Chapter 9. However, briefly: The phenomenon of radiation seeds became popular about twenty-five years ago, for the same reasons given above. Unfortunately, it didn't work then, and many men who were potentially curable died from prostate cancer. We are being told once again that this form of treatment works. And it may. However, to know whether any form of treatment works for localized prostate cancer, you have to follow patients for ten or fifteen years. This hasn't happened yet, and only time will answer this important question (see Chapter 10).

But what if you're in the "gray zone"? What if you're in your sixties, in reasonably good health, and a good candidate for either treatment? You're certainly in good company; thousands of men fit this description. How do they—and how should you—determine the better of these two good options? Here, after weighing all the facts, is where your own judgment matters most.

It may help to think of the worst-case scenario for each option. Picture yourself five years from now: What if you opted for surgery, and you're still experiencing complications? Your cancer was cured, but you've had significant long-term problems with urinary control, or maybe your sexual function has never come back. How would you feel?

Or, what if you selected radiation therapy, and you feel great, but your PSA level has started creeping back up? Could you live with your decision?

Which of these two situations would bother you the most? You may find—by imagining the worst, in addition to the best possible outcome—that you'll learn the most about yourself and how you should be treated.

Why Not Have Both Treatments? A Word on Combined Approaches

Although some men appear to have clinically localized cancer, there's a good chance that their cancer has spread beyond the prostate. For these men, the combination of radiation and surgery might sound like a promising option. However, it is not yet certain whether radiation after prostatectomy is ultimately helpful. (Note: Radical prostatectomy is definitely not very successful in men who have undergone radiation treatment, and in the minds of many urologists, surgery after the fact is not an option. However, men who have undergone radical prostatectomy *can* go ahead and have radiation therapy later.)

Some surgeons recommend hormonal treatment to shrink the prostate (and, they hope, the tumor) before radical prostatectomy, believing that this will make the cancer more curable. But hormone therapy is not a vacuum cleaner—it can't whisk the cancer cells back into the prostate once they've escaped. There is no reason to believe that hormone treatment before radical prostatectomy will make it possible for surgeons to retrieve and eliminate cancer cells that have strayed from the prostate. Also, this approach may mislead a surgeon into thinking the cancer picture is rosier than it actually is, and thereby encourage a less-aggressive cancer operation.

The findings in surgery determine the course of the operation— more or less tissue is removed, depending on what the surgeon sees and feels when the body is opened up. If, for example, there is any hint that the cancer has escaped the prostate along the nerve bundles that lie on either side of it, these nerves should be "widely excised"—cut out, along with as much nearby tissue as possible. But if a man has received hormonal treatment, the surgeon may be reassured—falsely—about the extent of disease. "Nah," a surgeon may think, "there's no way the cancer could ever reach out this far, not after that hormone treatment I started. I'll leave these nerve bundles in and give this guy a break—now he can keep his sexual potency." As a result of such well-meaning thinking, the surgeon may leave malignant cells behind instead of doing what any good surgeon normally does in a cancer operation—cutting out as much tissue as possible in an aggressive, no-holds-barred attempt to cure the disease. Indeed, one study from Canada found that men who received hormonal therapy before surgery actually had a higher rate of PSA returning after surgery than men who did not receive hormones.

There's another extremely important fact you should know about hormone therapy: It's effective *only while a patient is on it.* The day you stop taking it is the day it stops working. Inevitably and almost immediately, the cancer cells begin growing again. If a surgeon has been timid or overconfident during surgery and not removed all the tissue that needed to be removed, the cancer is going to come back— hormones didn't kill it.

However, *hormonal therapy before radiation may actually improve the results.* Several studies suggest that if a man receives hormonal therapy before beginning radiation therapy and stays on hormones for several years afterward, his chance of beating prostate cancer is better than that of a man who receives radiation therapy alone.

So What Do I Do?

First, educate yourself. Learn everything important there is to know about your own cancer—your clinical stage, PSA level, and Gleason score. Consult the Partin Tables in Chapter 6. Explore all your options—we've done our best to cover them all in this chapter, and specific forms of treatment are covered in greater detail in the next chapters. Get a second opinion, and a third if you need it, and talk to patients. If you can't get some names from your doctor, call a prostate cancer support group (see "Where to Get Help" at the back of this book) or another organization that specializes in prostate cancer. Be your own advocate, and take heart: There is much you can do to make sure you get the best treatment possible.

The Partin Tables can be extremely helpful to you and your doctor in making the decision about treatment. In the best cases, they can identify men who are likely to be cured. But what if the probabilities in the tables suggest that cure is unlikely? Say a man has a PSA between 10 and 20, a palpable tumor involving one entire lobe of the prostate (stage T2b disease), and a Gleason score of 7. What should this man do? Here, age plays a major role. Say this man is in his early fifties. Even though cure is not certain, it's possible, and it's clear that *if he does nothing* he will probably die of his disease. Because the side effects of surgery are much milder in men this age, surgery is certainly a reasonable option, and it does offer the possibility of cure.

On the other hand, say he's in his seventies. The question here is whether a man *who may not live long enough to die of prostate cancer* should be put through an operation with an uncertain likelihood of cure. Surgery has more side effects on people in their seventies. So, for this man, radiation therapy is a better, more reasonable option.

OPTIONS IN THE TREATMENT OF PROSTATE CANCER

Clinical Extent of Disease	Stage	Options
Localized	T1, T2	Radical prostatectomy Radiation therapy Watchful waiting
Locally extended beyond the prostate	T3, T4	Radiation therapy Hormone therapy
Metastasized to lymph nodes and bone	N+, M+	Hormone therapy Non-hormonal approaches and chemotherapy Spot radiation for pain

---

Final Thoughts on Treatment

What if you don't like any of the options? Maybe you're worried about the complications of surgery, and the efficacy of radiation therapy. Maybe you're also questioning whether your cancer really needs to be treated, because right now you feel terrific. And what about all the health stories in the newspaper and on TV? Every day, there's another new breakthrough on cancer. Look at the Human

Genome Project—maybe those scientists will discover the "prostate cancer genes" next week. Maybe some new form of treatment will come along—maybe gene therapy. After all, it's working in other diseases—it's just a matter of time before it works in prostate cancer, too. What if you bite the bullet, and undergo one of the "mainstream" treatments for prostate cancer, and open up the newspaper the next morning and see the headline: "Cure for Prostate Cancer Discovered—No Side Effects!"

Or maybe, like some men, you think you can achieve a time-out by putting your prostate on a "block of ice" for a while, by taking hormones. The problem there is, as we'll discuss later in this book, some prostate cancer cells respond to hormone therapy. But others don't—and unfortunately, it is the cells that don't that eventually could kill you. So if you take hormones, your PSA will plummet—even though, as we'll discuss later on, this is not the same as making the cancer go away completely—and the tumor may shrink clinically. But the cells that can eventually prove fatal *aren't affected at all.* So taking hormones does not cure you, and it doesn't really put the problem on hold. It doesn't stop the clock in the cells that are immune to it.

But what about the miracle cure that could come along any day now? Again, there's the "test of time" issue. Even if a new form of treatment were developed today, it would take fifteen years before we knew whether or not it really worked. That's the problem with prostate cancer. Localized disease progresses very slowly; this is why we can't tell if a treatment is working right away. And this is why you won't hear anything in the near future about a new form of treatment that is *proven* to work. This problem also comes up any time a treatment is changed. In order to reduce side effects, treatments are sometimes modified—but this can potentially reduce their effectiveness.

So, as nice as it would be for a new form of treatment that cures cancer without side effects to come along tomorrow, the truth is that this can't happen. Because there is no way to know whether or not that treatment will actually cure prostate cancer. The answer to that question, every time it's asked, takes many years.

How do you think calmly when you're riding a roller coaster? Most men who find out they have prostate cancer feel physically great. They have no symptoms. They're taking some doctor's word for it—not only that there's a cancer growing inside them, but that the cancer could kill them if they do nothing. Or, unfortunately, as is the case with some doctors (discussed earlier in this chapter)—men are being told the opposite: They're given false assurances that the cancer will grow slowly, and it's okay if they don't do anything but watch its progress.

Throughout this book, we've emphasized that the position of strength here, your best hope of surviving prostate cancer, is to educate yourself, to learn all you can about a disease that's deceptively simple—but which is actually so complicated that many doctors don't understand it.

Now we're at the crossroads. *Educating yourself is just half the battle—the half you can control. The other half involves a leap of faith: You must find a doctor you can believe in, and then you must be able to accept that doctor's advice.* We talk about finding a good surgeon in Chapter 8, but this is more than that—your doctor must be adept and knowledgeable, but must also inspire your trust. Ultimately, in matters of illness, this is something everybody must do. Even we doctors (keeping in mind the old adage, "the doctor who treats himself has a fool for a patient") must put our trust in the hands of another physician when we get sick. This is because—as educated as you may be, or as much as you've learned about this disease, or as accustomed as you are to taking charge of your life—you can't be objective, and somebody needs to be. Make sure this somebody is the best you can find, and then be prepared to follow the plan this doctor believes is best.

Getting through any course of treatment is a hard job. Every form of treatment takes its toll. It's a lot harder if you're spending precious energy and strength fighting—disagreeing with your doctor, or nit-picking and double-checking even the simplest morsel of advice. The time for questioning is now. Get it all out there—every question, every complication you can think of. Write it all down, meet with your doctor, and don't start anything until you're satisfied that you're doing the right thing. And then, once you've done this, release the burden from your shoulders. Let go and let the doctor take over. Spend your energy and strength following that advice, recovering from treatment, and beating this disease.

8

RADICAL PROSTATECTOMY

Read This First

Never underestimate prostate cancer. It is a formidable adversary, which springs up in several places at once inside the prostate. A cancerous prostate has, on average, seven separate tumors growing inside it. Thus, to cure the disease, we can't just take out a few of these spots of cancer; we must eliminate the entire prostate. *If cancer is confined to the prostate, there is no better way to cure it than radical prostatectomy.* The goal of all other forms of treatment for prostate cancer is to be as good as the "gold standard," radical prostatectomy. Today, radical prostatectomy cures the vast majority of men with cancer confined to the prostate, even if it has penetrated the wall, or capsule, of the prostate. And if the operation is performed by an experienced surgeon, preserving potency is common, and few suffer from serious incontinence.

Having said that, we must add right away that radical prostatectomy is not for everybody. It is intended for the *younger man with curable disease*, the man otherwise healthy, who can reasonably expect to live for at least another fifteen years. In other words, it is for the man who is not only curable, but who's going to live long enough to *need* to be cured. It is not something that an older man, or one burdened by other health problems, should have to put himself through.

The radical prostatectomy operation that's performed today has evolved over the last twenty years. My role in this operation began in the early 1970s. I wondered why so many side effects were occurring, and whether it was possible to avoid them. To solve this problem, I took an anatomical approach, and soon learned why these complications were so common. Surgeons did not understand the "periprostatic" anatomy, the terrain surrounding the prostate—the location of the nerves, arteries, veins, and sphincter muscles. Eventually, I was able to chart the course of the veins as they traveled over the top of the prostate. It became clear that there was a relatively narrow trunk that could be tied off over the urethra to control the major bleeding during surgery. With this "bloodless field," it became easier to see and save the anatomical structures that previously had been unrecognized and damaged during surgery.

During radical prostatectomies, I noticed that there was a cluster of arteries and veins, consistently located in the same region in adult men. I speculated that these blood vessels might be the key to preserving potency in surgery. On April 26, 1982, I performed the first purposeful "nerve-sparing" radical prostatectomy on a fifty-two-year-old professor of psychology. This man regained his sexual function within a year, and has remained complication-free, and cancer-free ever since. Today, the neurovascular bundle is widely recognized as the landmark used in nerve-sparing surgery.

Over the last twenty years, I have continued to refine the procedure, making certain that it is an excellent cancer operation, and attempting to speed up the recovery of urinary control and sexual function. Most recently, I have used the review of intraoperative videotapes—much like football coaches watching the "play by play" of last week's game—to see whether I could identify any differences in men who are continent and potent immediately after surgery, versus men who aren't. This has proven to be another good tool in improving the quality of men's lives after surgery.

In this chapter, we cover everything about radical prostatectomy and the complications that can occur in the months after the operation. But what about the long-term outlook, and the biggest question of all—has your cancer been controlled? For a detailed discussion of the results of all forms of treatment for localized disease—surgery, radiation, and cryotherapy—see Chapter 10.

Radical Prostatectomy—the "Gold Standard"

Never underestimate prostate cancer; it is a formidable adversary. In its own way, prostate cancer is much like the Hydra, the many-headed, hard-to-kill monster of Greek myth. It's what scientists call "multifocal"—which means it springs up in several places at once inside the prostate. A cancerous prostate has, on average, seven separate tumors growing inside it. Thus, to cure the disease, we can't just take out a few of these spots of cancer; we must eliminate the entire prostate. *If cancer is confined to the prostate, there is no better way to cure it than radical prostatectomy.* The goal of all other forms of treatment for prostate cancer is to be as good as the "gold standard," radical prostatectomy. (Note that when we talk about radical prostatectomy in this book, unless otherwise stated, we are referring to the anatomic radical retropubic procedure.)

Having said that, we must add right away that radical prostatectomy is not for everybody. It is intended for the *younger man with curable disease*, the man otherwise healthy, who can reasonably expect to live for at least another fifteen years. In other words, it is for the man who is not only curable, but who's going to live long enough to *need* to be cured. It is not something that an older man, or one burdened by other health problems, should have to put himself through. What if you're somewhere in the middle of these two ends of the spectrum? What if you're a young, otherwise healthy man, and the Partin Tables say there's a 50/50 chance your cancer can be cured? If surgery is the best way to cure you, then you should do it. What if you're a man in his early seventies, in excellent health, with curable disease and a family history of longevity? There is no question that older men are more prone to side effects after surgery than younger men, and you must consider the quality of the years added to your life. How would you feel if you never regained full control over urination? Also, what if you had complications and were not cured—remember, from Chapter 7, that older men often have more advanced disease, because it has been there longer. On the other hand, if you select a less effective form of treatment, have a long life, and your cancer comes back, you may end up asking yourself "what if"—what if you had gone for the best treatment the first time around? For older men, this can be a tough decision.

Today, radical prostatectomy cures the vast majority of men with cancer confined to the prostate, even if it has penetrated the wall, or capsule, of the prostate. And preserving potency—by *not* removing one or both of the nerve bundles adjacent to the prostate, which are responsible for erection (surgeons didn't even realize these bundles existed two decades ago)—does not compromise cancer cure; a recent study found that the odds of cure are just as high. Today, serious bleeding is very rare, and if the operation is performed by an experienced surgeon, preserving potency is common, and few suffer from serious incontinence.

Evolution of an Operation

Surgery to remove the prostate as a treatment for cancer was first performed in 1904, at Johns Hopkins by a urologist named Hugh Hampton Young. Young's procedure, called a radical perineal prostatectomy, was a success: Six and a half years later, when the patient died of other causes, an autopsy showed that his prostate cancer had been cured.

In the late 1940s, another approach called the radical retropubic prostatectomy was developed, and like Young's operation (which still is used today, although not as often as the retropubic approach), it proved extremely effective in stopping prostate cancer in its tracks— if, that is, the cancer was confined to the prostate.

Both the radical perineal and retropubic operations had a definite downside—two devastating side effects, incontinence and impotence. *Every man who had a radical prostatectomy was impotent, and as many as 25 percent had severe problems with urinary control.* Worse was the extreme, often life-threatening bleeding that went along with radical retropubic prostatectomy. It's no exaggeration to say that the operation used to be performed in a sea of blood. In this era, many men believed that the side effects from surgery were almost worse than having the disease. So understandably, when radiation treatment for prostate cancer was introduced in the 1960s and popularized (see Chapter 9), doctors as well as patients welcomed this alternative therapy. Although doctors realized that it probably did not cure prostate cancer as well as surgery, it certainly had fewer side effects.

The harshness of the procedure and its after-effects were the catalysts for change, inspiring the anatomical discoveries that have drastically reduced these side effects. As a result of these discoveries, when radical prostatectomy is performed by an experienced surgeon, most men should remain potent, and few men should have serious problems with urinary control. Today, radical prostatectomy is the most certain way to cure men with cancer that's confined to the prostate.

Crafting a kinder, gentler, better operation: How did radical prostatectomy change? My role in this operation began in the early 1970s. Like many urologic surgeons, I was appalled by the blood loss in these men. With the goal of finding surgical methods to lessen the bleeding—so we could actually see what we were doing instead of blindly feeling our way—I studied the anatomy of the venous drainage surrounding the prostate, and developed some new techniques, which did two things: First, with less bleeding, the operation became safer. And with what we call "a bloodless field," critical structures—which previously had been unrecognized and damaged, simply because there was too much blood in the way—could be looked for and saved. More precise dissection and reconstruction reduced the likelihood of significant urinary incontinence to 2 percent, and even those 2 percent are not incontinent all the time. (We're still working to improve this—more below.)

Breakthrough in Understanding Potency

But what about impotence? It had been widely assumed that penile nerves inevitably were damaged by the radical prostatectomy. Previously, many doctors thought the nerves that controlled erection ran through the prostate and would be destroyed as a necessity if you removed the prostate—the idea of "to make an omelet, you have to break a few eggs." These nerves were the "broken eggs"—an unavoidable hazard, the price of curing cancer.

It didn't make sense to me that the nerves from one organ would run through another organ. But this had always been the assumption, even in medical textbooks. One highly respected anatomy textbook, for example, stated merely that the nerves that enable erection were "extremely small, difficult to follow in the adult cadaver," and that their location was known "merely through experimental studies."

Around this time, something unbelievable happened: In 1977, one of my patients returned for a follow-up visit three months after surgery and reported that he was totally potent. To me, this news was staggering—how could this man be potent, if the nerves that control potency were inside the prostate that I had removed? Furthermore, if this could happen to one man, then why *only* this one? Why weren't *all* men potent after radical prostatectomy? The key was finding these elusive nerves. If we could just figure out where they were—and then find a way to save them but still cure prostate cancer—then men would no longer be faced with an either-or situation. They could be cured of cancer, *and* remain potent.

If this were a detective novel, then here's where we would say something like: "The place: Leiden, the Netherlands. The year: 1981. Here's where the whole case blew wide open." And really, it did—thanks to a urologist named Pieter Donker. I was in Leiden for a conference; Donker, who had recently retired as professor of urology there, was studying anatomy, and tackling unanswered questions. No one had successfully dissected the nerves to the bladder, because they were difficult to identify in adults. However, these nerves are not nearly so obscured in infants. I asked to see the laboratory where he was working to trace these nerves, in a cadaver of a stillborn male infant. I asked Donker if he knew what happened to the other end of this plexus of nerves—the ones that controlled penile erection. "I've never looked," he said. We got to work. Four hours later, we were jubilant: We could see clearly that the nerves were *outside* the capsule of the prostate—and that, indeed, it was possible to completely remove the prostate and preserve sexual function!

Over the next year, we worked together on this project long-distance, and then we met again. In the infant cadaver, the location of these nerves had become clear. But how could we apply our findings in stillborn infants (which are easier to see for many reasons, including the fact that infants have less fatty fibrous tissue than adults) and find these tiny, microscopic structures in the deep, complicated recesses of the pelvis in adult men? It was like having a schematic drawing, and trying to identify a burned-out transistor in your television set. During this year, I had noticed something important: There was a cluster of arteries and veins that traveled along the edge of the prostate in the exact location where these nerves were found in the infant cadaver. Perhaps these blood vessels acted as they do elsewhere in the body—maybe they provided a scaffolding for these microscopic nerves. And maybe we could use these bundles as landmarks. Donker agreed. I returned to Baltimore and tested this theory while performing an operation called a radical cystectomy, removal of the prostate and bladder, in a sixty-seven-year-old man. I had never seen or heard of a patient who had been potent after this operation. But ten days after surgery, this man stated that he awoke in the morning with a normal erection.

A month later, on April 26, 1982, I performed the first purposeful nerve-sparing radical prostatectomy on a fifty-two-year-old professor of psychology. This man regained his sexual function within a year, and has remained complication-free—and cancer-free—ever since.

Better understanding of the anatomical terrain also led to several important observations. Now that we've learned exactly where the scalpel can and cannot go, depending on the extent of a man's cancer, it has become possible either to save these nerves deliberately, or to remove more tissue by cutting these bundles away—in surgical terms, to create "wider margins of excision"—than we previously had believed possible. It used to be that surgeons never excised these nerves, because they were adherent to the rectum; instead, surgeons just cut the nerves and unknowingly left them in place. However, with these anatomical techniques, we now have a *better chance of removing all the cancer.* Many people call this a "nerve-sparing" operation, but a more accurate description is that it's an "anatomic radical prostatectomy," because there are actually two things going on here: one is preserving the nerves; the other is creating wider margins—by excising them when necessary, removing as much tissue as possible around the cancer—making this a better cancer operation.

At the same time these discoveries were taking place, an anatomist provided an entirely new insight into the location of the sphincter responsible for urinary control. Previously, we believed that the pelvic floor muscles opened and closed like sliding doors. But this was not the case; it turns out that the sphincter is a tubular structure, embedded in the veins that had once bled so much during surgery. This observation explains why the anatomic approach improved the results of urinary continence: In controlling the venous bleeders, and making the "bloodless field," we did a better job of preserving this sphincter.

Today at Johns Hopkins (the hospital is noted here because results vary worldwide, depending on a range of factors, including the surgeons' skill and the selection criteria for patients), 86 percent of men who undergo surgery are potent, only 2 percent wear a pad that they change more than once a day, and the cancer control rates are used as the "gold standard," to which all other forms of treatment are compared.

Overall, in men treated since 1989, at ten years or more after surgery, only 2 percent have developed local recurrence of cancer and only 8 percent distant metastases; and 80 percent have an undetectable level of PSA. (For more on cancer control, see Chapter 10.) Important determinants in the return of sexual function include age, the extent to which the cancer extends outside the prostate, and the extent of nerve loss—whether one or both nerve bundles remain, or whether they had to be removed during surgery.

We tell our patients that we have three goals: removing all of the tumor, preserving urinary control, and preserving sexual function. *Sexual function is number three, because if it is lost there are many ways to restore it.*

Men who are impotent following radical prostatectomy have normal sensation, normal sex drive and can achieve a normal orgasm. The one element they may be lacking is the ability to have an erection sufficient for intercourse, and that can be restored by drugs such as Viagra, or by other means. (For more on erectile dysfunction, see Chapter 11.)

WILL I BE FERTILE AFTER SURGERY?

For most couples, there is good news after a radical prostatectomy: You can safely discontinue birth control measures. That's because the vas deferens (see Chapter 1), which carries sperm, is completely divided, and there is no way that a woman can become pregnant during intercourse. However, many men who undergo radical prostatectomy today are younger, and may not have completed family planning. If you're not ready to close this door forever, the safest thing to do is store sperm before surgery (a process called cryopreservation). This is the most cost-effective way to ensure that you can have a baby someday, if you choose. There is a "plan B" here, for men who have already undergone radical prostatectomy and then decided that they want to have children. This is a process called ICSI (intracytoplasmic sperm injection). It's somewhat complicated, and expensive. Basically, it involves using a tiny needle to harvest sperm from the testis or epididymis. These sperm are then injected directly into eggs that have been harvested from the patient's wife. After a period of incubation, they are then implanted. But the best bet, if there's even a remote chance that you may want more children after surgery, is to plan ahead, and store your sperm.

Perfecting the Radical Prostatectomy

Baseball pitchers use videotape to perfect their fastball; tennis players use it to get a better spin on their serve. The video camera is a staple for most athletes, in fact: No respectable football coach would dare contemplate next week's game without spending hours seeking wisdom from hindsight, going over the this week's effort on the gridiron, play by play.

So why don't surgeons do the same thing? How are we ever going to improve our technique if we don't analyze our own work this way?

Over the years, I have come to believe that very small differences in surgical technique can have a major impact on outcome. Recently, I put this theory to the test, watching my own operations. Using a high-quality, three-chip video camera, I videotaped the operations on the men discussed below (see "Continence and Potency: Quality of Life After Radical Prostatectomy"). Then, eighteen months after that study began, I reviewed these tapes. My goal was to make a good operation even better, by minimizing the operation's two major side effects—incontinence and impotence. This is what I wanted to find out: When a patient is continent and potent immediately after surgery, *what made the difference* in this man? I spent my summer vacation examining these videotapes, sometimes stopping them frame by frame looking for insight. (Another bonus of the video camera is that it allows surgeons a view of the entire operative field, and not just the small area where we focus as we operate.) It took many hours of intense scrutiny to watch sixty two-hour operations, but gradually I was able to identify four slight variations in my technique—in controlling bleeding from the dorsal vein and dividing the sphincter—that appeared to make the difference in the men who recovered sexual potency the soonest.

Perhaps most exciting was that a new finding came out of this research: It turns out that some men have a significant anatomical variation. Previously, everyone believed that the neurovascular bundle took a rather straight pathway from its origin in the sacrum along the lateral surface of the prostate to the urethra. But I learned that in many patients the bundle curves around the apex of the prostate, and is tucked just beneath the sphincter and held there by a small group of vessels. And that, if one attempts in good faith to preserve as much of the sphincter as possible, the neurovascular bundle can be damaged, and recovery of sexual function delayed. Indeed, the eight men who at eighteen months had not yet recovered full sexual function all seemed to have this variant curve.

Part two of this project was to make the study " blind." I went back over the operations again—this time without identifying the patient or the outcome—to see if the steps I had identified checked out. Fortunately, they did.

Incontinence is a long-term significant problem for only about 2 percent of our patients at Johns Hopkins, and I was unable to find evidence that anything I did or did not do during surgery would make a difference there. Clearly, it had nothing to do with preservation of the sphincter. There was one man with perfect preservation of the sphincter who was still wearing a pad one year after the surgery. For this reason, I am now taking a different approach, by working to refine the procedure for reconstructing the bladder neck during radical prostatectomy.

To the best of my knowledge, this is the first time that any surgeon in any field used retrospective reviews of intraoperative videotapes to improve any surgical technique. I believe many surgeons could benefit from regularly reviewing their operations in this way. Because many surgeons use different techniques, it's likely that each surgeon may be able to identify other important, arbitrary variations that may help patients. Also, for surgeons whose patients seem prone to more side effects than usual, the review of early successful cases may help them identify ways to modify their technique, and improve the outcome of future patients. If I had videotaped that first successful operation in 1977—after which the man was potent immediately—I would have discovered the location of the nerves four years sooner.

Are You in Good Hands?
What to Look for in a Surgeon

Doctor A is a nice, personable young doctor, whose empathy for your condition appealed to you immediately.

That's great. Now what else do you know about him? He's got a terrific bedside manner, but is he a board-certified urologist? What training has he had? Does he know—and use—the nerve-sparing techniques, the anatomical approach to radical prostatectomy? How many of these operations does he do a year? What success has he had in preserving potency and continence? (If he can't or won't give you his rate of success as compared to reports from other surgeons, or to results published in medical journals, this may be a red flag, and perhaps you should look elsewhere.) You should be able to get a good idea of his success rate, in numbers or percentages. And if he hasn't done very many of these operations—ideally, hundreds—you might want to find a more experienced surgeon. Look at it this way: *Do you want to be one of the patients he's learning on?* Do you want to be part of someone's learning curve?

When you're looking for a surgeon, you don't necessarily want some name-brand academician or a specialist in other areas of urologic surgery. You want to find a doctor who performs this particular operation. *Often.* Preferably, a doctor who does this operation several days a week. Even better, a surgeon who has dedicated his or her life to doing this one operation.

Doctor B is another nice doctor, a respected, fatherly man who's been operating in your town as long as anybody can remember. Just looking at him inspires confidence.

Swell. But does he also keep up with the latest research? Does he continue his education regularly, brushing up on old surgical skills as well as mastering new techniques?

Does he operate on nearly every man who has prostate cancer? (This is not a desirable quality in a surgeon.) Or does he screen his patients carefully, making every attempt to spare any man with cancer that *can't be cured by surgery* the unnecessary ordeal and side effects of an operation?

There's no getting around it: Radical prostatectomy is a tricky operation, one of the most difficult in medicine. There can be tremendous, at times life-threatening, blood loss. Does your surgeon have the proverbial "nerves of steel"? A good surgeon can handle unexpected or excessive bleeding without panicking, but also—thinking of your long-term quality of life—won't damage the microscopic nerves necessary for erection. An experienced surgeon knows how to preserve these nerves, and *when it's safe to do so.* You don't want someone whose knee-jerk reaction to the biopsy is to cut, cut, cut. For example, if the biopsy is positive on the right side, and your surgeon says, "We'll take out the nerves on the right side, and on the left, too, for good measure—I'm interested in getting out all the cancer," then you should find another surgeon. For one thing, just because the biopsy is positive on the right side doesn't mean the nerves on the right side are involved in the cancer. For another, it's unlikely that such a surgeon will actually remove the nerves on either side—a more probable scenario is that he'll cut the nerves, and leave most of them in place. Excising these nerves widely is as difficult as preserving them, because they're adherent to the rectum, and it takes great skill to cut them out completely. Or there's also the surgeon who says, "We don't care about side effects; I'm just there to get out all the cancer. We can always put in an artificial sphincter [for control of incontinence], and give you shots or a penile prosthesis [for impotence]." Again, probably not the right surgeon for you. Your ideal surgeon should get out all the cancer *and* make every effort to minimize side effects.

Remember: *You don't want a surgeon who's "pretty good"* at removing the prostate. And you can't assume that every urologist does this well. There are no second chances here; this is a one-shot operation. *You are looking for the one surgeon who will perform the one rad-*

ical prostatectomy you will ever receive in your life, the one operation that will cure your cancer. You want a surgeon who isn't going to leave some cancer behind, who knows how to minimize trauma to your body during surgery so you don't wind up incontinent, impotent, or both. (Note: Unexpected trouble can crop up in any operation; nobody can help that. But the unexpected is less likely to happen with an experienced surgeon.) So ask questions, like:

- How many of these operations do you do a week?
- Do many of your patients have positive margins?
- How do you collect data on your patients? Do you know their long-term outcome? If the answer is something like, "Only if they let me know," then find someone who keeps better tabs on his or her patients. Urologists who don't know their own results may not realize that their technique should be better. And, if the urologist can produce statistics, but you don't like those results, get another opinion.
- How often do your patients require radiation therapy after surgery, or treatment with hormones? If the number is greater than 15 percent, this suggests that the doctor either doesn't do a very good job selecting surgical candidates, or is not completely removing all the cancer during surgery. It also suggests that you need to get a second opinion. But you should get a second opinion anyway. *Always get a second opinion.*

Finally, ask to talk to the urologist's patients. Find out how they're treated—how hard is it to get the doctor when you have a question, or need help? If they've had post-surgical complications, how did the doctor treat them?

Finding the right physician may mean that you must travel to a major medical center in another city. This may mean that you'll be away from home for four days. But after that, even though you will be wearing a catheter for a week or two (see below), the recovery from this operation is usually speedy, and follow-up communications can usually be carried out over the telephone (for example, if you have your follow-up PSA tests done in your hometown, you can have them sent to your surgeon, and discuss them—or any complications or troubling issues, such as incontinence or impotence—over the phone).

HOW COULD THE STANDARD OF CARE BE
IMPROVED NATIONALLY?

Why are results of radical prostatectomy so uneven across the country? In the hands of an expert, the complication rate from this operation is low. But many of the patients with bad results—lifetime incontinence, for example, or worst of all, an immediate return of cancer—are men who should never have undergone the operation in the first place, because they were not good surgical candidates, and/or because their cancer was not curable when it was diagnosed. It's unfortunate that so many men with prostate cancer must adhere to the phrase "caveat emptor"—Buyer, beware.

The burden of making sure the doctor is competent shouldn't have to weigh so heavily on the patient's shoulders. For example, it seems absurd that a would-be buyer at an Internet auction house can instantly learn the track record and customer rating of a seller before committing to doing business, but a man who is looking to place his life in the hands of a surgeon must do his own research—and even then, hope he's asked all the right questions, and left no important stone unturned. There should be a similar mechanism to monitor the performance of urologists, and all physicians.

The information is already out there: Insurance companies know how long a surgeon's patients are in the hospital, how many must be readmitted for complications, how many eventually need placement of an artificial sphincter to control incontinence, how many need postoperative radiation, or immediate treatment with hormonal therapy. If the insurance companies and managed care organizations were really interested in seeing that their patients received the best care, they could identify surgeons who have the highest volume of patients and lowest rate of complications. This might stimulate the physicians whose patient outcomes were not as good to improve their skills—or, to decide that performing one operation a month was not the best thing for them or their patients.

The next step would be for an organization to collect patient-reported outcomes. Again, this is something insurance companies could do—find out exactly how patients are doing, and then put together a roster of surgeons who provide the best service. To some, this might seem like unnecessary interference; after all, the idea of "letting the market decide" is a cornerstone of private enterprise, capitalism, and the American way. But this is different from buying a car that turns out to be a lemon. If you have winced at the results of a botched operation, feeling at once sorry for the patient—who came to you, hoping you could repair the damage—and outraged that medical care in this country is so variable, you might agree that the system ought to be improved. For every procedure, and for every illness—not just radical prostatectomy, and not just prostate cancer. What about the surgeons whose work is not up to the national standard? One obvious solution is that they could work to improve their technique. It's never too late to learn. (See "Perfecting the Radical Prostatectomy.")

Undeniably, the results of surgery are best when patients are in the hands of experts. For the sake of men with prostate cancer—and their families—it's time for this information to be made available to everyone.

The Anatomical Retropubic Prostatectomy

Questions You May Have before Surgery

Why do I have to wait several weeks for the operation? There should always be a delay of about six to eight weeks between the time a man's prostate cancer is diagnosed and the time he can undergo surgery. Many men are frustrated by this. They think, "I've got cancer, it's curable, I want it out of there right now!" They see the delay as an operating room equivalent of an overbooked airport, with planes stacked up waiting to land, and interminable layovers. But this is not the case. The main reason for the six- to eight-week lag time between diagnosis and surgery is not to accommodate a busy hospital's schedule; it's so you can have a *better cancer operation.*

Immediately after the needle biopsy, which often involves a dozen punctures of the rectum, your body reacts—as it does to any injury—with inflammation and bleeding. Now is not the ideal time for surgery. A biopsy is what doctors call an "insult" to the body, in this case, to the wall of the rectum, which is riddled with tiny holes, and weakened (think of how much easier it is to tear perforated paper than regular, intact paper). The body needs time to recover from this relatively minor insult, so it will be ready for the really big one—major surgery. Even after two weeks, the punctures may have healed, but the prostate is now adherent to the rectum; it remains stuck to the rectum until the inflammation resolves. If surgery were attempted at this point, it would not be easy to release the rectum from the prostate—and the last thing the surgeon wants to do is make a hole in the rectum. In an attempt to protect the rectum, the surgeon may cut too close to the prostate, possibly leaving cancer cells behind. But give it a few more weeks, the inflammation heals, and the prostate is no longer "sticky." The normal anatomy is restored, and it's easier for the surgeon to see the terrain.

Before surgery, when you give the doctor your medical history, be sure to say so if you've had any unusual problems with bleeding in the past (from dental work, for example). Aspirin and drugs such as ibuprofen (Advil, Motrin) can cause excessive bleeding; *if you are taking aspirin or a similar drug regularly, make sure you stop at least ten days before the operation.* Also be sure to tell your doctor if you are taking vitamins—particularly, vitamin E—herbal compounds, or other dietary supplements. These supplements still count as medications, even if they "just came from the health store," and they can affect blood-clotting mechanisms; thus, you should stop taking them as well.

What about donating my own blood? This is another point to discuss with your doctor: Many men who undergo radical prostatectomy need a blood transfusion during the procedure. The best blood for you to get, obviously, is your own; if your hospital allows this, it's a good idea to donate several units of your blood ahead of time. (This is another good reason for the six- to eight-week delay; it gives you plenty of time to make up your own blood bank.) However, there is some difference of surgical opinion here. Some surgeons say that their patients never lose any blood, and therefore don't need any blood transfusions. For these physicians, the most important thing during the operation is to clamp, ligate, and clip every little bleeder—every blood vessel that bleeds. My philosophy is somewhat different. The nerves that control erection are surrounded by blood vessels; in fact, that's what the neurovascular bundle is, a knot of blood vessels. To expose these vessels, there is often bleeding, and if a surgeon aggressively clamps every bleeder, it is unlikely that the nerves will survive. So, with the patient's long-term outlook—controlling cancer, *plus* maintaining quality of life—as my main goal, I must sometimes "spend" a little bit of blood. If I see something bleeding, I may wait until I've completely released the tissue surrounding that bleeder to see what's beneath it—and then control just that bleeding vessel, leaving the nerves beneath it intact. If a patient gives his own blood and receives a unit or two of it during surgery, there is no harm; in fact, it may improve his quality of life immediately after surgery.

The reason for this is something called hematocrit—the percentage of blood that's occupied by red blood cells. Normally, this percentage is around 45 percent. A number of studies have suggested that the hematocrit can fall to as low as 21 percent and still be adequate to reduce the patient's risk of having a heart attack after surgery. But would men feel better if they went home with a hematocrit of 31 instead of 21? Again, there's a difference in philosophy (and that's about all it is, because there has been no scientific study of quality of life in men with different hematocrit levels after surgery). Some surgeons just don't want to transfuse any blood, and feel that the man who goes home with a hematocrit of 21 will do just as well as the man with a hematocrit of 31. Also, many argue that bank blood today is very safe, and that the main risks of a transfusion (getting the wrong blood or infected blood) are not avoided by donating your own blood. Advocates of giving your own blood disagree. So you need to ask yourself—if you will need a transfusion, whose blood do you want—your own, or someone else's?

You can give one unit of blood a week for three weeks before surgery. The day you start giving blood, take one iron tablet three times a day, and continue until the day of your last blood donation. And while you're giving blood, don't take aspirin, ibuprofen, vitamin E, or any similar medication; if this blood will be going back into your body during surgery (presumably because you've lost enough to need it), the level of these drugs may be high enough to interfere with the clotting of your blood during surgery.

Does it matter if I've had previous prostate surgery for BPH? This is how some men find out they have prostate cancer—when the prostate tissue removed in a TURP procedure or open prostatectomy (another procedure for BPH) is evaluated by a pathologist. It's more difficult for surgeons to perform a radical prostatectomy after an open prostatectomy, but that doesn't mean it can't be done. It often is, and with great success. You may need to wait about twelve weeks after a TURP procedure, until the inflammation from this operation has gone down.

ARE YOU IN SHAPE FOR SURGERY?

In any man, the prostate is not terribly accessible. It's way down there, deep in the pelvis, and in the retropubic procedure (as opposed to the perineal approach, discussed later in the chapter), the surgeon must go through the lower abdomen to find it. This is not only much more difficult in a man who is overweight; it can also interfere with performing a good cancer operation, preserving urinary control, and preserving potency.

If you are overweight, your surgeon may only operate on the condition that you lose weight beforehand. It is in your best interest to meet this challenge—it may be that your life will be saved twice, because men who are overweight are medical time bombs. Heart disease, stroke, diabetes— you're at high risk for all of these, and if you smoke, or have high cholesterol, the risk skyrockets. In blunt terms, what's the point of curing your cancer if you're not going to live long enough to benefit from it?

Here, as an example of what can be done in just two months, is a diet plan developed by one of my patients, who was diagnosed with prostate cancer at age fifty-three. I agreed to operate on him under the condition that he lose at least thirty pounds. Here's how he explains it: "I needed to lose the weight for my own health benefit, and a leaner patient would simplify the surgical procedure, improving prognosis for success. I dropped from 224 pounds to 189 pounds, between November 8 and January 8. I had surgery January 15, stronger and leaner. Here's how I did it:

- "Goal setting and plotting expectations kept me motivated to lose weight continually.
- "Actual weighing-in only took place twice a week, Monday and Thursday. There is too much weight shift due to water retention to recommend everyday weighing. I wanted to avoid setbacks. Every weigh-in should result in a legitimate loss.
- "I didn't starve! It took only four days to get used to a daily diet which roughly followed this pattern: Breakfast—Ultra Slim Fast; tea or coffee. Lunch—salad (I was creative, using a variety of vegetables), cup of soup; Dinner—tossed salad, Stouffer's Lean Cuisine. These are delicious, come in many varieties, and provide a 'unit dose' of calories, about 230 to 290. I favor the spicier ones.
- "I wrote down everything that I ate or drank, meal by meal, in a daily journal. Having to confront my sins in black and white kept me from committing them.
- "Exercise played a key role. I worked out daily, varying the thirty- to forty-five-minute exercise between NordicTrack, treadmill, jogging, and briskly walking my dog. This burned off one of the meals, so I netted out at two meals per day."

Countdown to surgery: One of the most important steps in recovering from a radical prostatectomy is the recovery of the gastrointestinal tract—mainly, this means the return of normal bowel movements. This return to normal happens much faster, and with fewer complications, if the bowels are empty when you undergo surgery. Thus, to help speed things along *after* surgery, you can work on improving your digestive tract *before* surgery. Be sure that your bowels are moving well for about two weeks before the operation; increase your daily intake of fiber, fruit, and liquids. Note: Iron supplements (which you should be taking if you are giving your own blood—see above) can sometimes cause constipation. If necessary, take a stool softener, or talk to your doctor about a bulking laxative (such as Citracel). Stick to clear liquids during the day before surgery. Then, on the night before surgery, take a laxative, and don't eat anything after midnight. On the morning before surgery, give yourself an enema.

Anesthesia: Your two best options are spinal or epidural anesthesia. The great advantage to both of these approaches, as opposed to general anesthesia, is that there is less bleeding during surgery. Also, both reduce the likelihood of blood clots forming in the legs after surgery (perhaps because there is increased blood circulation in the legs during surgery). With both forms, you can remain conscious and aware of the procedure if you like, even though you can't feel it. For many patients, this is a cause of concern; they say, "I don't *want* to know what's going on." Don't worry: You can be sedated (with a mild drug such as Valium, which will make you sleep), as well as anesthetized. Most men don't remember anything about the operation. In *spinal anesthesia,* a tiny needle is used to inject a local anesthetic into the small of your back through the dura, the membrane lining the spinal cord, and into the spinal fluid. Within minutes, you'll feel numb, relaxed, and heavy from your waist to your toes. After surgery, you'll be asked to lie flat in bed until the numbness goes away and you can move your legs again. *This is important; sitting up too soon can cause a severe headache.*

Epidural anesthesia is like having an IV tube hooked up to your back, instead of to a vein in your arm. A local anesthetic enters the body through a tiny plastic tube, inserted between the vertebrae of your spine near the small of your back. The epidural anesthetic (often used to provide pain relief in pregnant women during labor) bathes the area outside the membrane lining the spinal cord, temporarily numbing the nerves in your lower body. Unlike spinal anesthesia, which comes in one dose, epidural anesthesia can be given continuously. The area of numbness can be adjusted; so can the degree of pain relief.

During surgery: What happens. First, let's review the territory. (It might help if, as you read this, you refer to Figures 8.1–8.8.) For a surgeon, this is precarious terrain indeed: The prostate (Fig. 8.1) is located deep in the pelvis, surrounded by structures that are fragile and vulnerable to injury—the rectum, the bladder, the sphincter responsible for urinary control, some large blood vessels, and the bundles of nerves that are responsible for erection.

The operation begins with an incision through skin that extends from the pubic area to the navel. Next, the muscles in the abdomen are separated in the midline and spread apart. They are not cut, and that's one of the reasons why men recover from this operation fairly quickly, with little pain, and with no long-term injury to their abdominal muscles.

The next step is the *staging pelvic lymphadenectomy* (discussed in Chapter 6)—dissection of the pelvic lymph nodes, to make sure they're free of cancer (Fig. 8.2). To do this, we remove a triangle of tissue on each side of the bladder; these triangles contain important lymph nodes. In the past, these lymph nodes were then rushed to a pathologist for what's called "frozen section analysis" (the tissue is frozen, then sliced into very thin sections and examined under the microscope). Today, we don't do that very often. In most men, these lymph nodes are usually removed as part of the operation, and sent along with the prostate to the pathologist, who then examines this entire "specimen," or bunch of removed tissue.

Today, staging pelvic lymphadenectomy (as a separate procedure, done several days ahead of time) is usually performed only in men with a Gleason score of 8 or higher. This is because for lower-grade, well- to moderately well-differentiated tumors —Gleason 7 or less— the long-term prognosis is different than that for men with high-grade, poorly differentiated tumors. With Gleason scores of 7 or lower—even when there is a tiny bit of cancer in a lymph node—60 percent of men without further treatment have no sign of metastases on bone scans ten years later. This doesn't mean the cancer won't eventually come back in these men, but that it can take years longer to return when the tumor is of a lower, better-differentiated grade. So, because these men can live for many years, they often benefit from having their prostate removed. Removing it now will help them avoid problems with urinary tract obstruction and bleeding later, if the cancer does return. Furthermore, we have some evidence that men in this situation who have their prostate removed live longer (see Chapter 7).

For men with Gleason scores of 8 or higher, it is very important to know the status of the lymph nodes before going ahead with a radical prostatectomy. Because frozen section analysis may miss small but important deposits of tumor in the lymph nodes, we prefer to carry out this procedure at least several days ahead of time. (As discussed in Chapter 6, this can be performed either laparoscopically, or with a modified procedure called a "mini-lap.")

Next (Fig. 8.3), the major vein system that overlies the prostate and urethra (this is called the dorsal vein complex) is divided and tied. This is a crucial step; control of these veins makes a huge difference in the surgeon's ability to see what's happening, and it's particularly significant for what happens next—cutting through the urethra (Fig. 8.4). If the urethra is cut too close to the prostate, some cancer might be left behind. This is the most common location for a "positive surgical margin," for the presence of cancer cells at the cut edge of the removed prostate specimen. Positive surgical margins are discussed later, but briefly, a positive margin can mean one of two things: It may mean that the tumor extends outside the prostate, to a point where the surgeon can't remove it all. But it often means simply that the boundaries of the prostate are indistinct, and the surgeon cut extremely closely along the edges of the prostate. This is the part of the operation where it's most difficult to see exactly where the prostate ends and the tissue outside it begins. If we err on the other side—if we cut too far away from the prostate—the urethral sphincter might be damaged, and such an injury can make a man incontinent. The surgical line here is literally not much more than a hairbreadth.

Next, depending on the degree of cancer, the surgeon must make a decision that will affect the patient's potency—to leave intact the neurovascular bundles, the wafer-thin packets of nerves that sit on either side of the prostate, or to remove one or both along with the prostate (Fig. 8.5). These are the nerve bundles responsible for erection.

Remember the three goals of radical prostatectomy: first is removing the cancer, then preserving urinary continence, and then preserving sexual function. In that order. The primary goal here is not to preserve potency; it's to *get rid of the cancer, in a careful but thorough way.* Fortunately, because prostate cancer is being detected early in most men, it is usually possible to preserve the neurovascular bundles on both sides. These bundles are outside the capsule of the prostate; even when cancer penetrates the capsule, it travels only *one or two millimeters*—not much more than the width of a pencil point—away from it before turning northward, toward the seminal vesicles. Because the neurovascular bundles are, on average, about *five millimeters* from the prostate, we can usually preserve both neurovascular bundles without creating a positive surgical margin. In a review of five hundred consecutive men who underwent radical prostatectomy at Johns Hopkins between 1997 and 2000, 87 percent of men had both bundles preserved, and 13 percent of men had one bundle preserved. Pathological study confirmed that the cancer was completely removed, with no evidence of cancer at the edge of the removed tissue (in "surgeon-ese," the margins were "negative") in 95 percent of these men. Only 5 percent had a positive surgical margin, and only 2 percent had cancer cells at the neurovascular bundle. In half of these "positive margins," the cancer was on the *opposite* side of where the biopsy had suggested (again, more evidence for caution before a surgeon should reflexively decide to remove the bundle on the side of the positive biopsy). As we discuss in Chapter 10, the vast majority of these men were eventually proven to be cured of their cancer.

Having said all that, we must now say that if it's necessary to remove one neurovascular bundle, it should go (Fig. 8.6). Remember, *men can remain potent even if one bundle is removed, and can still have normal sensation, sex drive, and orgasm even if both bundles are removed.* And frankly, there are plenty of older men out there who *haven't* had prostate surgery who still have problems with erection. This is an inevitable problem for many men, one of those things that come with the territory of aging; in other words, it may be a bullet you couldn't have dodged anyway. Having said that, however, it's also important to repeat that *there is plenty of help available, and you can still have a normal sex life.* (See Chapter 11.)

There is no way for the surgeon to know for certain before the actual operation whether or not the bundles can be spared. *Only during surgery is it truly possible to see where the cancer is.* Some urologists believe that the neurovascular bundle must always be excised on the side of a positive biopsy—in other words, if your biopsy showed cancer cells on the left side, then that bundle's got to go. This is not the case, and although well intentioned, is a bit of a knee-jerk reaction. Actually, the most common site of positive surgical margins is the apex of the prostate (where the sphincter meets the urethra), followed by the posterior (next to the rectum), and lastly, the posterolateral area, near the neurovascular bundle.

Experienced surgeons don't make any decisions beforehand. We wait, and assess the extent of a tumor during surgery. We can see it, and more importantly, we can *feel* it. During surgery, if we feel cancer on the edge of the prostate, the neurovascular bundle should be removed. It should also be removed if, at any point during its release (when we slowly peel it away from the prostate), it seems adherent, or sticky. Red flag—this is often a sign that the cancer is beginning to escape the prostate. However, if no firmness is felt, and the neurovascular bundle falls away from the prostate, it's safe to preserve it. As a final precaution, we double-check the bundles later in the operation. Once the prostate has been removed, the surgeon carefully examines the specimen, feeling every inch of it for hardness. If there is any suggestion that we need to go back and remove a bit more tissue, we can remove the bundle at that time.

If the surgeon decides to preserve the nerve bundles, the tiny branches that connect the nerves to the prostate are divided carefully. If, however, one or both bundles must be widely excised, the nerve bundles are cut near the urethra and beside the rectum.

Next, the surgeon goes to work on the prostate, making a cut to separate it at the bladder neck, which links the bladder to the prostate (Fig. 8.7). The seminal vesicles are removed, along with the vas deferens on each side (for more on the anatomy, see Chapter 1). The goal here is to remove as much surrounding tissue as possible along with the prostate. Finally, the surgeon must carefully rebuild the urinary tract, hooking up the bladder once again to the urethra and urethral sphincter, which is responsible for urinary control. This reconnection is called an anastomosis. Note that the gap between the bladder and urethra—where the prostate used to be—is now filled by the bladder. Some men worry that the penis will be shortened—that the surgeon will pull it up to meet the bladder. This doesn't happen; instead, the bladder is mobile, and can easily be pulled *down* to meet the urethra. The surgeon uses sutures, or stitches, to narrow the bladder neck so it matches the size of the urethra (Fig. 8.8). The Foley catheter is left in place after the operation, to drain urine until the connection has healed and is watertight.

THE NERVE GRAFT BANDWAGON

Some urologists believe they'll have a better chance at curing cancer if—just to be on the safe side—they cut out both neurovascular bundles, and put in nerve grafts to restore the potential for erection they just cut out. Hey, there's a great idea! Except that in the PSA era, where most cancer is diagnosed at a curable stage, it is hardly ever necessary to cut out both neurovascular bundles.

If a man has "bilateral" capsular penetration (cancer on both sides of the prostate) to the point where it's necessary to remove both neurovascular bundles, then this man is probably not curable with surgery, because cancer has already spread to distant sites. Out of 2,700 radical prostatectomies I performed between 1986 and 1999, only seven potent men had both neurovascular bundles removed. Four of these men were not cured, because they had positive lymph nodes, positive seminal vesicles, or a positive margin elsewhere; in the other three, it was not necessary, because there turned out to be no capsular penetration on that side. Because of this, I have come to believe *it is almost never necessary to remove both neurovascular bundles.* A man who needs both bundles removed probably shouldn't be undergoing the surgery anyway, and a man who doesn't need them removed is going to be a lot better off with nerve-sparing—preserving what he's already got—than with a nerve graft—trying to replicate what should have been left alone to begin with.

Now, having said all that, I should add that the idea of nerve grafts in radical prostatectomy patients—although recently revived—is not that new. In fact, the first experimental work on nerve grafts to restore sexual function was reported from the Brady Urological Institute at Johns Hopkins in 1989. We found an ideal animal model. In the rat, the nerves responsible for erection are relatively large, distinct structures, compared to the tiny cluster of nerves and blood vessels in men. The experimental studies in rats were encouraging, and in the early 1990s, collaborating with a neurosurgeon, I carried out a study of nerve grafts in patients who underwent wide excision of the neurovascular bundle. We followed the patients for more than five years, and unfortunately, there was no difference in the recovery of sexual function in men who received a nerve graft and those who did not. At the same time, another trend was emerging; with the widespread use of PSA testing, more men were being diagnosed with localized cancer, and as a result, fewer men needed to have a neurovascular bundle removed.

Recently, surgeons have been taking another look at nerve grafts.

Some urologists have reported that in men who had both neurovascular bundles removed and received nerve grafts (using small nerves taken from the side of the foot), 30 percent had recovery of sexual function. However, in reviewing these surgeons' results, I found that 58 percent of the patients who underwent nerve grafts had no evidence of capsular penetration on either side—and thus, they didn't need to have either nerve bundle removed in the first place. Also, it is not clear whether the men who recovered sexual function were the ones who actually needed the nerve bundle removal—the men with cancer that needed to be cut out—or the men with organ-confined cancer—who had less disease, and whose nerve bundles should have been spared anyway.

What about nerve grafts in men who have one bundle removed? This same group of surgeons states that when they remove one neurovascular bundle, only 25 percent of their patients are potent. If they could improve these results by 30 percent, then almost 50 percent of their patients might expect recovery of sexual function. If only 25 percent of a surgeon's patients are potent after one neurovascular bundle is removed, then this surgeon's patients might benefit from this extra procedure.

However, at Johns Hopkins—without a nerve graft—*64 percent* of the patients who have one neurovascular bundle removed are potent. Would a nerve graft improve these results even further? The argument is not terribly convincing. In a study done at Johns Hopkins several years ago, we analyzed the factors that influenced a man's recovery of potency after surgery. It turned out that men who had more extensive disease—capsular penetration, or cancer involving the seminal vesicles—were less likely to have recovery of sexual function, even if *both* neurovascular bundles were preserved.

Also, nerve grafts are not without their own risks. Potential side effects include the development of numbness or nerve damage on the side of the foot (at the site where the to-be-grafted nerve is removed), and the possibility of a delay in walking after surgery. Also, removing a nerve, closing that site, and then grafting the nerve in the pelvis prolongs the surgery, and may cause men to lose more blood. Before nerve grafts become an added component to many radical prostatectomies, they need to be studied in many men, in a randomized, controlled study.

The bottom line: Men with more extensive localized disease—cancer that spreads slightly outside the prostate—are less likely to recover sexual function regardless of the status of their nerves, and are unlikely to be helped by placement of a nerve graft. If it is likely that a man will need to have one neurovascular bundle removed, the best thing he can do to ensure his recovery of sexual function is to find a urologist who can do a good job of preserving the nerve bundle on the other side. (Note: Again, *this does not mean that a man can't still have a normal sex life;* see Chapter 11.)

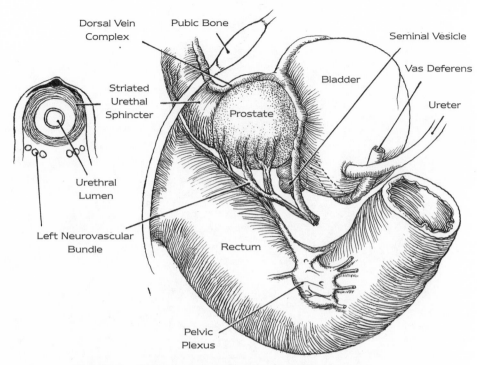

FIG. 8.1 The Radical Retropubic Prostatectomy, Step by Step

You're looking at the prostate and surrounding terrain—the rectum and bladder, key nerves, veins, and the urethral sphincter, a tube-shaped structure that helps control urine. You can also see one of the two neurovascular bundles, the package of nerves critical for erection, which sit on either side of the prostate. [Figures 8.1–8.8, by Leon Schlossberg, reprinted from Patrick C. Walsh, "Radical Prostatectomy: A Procedure in Evolution," *Seminars in Oncology* 21 (1994): 662–71. Used by permission, W. B. Saunders Company.]

The Radical Retropubic Prostatectomy, Step by Step

After surgery: A drain will be left in the abdomen until nothing flows through it (this usually takes a day or two), and a Foley catheter, inserted in the penis and anchored by a tiny balloon in the bladder during surgery, will remain in place for three to twenty-one days. Note: To minimize your risk of getting a urinary tract infection, which often happens in men who have a catheter, you should begin taking an antibiotic such as ciprofloxacin or levofloxacin the day before the catheter is scheduled to come out, and keep taking it for five days. On the day the catheter is due to come out, be sure to drink extra fluids. Your doctor will want to make sure that you are urinating with a

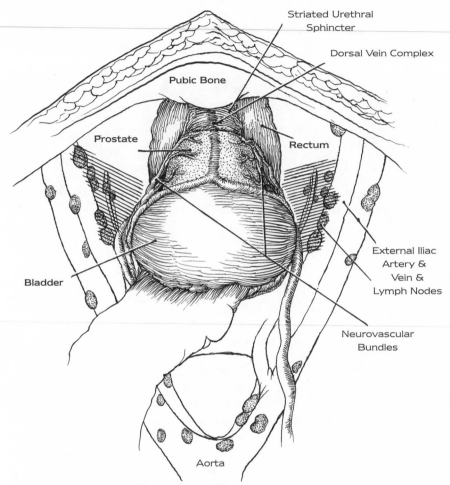

FIG. 8.2 The Radical Retropubic Prostatectomy (Continued)

This is a schematic look at the prostate, bladder, and lymph nodes. It's the view the surgeon has after the abdominal incision has been made. Inside the shaded area are the lymph nodes removed during a staging lymphadenectomy.

strong stream. (Note: The time it takes to recover urinary control varies, and it is not likely that your urinary control will be perfect immediately. Your doctor just wants to make sure there is no urinary obstruction.)

The main reason for the catheter is that it allows the anastomosis (the site where the bladder and urethra have been connected) a chance to heal. The drain is there to evacuate any urine that might leak from the anastomosis as it's healing; it must stay in place until

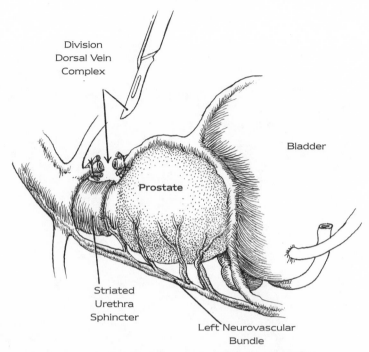

Division
Dorsal Vein
Complex

Bladder

Prostate

Striated
Urethra
Sphincter

Left Neurovascular
Bundle

FIG. 8.3 The Radical Retropubic Prostatectomy (Continued)

This is how the surgeon helps create the critical "bloodless field"—carefully cutting the dorsal vein complex, which travels over the urethra and prostate, and carries a great deal of blood.

nothing more flows through it. *It is critical that the Foley catheter stay in place.* If it is inadvertently pulled out or removed too soon after surgery, this can be disastrous, and may lead to permanent incontinence. Your catheter should be securely taped to your thigh, and you should examine its mooring often. The catheter may take some getting used to, but remember—it's only temporary, and its presence is helping the body heal. While you're at home, keep the catheter connected to a large drainage bag most of the time, and use the leg bag only if you plan to go out of the house. The reason many doctors suggest this is that the leg bag doesn't hold as much urine, and if the bag becomes full and the patient doesn't realize what's happening, the urine can back up into him because it has no place else to go. Depending on your surgeon's preference, the catheter will be left in place from less than one to three weeks.

Bleeding around the catheter: This looks scary, but it's pretty

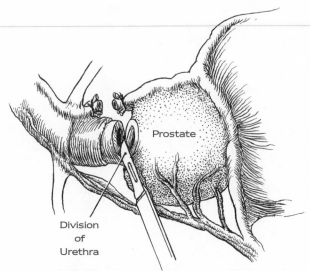

FIG. 8.4   The Radical Retropubic Prostatectomy (Continued)

The surgeon is now cutting the urethra, which runs through the prostate. This is another delicate procedure: Cutting the urethra too close to the prostate might mean some cancer is left behind; but cutting it too far from the prostate might mean damaging the urethral sphincter, which helps control urine. With great care, the prostate is separated from all the tissue and blood vessels that are connected to it.

common, especially if you strain to have a bowel movement. Don't worry; it will stop. Also, don't worry if you see some blood in the urine. This usually has no significance, and almost always resolves on its own—usually by the time the catheter is removed. Sometimes this bleeding happens spontaneously, sometimes it's due to overexertion (walking too briskly, for example), or a result of taking aspirin or Motrin. If you see blood, flush it out by drinking a lot of fluids. This will dilute the blood, so that it won't clog the catheter, and it will also help stop the bleeding.

Leakage around the catheter: Another scary phenomenon, this, too, is usually nothing to worry about. Leakage can occur when you're up walking around, or when you're having a bowel movement. It can usually be managed with the use of diapers or other absorbent materials. Important: If your catheter stops draining completely, lie down flat and drink a lot of water. If after one hour there is no urine coming through the catheter, it is possible that your catheter has become clogged or dislodged. Call your doctor right away.

Urinary sediment: Another common, disconcerting problem. This

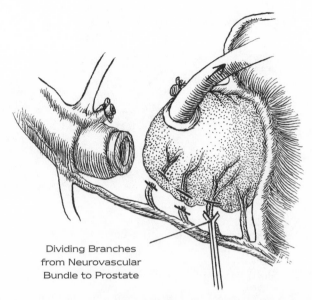

Dividing Branches
from Neurovascular
Bundle to Prostate

FIG. 8.5   The Radical Retropubic Prostatectomy (Continued)

If it's possible—and for most men today, diagnosed with curable cancer, it usually is—the surgeon can preserve the neurovascular bundles on either side of the prostate. To do this, the surgeon gently separates each branch of these nerves and vessels from the prostate.

can manifest itself in several ways. You may see some old clots, which appear as dark particles, after you have had bloody urine. These usually go away on their own. Also, the pH balance of the urine (its acidity) changes throughout the day. After a meal, for example, urine often becomes alkaline. There are normal substances in the urine called phosphates. These can precipitate if the urine has too little acid, and can cause cloudy masses to appear in the urine. (The urine also may appear cloudy if you have a urinary tract infection—see below.)

Bladder spasms: This can be extremely painful. Fortunately, bladder spasms are not very common. The men most likely to have them are those who have been troubled by urinary symptoms before surgery (usually, men who have had BPH), who have developed a thickened bladder wall, and a "hair-trigger" bladder that is easily irritated. In this case, the irritant is huge—the catheter—and the bladder is trying its best to push it out, with contractions. The spasms may happen at random, or they may be provoked by an activity, such as having a bowel movement, or after going for a walk. If you have a bladder spasm, lie down until the contractions improve. If you have

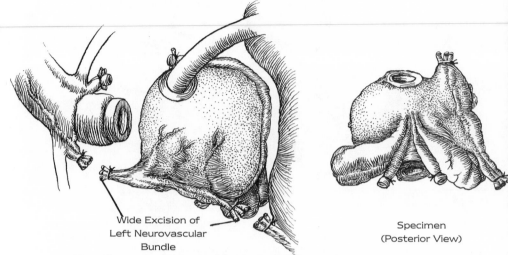

Wide Excision of
Left Neurovascular
Bundle

Specimen
(Posterior View)

FIG. 8.6 The Radical Retropubic Prostatectomy (Continued)

If it is not possible to preserve these nerve bundles—if they have been reached by cancer—then the surgeon removes them along with the prostate. This is called "wide excision." The surgeon cuts out as much tissue as possible surrounding the prostate in an aggressive attempt to get every last bit of cancer.

frequent spasms, you may be helped by medication. Nonsteroidal analgesics (such as Motrin) work quite well, because they relax smooth muscle. For persistent spasms, tranquilizers (such as Valium) are usually able to control the problem.

Pain: You'll be dealing with the catheter mostly at home; the economic trend these days is for patients to leave the hospital as soon as possible after any procedure, and prostate surgery is no exception. Fortunately, radical prostatectomy patients are actually *able* to go home and generally be more active sooner than ever. It used to be that men would have to stay in the hospital for a week after radical prostatectomy, because they were unable to eat. We always blamed this on the operation, assuming that, somehow, the surgery caused the intestines to hibernate. It took between two and four days for men to resume normal bowel activity. As it turned out, this slowdown was caused by the pain medications—the narcotics we routinely gave after surgery. Today, we administer pain medication more judiciously. For the first twenty-four hours or so after surgery, men receive intravenous painkillers. (At Johns Hopkins, an automated delivery system provides a baseline level of pain relief, and if a patient needs more, he

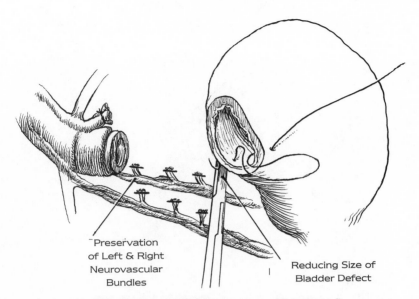

Preservation
of Left & Right
Neurovascular
Bundles

Reducing Size of
Bladder Defect

FIG. 8.7   The Radical Retropubic Prostatectomy (Continued)

This shows the situation after the prostate has been removed. Note how big the opening in the bladder is in comparison to the urethra. This must now be narrowed in size, so the two can be connected.

can press a button and adjust the dosage.) Afterward, patients are switched to oral pain medication. This is because we've learned that for most men, the less pain medication you take after surgery, the better you'll feel, and the sooner you'll be up and around. For most men, the nausea caused by the pain medication is worse than the pain caused by the operation. The day after surgery, you should be up and walking around. As soon as your pain is under control with oral medication, you have no fever, and you are able to eat—probably within the next one or two days—you will get to go home. You probably won't feel the pain where you would most expect it—right along the incision. Instead, it's usually on one side or the other; it rarely hurts equally on both sides. The pain comes from irritation of the abdominal muscles; sometimes it occurs where the drainage tubes stick out of your body. It will go away on its own.

Again, it wasn't always this way; we used to keep men in the hospital for a week or more. But we've learned that by sending men home earlier, they become more independent, are more active, and have fewer complications.

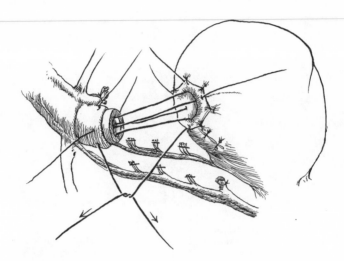

FIG. 8.8   The Radical Retropubic Prostatectomy (Continued)

The operation's almost over now. Here the surgeon rebuilds the urinary tract, pulling the bladder down to bridge the space connecting the urethra and urethral sphincter.

After surgery, as soon as your doctor says it's okay, you can eat and drink whatever you wish—even alcohol, in moderation. The main thing is that you avoid becoming constipated. Remember, the prostate sits on top of the rectum; when it's removed, this part of the rectum is thin, fragile, and particularly vulnerable to injury for the first three months after surgery. Therefore, it is critical that you *do not have an enema* or your temperature taken rectally any time soon. And, it's absolutely essential that you have a bowel movement every day. For many men, this is easier said than done; pain medications, inactivity, slight dehydration (from not getting enough fluids before or after surgery), all can add up to constipation. To help keep things moving, you'll probably be given stool softeners or laxatives for several days. If you do become constipated, take mineral oil and milk of magnesia (but again, do not use an enema—you could perforate your rectum).

Caring for the incision: You can take a shower as soon as you are discharged from the hospital. Your surgeon will probably remove the "skin clips" (the surgical equivalent of staples) before you leave the hospital, and put "steri-strips" in their place. These are surgical tapes that hold the edges of the incision together nicely—they'll probably be kept on for about a week—until the body's own healing process gradually takes over. (Their presence seems to encourage a thinner scar to form.) To protect these strips, tape some Saran Wrap over the incision before you shower. Some men develop an infection in the incision several days after they get home from the hospital. This is usually manifested by some drainage—either a clear fluid, or an unsightly mixture of blood and pus. Don't worry; this can be treated simply, with some hydrogen peroxide and a Q-Tip. Soak the cotton swab in hydrogen peroxide, and stick it through the opening in the incision.

Urinary tract infection: Having a catheter often means getting a urinary tract infection; the two seem to go together. If you develop an infection while the catheter is still in, you may notice that your urine becomes cloudy, or you may see some pus in the drainage around the catheter. Talk to your doctor, who will probably prescribe an antibiotic such as levofloxacin or ciprofloxacin.

Other things you should do, or not do: Avoid lifting anything over ten pounds for six weeks from the day of surgery, including grandchildren and the family pet. Also avoid strenuous exercise (calisthenics, golf, tennis, jogging, even vigorous walking). This is because, for the first six weeks, only stitches are holding your incision together. After this time, the body's own mending device, firm scar tissue, will protect the incision. Heavy lifting too soon can cause a hernia to develop in the incision. Also, lifting or other strenuous activity may hurt the anastomosis connecting your bladder and urethra, and this could lead to long-term problems with urinary control. Keep telling yourself that this isn't forever—after six weeks, you can do anything you want.

And even during this healing time, you can eat and drink whatever you want, take long (but not strenuous) walks, and make as many trips as you'd like up and down stairs. Also, you can drive a car and go back to work three to five weeks after the surgery. (Exactly how soon you resume daily work activities will depend on how quickly you seem to be recovering.)

Expect to have some incontinence (see below). This is normal, and it, too, is not permanent. It will go away eventually—don't be discouraged. Also, expect to have some trouble with erections (see Chapter 11).

Finally, you'll be encouraged to sit in certain positions, do leg exercises to boost your circulation, and to walk around almost immediately. This also is crucial—among other things, it can help reduce your risk of developing blood clots (see below).

Other Procedures: The Radical Perineal Approach and Laparoscopic Radical Prostatectomy

In the *radical perineal prostatectomy*, the prostate is removed through a small incision in the perineum, the space between the scrotum and rectum. (This is the original operation devised by Hugh Hampton Young, the Johns Hopkins surgeon who pioneered radical prostatectomy in 1904.) Similar to the retropubic procedure (in which surgeons reach the prostate through the abdomen) in terms of before-surgery preparation and recovery, the radical perineal approach offers some advantages over that technique: There's less bleeding, because the major vein system that overlies the prostate (the dorsal vein complex) is not removed with the prostate. However, this also means that surgeons aren't able to cut out as much tissue as in the retropubic approach—so if the cancer has penetrated the prostate wall, "positive surgical margins" may be more likely here than in the retropubic approach. If the likelihood of cancer appearing in the pelvic lymph nodes is low (see the Partin Tables in Chapter 6), there's no need for an abdominal incision. Many men, however, do have a laparoscopic lymph node dissection before getting a perineal prostatectomy just to be sure cancer hasn't reached the lymph nodes. There are also reports that the return of PSA after surgery may be higher with the perineal procedure than with the retropubic approach. Thus, if you are at high risk of having "capsular penetration," or cancer reaching the wall of the prostate, you should have the retropubic procedure.

Some studies suggest that the odds of incontinence with the perineal approach are lower than with the retropubic technique, although there is a higher risk of another complication, fecal incontinence, because the anal sphincter is stretched. One study suggested that as many as 9 percent of patients had fecal incontinence during an average week after the procedure.

Another drawback with this approach is that it's more difficult for surgeons to see—and thus protect—the neurovascular bundles, the thin packets of nerves that sit on either side of the prostate and are essential for erections. Therefore, preserving potency is not as certain.

The operation is not ideal for heavyset men, particularly men with a large "barrel" abdomen. Also, for the surgeon to get at the perineum, it's necessary for the patient to be folded up, almost like a pretzel, with his legs held up in stirrups. This can lead to compression of nerves, a condition called neurapraxia (the same problem that can affect the nerves that control erection, if they are injured during surgery), and can sometimes cause sensory or motor problems in the leg and foot. A study by researchers at Duke University Medical Center found that neurapraxia developed in 21 percent of 111 men who underwent radical perineal prostatectomy. In almost all of these men, the symptoms were temporary. The researchers concluded that this problem could be prevented if the time the patient spends in the position (called the "exaggerated lithotomy position") is limited.

During surgery: What happens. You will be given general anesthesia, which means you'll be unconscious during the procedure. To reach the prostate, surgeons make an incision just above the rectum. The prostate is gradually separated from the rectum, bladder, urethra, and vas deferens. The seminal vesicles are removed along with the prostate, and then the bladder is linked once again with the urethra.

Laparoscopic radical prostatectomy: The idea behind any surgical procedure using a laparoscope (a lighted tube that enters the body through a tiny hole, through which a surgeon can thread a scalpel) is that "less is more"—smaller incision, fewer side effects, shorter recovery time. Laparoscopic versions of other operations—such as removal of the gallbladder—have turned out quite well, and the promise of fewer side effects has proven true.

What about laparoscopic removal of the prostate? Just a few years ago, laparoscopic radical prostatectomy offered no clear benefits; fledgling attempts at this operation were disastrous because of excessive bleeding and difficulty creating the anastomosis, resulting in marathon operations that lasted as long as twelve hours. However, new suturing techniques, popularized by surgeons in Europe, have led to a revived interest in the laparoscopic procedure. Now, European surgeons have reduced the operating time to less than three hours, and say that the procedure offers several advantages—less bleeding, and the ability to make a watertight anastomosis.

The surgeons promoting this procedure are enthusiastic. However, it is not as clear whether the long-term cancer control rates will be as good as the "gold standard"—the anatomic radical retropubic procedure. Here's why: During open surgery (as discussed above), surgeons can find out much by *feel*. Tactile sensation—feeling subtle differences in tissue with our gloved fingers—shows us exactly where to cut; it tells us whether the neurovascular bundle should be preserved or widely excised, and whether the structures next to the prostate are suspiciously adherent to it. Here, the laparoscopic surgeon is operating at a distinct disadvantage; one important avenue of information and feedback is lacking.

The true long-term benefits of this procedure over the open procedure are still arguable. With the open surgery, no muscles are cut, most men leave the hospital in two or three days with little discomfort, and are able to return to work in three to four weeks, with no heavy lifting for six weeks. It is not clear whether the pain and recovery time after the laparoscopic approach are that much better than that for the radical retropubic prostatectomy. Also, even with the laparoscopic procedure, an incision has to be made so the surgeon can haul out the prostate; thus, men who have the laparoscopic procedure can't do any heavy lifting for six weeks either. At this point, the laparoscopic approach is still in its infancy, and much more experience must be gained before we will know its true value.

Complications

Early complications: Like all surgery involving anesthesia, radical prostatectomy carries the risk of death, but *this is extremely rare.* In a Johns Hopkins study of more than 2,800 patients, there were three deaths—one man had a heart attack before surgery as the anesthesia was beginning, and two men died after surgery (one at ten days, one three weeks afterward) from a blood clot to the lung. (For important tips on how to recognize symptoms of this, see below.)

The most common complication during surgery is excess bleeding, usually a result of a blood vessel being injured during the operation. That's why it is absolutely critical that your surgeon has mastered the techniques for ensuring a "bloodless field" (described above; see also "Are You in Good Hands? What to Look for in a Surgeon," above). Less common complications during surgery include injuring the rectum or ureters; such injuries can be repaired during surgery, and extra surgical precautions can be taken to avoid permanent damage.

Complications shortly after surgery include:

Blood clots: These are among the most common—and potentially most serious—complications of radical prostatectomy. One of the body's most effective defense mechanisms after any trauma is something called the "clotting cascade"—a chain of events that causes the blood to coagulate. This can help stop bleeding if you skin your knee, or even help save your life if you're in a car wreck, but this helpful system can also be activated when it's least welcome—after surgery— and can do more harm than good. Blood clots that form in the legs' deep veins (this is called deep venous thrombosis) can be, at best, painful. At worst they can be fatal. The leg veins are, basically, a straight shot to the lung; the nightmare scenario here is for part of a blood clot in the leg to break free and shoot up to the lungs.

Blood clots in the legs and pulmonary embolism, or blood clots in the lungs, occur in an estimated 2 percent of men. At Johns Hopkins, two men out of the first 1,300 patients who had the anatomic radical retropubic prostatectomy died of a blood clot. In the more than 1,500 operations since that time, none of our patients has died of a blood clot. (Note: Both of these men had major underlying heart disease— and this underlines what we have discussed earlier, that this operation is not always the best choice for men with significant health problems. If you have serious heart disease—even if your cardiologist gives you the "green light" for surgery—you may be more likely to experience complications, and may not tolerate them as well as other men.)

Clearly, the best way to deal with this problem is *to prevent it from ever happening.* Some doctors do this by administering blood-thinning medications such as mini-dose heparin. Some doctors also give their patients compression devices—various forms of heavy-duty support hose—for the legs. One of these looks like a pair of long johns, and is designed to force all blood into the deep veins, and keep the flow powerful and continuous. (Sluggish blood flow leads to clot formation.) Other hose have special compression chambers that control blood flow, and are designed to "milk" blood up the leg.

Important: If you have ever had a blood clot, make sure your doctor knows about it. This could influence the way your anesthesia is administered. Also, men considered at higher risk of developing a blood clot may have a stronger blood-thinning medication administered by IV throughout their stay in the hospital.

These preventive steps are very important, but they're only part of it: The rest falls squarely on your shoulders. Make sure you and your family members know the warning signs of a blood clot, and if you think you have any of them, seek treatment immediately. A blood clot is a problem that can be treated easily, with anticoagulants ("blood-thinners" and clot-dissolving medications), if it's caught early. But if diagnosis—and therefore, treatment—is delayed, a blood clot can be fatal.

You may have a clot if you have:

• Swelling or pain in the leg, especially in the calf.
• Sudden chest pain—especially if it gets worse when you take a deep breath—or coughing up blood, shortness of breath, the sudden on-set of weakness or fainting. *If you have any of these signs—even if you don't feel anything unusual in your legs—you could have a blood clot in your lungs. Call your doctor immediately!* Don't wait for your doctor's office hours if this happens in the middle of the night! If you can't get to your doctor, go to an emergency room and tell the doctor there that you need to be evaluated for deep venous thrombosis or pulmonary embolism, with ultrasound of the leg veins or a spiral CT of the lungs.

Exercise is another crucial factor in helping to avert blood clots. Walking is good; it pumps blood back to the heart. Walk as soon as you're allowed to after surgery. If you stand up, don't stand still for longer than a few minutes at a time—move around. The only way the blood that's in the veins in your legs gets back up to the heart is by the pumping action of the muscles. Your doctor will probably encourage you to do dorsiflexion exercises—pumping your feet up and down to exercise the calf muscles. Do these often, about one hundred times an hour in between naps. Also, it is essential that you *do not sit upright in a chair* (with your legs hanging down) for more than an hour at a time during the first four weeks. Try to sit with your legs elevated on a sofa, reclining chair, or comfortable chair with a footstool, as much as possible. This accomplishes two goals: One, because it raises your feet, it improves the blood flow from the veins in your legs. Also, it protects the area of surgery from bearing your full weight.

Note: Because patients are in and out of the hospital so fast these days, it's likely that any post-surgical trouble you experience will be when you're at home. That's why it's essential that you and your family be aware of the warning signs of a clot in the leg or a clot that has gone to the lung.

CALL YOUR DOCTOR!

Particularly if you have any of the warning signs of a blood clot. This is all part of being your own advocate. It doesn't mean that you have to be militant, or obnoxious, or that you should call your doctor in the middle of the night just to chat (please don't!).

What it *does* mean, however, is that you have certain rights. If you have a question or problem during office hours, by all means, go ahead and call; you may not always get the doctor, but you'll get somebody who can help.

And if you have a problem that you don't think can wait until morning, call at night. Most doctors have twenty-four-hour answering services; many doctors have partners who share "on-call" time—they split it up, each taking a certain number of nights, weekends, and holidays a year. They do this because they *expect* to get some calls at night, because they know from years of training and experience that medical emergencies don't always happen during office hours.

This won't be the first phone call your doctor gets in the middle of the night, and it certainly won't be the last. What would you rather do—wind up in the hospital as a result of a serious complication that should have been treated hours ago, or "bother your doctor"?

Bladder neck contracture, or constriction of the bladder neck: This is scar tissue that forms where the bladder neck is sewn to the urethra, and it has been reported in between 1 and 12 percent of men after surgery. Its symptoms are usually manifested by persistent incontinence, and a very slow or dribbling urinary stream when—this is the tip-off—the bladder is full. Remember, incontinence immediately after surgery is a very common problem. In the early days after surgery, many men who are having incontinence also worry about having a slow urinary stream. But it's hard to achieve a good stream if there's not much in the bladder—and it's impossible to store up urine in the bladder if it keeps leaking out. Bladder neck contracture is different; the bladder is full, but the best you can manage is a dribble, because the scar tissue is blocking the flow, like a stuck washer in a faucet.

If you are having prolonged incontinence, you should be evaluated with cystoscopy and cystometry, a test that measures bladder progress and function by passing a small catheter through the urethra into the bladder. Changes in pressure are monitored as the bladder fills with water. If scar tissue is causing the trouble, it can be reopened in a simple outpatient procedure as a urologist, using a cystoscope (a tiny tube inserted through the tip of the anesthetized penis, through the urethra and into the bladder), makes a few tiny cuts to relax the tight scar tissue.

To keep the area open, your urologist may recommend that you pass a small catheter through the urethra every day for a month or so after the procedure. This way, the scar tissue won't re-form, and the normal lining of the bladder and urethra will cover the opening as it's supposed to. If the scar tissue is particularly stubborn, your doctor may inject a powerful steroid called triamcinolone into the area of the contracture; this can be effective in preventing the scar tissue from returning.

Long-Term Issues: Urinary Continence and Sexual Potency

Urinary continence: Before surgery, many men focus on impotence as the major complication of radical prostatectomy. They're wrong. Recovery of urinary control is far more important and—if it happens slowly, or doesn't happen at all—casts a far greater shadow on your life. If something's wrong with your ability to urinate, you'll be reminded of it several times a day—or worse, several times an hour—not just a few times a week or month. And frankly, having to change your adult diaper because you just involuntarily urinated in it can dampen—literally—any romantic thoughts that you do have. Thus, before you go "under the knife," you and your urologist need to talk about the risk of incontinence. (See "Are You in Good Hands? What to Look for in a Surgeon," above.)

Why does incontinence happen after radical prostatectomy? Let's take a moment to review the male plumbing. Men are equipped with three separate anatomical structures that control urine—a sphincter at the bladder neck, the prostate itself, and the external sphincter (also called the striated sphincter). Radical prostatectomy knocks out two of these—the sphincter at the bladder neck and, of course, the prostate—leaving only the external sphincter to do the work of three.

Because of the powerful structures upstream, this external sphincter is never tested or even used much in most men. Thus, we have no way of knowing before radical prostatectomy how strong this sphincter really is. In some men, it's extremely well developed; in others, it's not. Like the rest of the muscles in the body, this sphincter loses its tone with age, and here's where older men have the disadvantage. Men over age seventy have more problems recovering perfect urinary control after surgery than do younger men. Here, too, is where men differ from women: Women only have this one sphincter. In consequence, they have very thin bladders. Men, in contrast, normally have thicker, more muscular bladders to begin with. Add any element of BPH (benign enlargement of the prostate, which often makes the bladder work harder and become muscle-bound), and a man's bladder can become quite thick. Thus, some men are left with a situation where a burly, thickened bladder is connected to a sphincter that may not have been that effective to begin with.

To make matters worse, at the time of surgery, the sphincter can be damaged, because the major blood vessels that can cause excessive bleeding are intertwined within it. This is why the skill of the surgeon is so important: One of the first steps in a radical prostatectomy is to divide this complex structure. If too much sphincter is taken out, or if the sphincter is injured during the surgeon's attempts to stop bleeding, urinary incontinence can result. Thus, it's vital that your surgeon understand the complicated anatomy, and know how to preserve the urinary sphincter and carefully rebuild the urinary tract. Urinary incontinence is a huge quality-of-life issue. You must think about it now, before surgery, and do your best—by choosing an experienced surgeon, and afterward, following the exercises described below—to minimize trouble later.

The return of urinary control: Some men are lucky. They are dry from the moment the catheter is removed. They can stop their stream on a dime, and start it whenever they want to. The great physician Sir William Osler once made a perceptive comment that applies here: "The man who is well," he said, "wears a crown that only the sick can see." Men who are continent immediately after radical prostatectomy are blessed. Most men, however, have variable amounts of urinary leakage. You may be one of the lucky ones; then again, you may not. Most likely, it will take some time for your control of urine to come back completely. For most men, this process happens in three distinct stages: Phase One is when a man can remain dry when he's lying down. In Phase Two, you're dry when you're walking around. If you can walk to the bathroom and not urinate until you get there, that's a great sign—it means that the sphincter is intact. And in Phase Three, you are dry when you stand up (using muscles that put pressure on the sphincter) after sitting.

At Johns Hopkins, about half of men are wearing no pads at three months after radical prostatectomy; 80 percent are wearing no pads at six months, 90 to 93 percent are dry at twelve months, and 93 to 95 percent at two years. (Note: At Johns Hopkins, we consider any man incontinent if he wears a pad—even if he just leaks a few drops of urine a day. Your doctor may have a different definition, which you should find out before surgery.) However, most men (even at three months) are not very wet, and when asked in a confidential questionnaire, 96 percent stated that leakage causes little to no bother. It's hard to believe, but urinary control does continue to improve over two years and, in an occasional patient, even longer than that.

Can you do anything to speed things along, and improve your urinary control? First, whatever you do, *do not wear an incontinence device with an attached bag, a condom catheter, or clamp!* If you use any artificial device, you will hurt yourself in the long run. You won't be able to recover your urinary control, because you won't develop the muscle control you need. Until your urinary control returns completely, wear a pad, such as a Serenity pad, or disposable diaper, such as Depends. You can get these at the pharmacy or grocery store. Some men prefer using a special kind of padded underwear called Confidens Briefs; your doctor should have good suggestions and perhaps even some samples for you to try.

Also, until your urinary control has returned to an acceptable level, don't force fluids. When the catheter is in, you're asked to drink a lot of fluids, to "flush out the system." However, once the catheter is out, you've got to slow the pace considerably. Avoid drinking excessive amounts of fluids, and stay away from caffeine in all forms—coffee, tea, even soft drinks. Caffeine, especially, is a powerful pharmacological agent that increases the frequency and urgency with which you need to urinate. (Note: If you are being treated for high blood pressure with an alpha-adrenergic antagonist such as Cardura, ask your doctor to put you on a different kind of drug. Cardura makes the sphincter relax, and can make incontinence worse.)

Exercises you can do: Next, every time you urinate, do it standing up. You can't practice the following exercises, which strengthen the external sphincter and speed up your recovery of urinary control, while you're sitting down. Start your stream, and once it's in full force, stop the stream by contracting the muscles in your *buttocks*—not your abdominal muscles, not the muscle "up in front" around the penis. Tighten your buttocks; imagine you're trying to hold a quarter between your cheeks. Hold the urine back for five or ten seconds, and repeat as many times as you can. Note: Only perform these exercises when you're urinating; if you keep contracting these muscles throughout the day, you'll overdo it—the sphincter tires easily—and you'll end up wetter than you would otherwise.

Remember, for many men, the recovery of urinary control is a slow process. The most important thing you can do during this time is not to get discouraged. If your doctor told you there was only a 2 percent chance that you would have a long-term, serious problem with urinary control, believe it. This means there's a 98 percent chance that you'll be back to normal someday, even if no crystal ball can say exactly when. It will help for you to discuss your progress at regular intervals with your urologist—even a phone call every so often can make a world of difference in how you see your progress. Note: It may also help for you to take part in a support group—so you can talk about the issues that are bothering you with other men who are in the same boat, going through the same process of recovery. You can do this online, from the privacy of your own home (this may be better for men who are uncomfortable talking about personal matters in front of others), or you can find a local prostate cancer support group. Ask your doctor.

If you are experiencing no progress, it's reasonable to consider whether something else—other than the natural, gradual return of urinary control—could be causing the delay. One possibility is a bladder neck contracture, the formation of scar tissue around the anastomosis (the reconnected bladder and urethra—discussed above). Incontinence after surgery falls into two basic categories: stress incontinence and urgency incontinence. *Stress incontinence* is caused by a weak sphincter; urine leaks out when you cough, sneeze, laugh, or run. *Urgency incontinence* (also called "urge incontinence") is when you know you have to go to the bathroom, but can't get there in time and some urine leaks out. Men with urgency incontinence leak right away, when they have the sudden urge to urinate and can't hold it back.

If you have stress incontinence, there are several medications that may help. For example, decongestants, used to treat a stuffy nose and cold symptoms, work by contracting smooth muscle in the nose. The urethra is surrounded by this same smooth muscle. Thus—if you do not have high blood pressure—you may benefit from taking a short-acting decongestant such as pseudoephedrine (Sudafed), or a long-acting agent combined with an antihistamine such as Claritin-D. However, some of these drugs can cause drowsiness and a dry mouth, and some men find those side effects worse than the urinary leakage itself. Another drug, called imipramine, has a two-pronged approach. It relaxes the muscle in the bladder, and also tightens the muscle tone of the external sphincter. This drug, too, can cause drowsiness and a dry mouth; however, some men find that if they take just one tablet at night, it lasts well into the next day. (Otherwise, the usual dose is 25 milligrams, up to three times a day.)

If you had an enlarged prostate before surgery, and experienced a lot of urinary frequency and urgency, you may have urgency incontinence resulting from a hyperactive bladder. Your doctor can check for involuntary bladder contractions with cystometry, a test that measures bladder progress and function by passing a small catheter through the urethra into the bladder. Changes in pressure are monitored as the bladder fills with water.

If you have urgency incontinence, you may benefit from treatment with an anticholinergic medication. A simple, over-the-counter one is Benadryl; another choice, available by prescription, is either of the long-acting drugs Detrol or Ditropan XL, which mainly target the bladder and have fewer side effects (including dryness of the mouth and eyes, headache, constipation, and rapid heart rate) than other drugs of their kind. Anticholinergic drugs have an antispasmodic effect—they can prevent involuntary bladder contractions, and help prevent urine leakage. Other drugs, classed as "antispasmodics" (which means they fight muscle spasms), can help relax an overenthusiastic bladder muscle that contracts too frequently. These include flavoxate

(Urispas) and dicyclomine (Bentyl). Antidepressants also may help, by strengthening the internal sphincter and relaxing the bladder.

Many doctors advise their patients to undergo something called "pelvic floor biofeedback." This includes a forty-five-minute biofeedback behavioral therapy session—a tutorial on how to use your pelvic floor muscles. Patches are placed on the perineal and abdominal muscles to be sure that you're performing these exercises correctly. Some men find this helpful. However, this is an expensive way for a man to learn how to start and stop his stream, and indeed, critical studies have demonstrated no great benefit to this elaborate and expensive procedure.

If it still doesn't get better: The gains made in recovering urinary control can be incremental, often frustratingly so. But there's a point at which it probably isn't going to get any better on its own. If incontinence persists beyond two years, there are several options for treatment.

Collagen: The sphincter can be "bulked up" by the injection of collagen—a procedure similar to that used by plastic surgeons to take away wrinkles in a patient's face. Before you consider collagen, you should have cystometry to rule out the possibility of involuntary bladder contractions. You should also be checked with a cystoscope (a lighted tube, inserted in the anesthetized penis and threaded through the urethra into the bladder) to make sure you don't have a bladder neck contracture, and to evaluate the anatomy, to see whether it's amenable to injection. Collagen injection is performed as an outpatient procedure. It may take three or four injections for you to receive maximal benefit. Some men feel an immediate improvement, which may ebb over the next few days, then return. It usually takes about a month before the collagen settles.

Before you consider it, you should know that collagen is not for everybody: For one thing, some people are allergic to it, so you should have a skin test, to see whether you react to this substance. For another, it is not helpful for men who have had treatment for a bladder neck contracture, or for men who have undergone radiation therapy. And it simply is not helpful for men who have severe incontinence—a few bits of collagen are like sealing wax. Their effectiveness is limited. At best, only about 60 percent of men who receive collagen injections have what they consider to be a good result. Also, because collagen is eventually reabsorbed by the body, even if the treatment is successful, it probably won't last forever; you may need repeat treatments every six to eighteen months. (Note: Collagen injections are not generally helpful in men after radiation therapy.)

Before you decide on collagen, you need to ask yourself some serious questions: Do I really need it? Am I that uncomfortable? The reason we're saying this is that some men have almost perfect control—almost. They wear a small liner in their pants, and they only have to change it once a day. But in an attempt to become perfect, they undergo collagen injections—and wind up wearing adult diapers that they must change two or three times a day. There's an old saying in medicine that "perfection may be the enemy of good."

Artificial sphincter: Men who have severe, prolonged incontinence should undergo placement of an artificial sphincter. In this procedure, a soft, sylastic (a material that's flexible and stretchy, like elastic) cuff is positioned around the urethra and connected by tubing to a reservoir for fluid that's installed in the abdomen. The placement of this reservoir is important. It's designed so that when a man coughs or sneezes, or does anything else to increase the pressure within the abdomen— activities that would otherwise result in stress incontinence—that pressure is instantly transferred to the cuff. This temporarily increases the pressure around the urethra, and blocks urine from leaking out. The artificial sphincter features a valve, placed in the scrotum, which is used to deflate the cuff and allow urine to pass. The device is somewhat elaborate, but it works very well for men with severe incontinence. The idea is that "the buck stops here"—urine comes out only when *you* decide it's time. In the past, artificial sphincters had two main complications—the risks of infection and of malfunction. Infection can cause erosion of the tissue that holds the device in place (in the urethra and bladder neck), may make incontinence worse, and may even mean that the device must be removed. If the infection is severe, this tissue damage may limit the success of any replacement sphincter. The device may need to be replaced if, for some reason, the original one is a dud. The good news here is that, as technology evolves, these devices keep getting better, and the odds of malfunction are going down all the time. In the future, it may be possible for surgeons to make a "natural" artificial sphincter, by reconfiguring a muscle from the thigh, and using magnetic energy to make it open and close.

Sexual potency: Chapter 11 is devoted to erectile dysfunction, so you should consider this just an introduction to this difficult subject. The first thing we need to do is make sure we're all talking about the same thing: What do we mean by potency? The medical definition is simple—"an erection sufficient for vaginal penetration and orgasm." Having said that, it's worth repeating that men who are impotent after radical prostatectomy have *normal sensation, normal sex drive, and can achieve a normal orgasm.* Their only problem may be in achieving or maintaining an erection.

Potency after radical prostatectomy can be affected by many things: a man's age and the stage of his cancer, the surgeon's skill, and the extent of tissue removed—in other words, whether one or both neurovascular bundles were removed during the operation.

In men younger than fifty, potency is similar (about 90 percent) in men who keep both neurovascular bundles intact, and in men who have one nerve bundle removed. This suggests that all that's needed for men to achieve erection is one of these nerve bundles, and that nature has provided a "spare." In men older than fifty, however, sexual potency tends to be better in men who have both neurovascular bundles preserved than in men who lose one bundle. When the relative likelihood of impotence after surgery is adjusted for age, the risk is higher if the cancer has penetrated the prostate wall; if it has invaded the seminal vesicles; or if one neurovascular bundle has been removed. Thus, the men most likely to remain potent are younger, with disease confined to the prostate. These also are the men who will benefit most from surgery. Again, for more on erectile dysfunction, see Chapter 11.

FIGHTING INFLAMMATION **DURING** *SURGERY* **MAY HELP MEN RECOVER POTENCY**

As we mentioned above, the nerves involved in erection are gossamer-thin, exceedingly fragile, and tiny—so small, in fact, that for more than seventy years, surgeons performing the radical prostatectomy routinely cut them and left them in place, never realizing they existed. Then came the "nerve-sparing" radical prostatectomy. Now, impotence is no longer considered an inevitable consequence of the operation: Surgeons know that if even one of the two bundles of nerves that are responsible for erection can be preserved during the surgery, it is still possible for a man to recover potency.

The problem is, even if *both* nerve bundles are preserved, potency—the ability to have and maintain an erection—is still not a certainty; also, the recovery of potency may take months. Two men the same age, with the same degree of prostate cancer, can have exactly the same operation, performed with the same skill by the same surgeon: Afterward, one or both of them may be potent. There is no guarantee, and no surefire means of predicting.

In any part of the body, whenever there is injury, there is an immune response. In an attempt to protect themselves, the tissues around the nerves fight back, with inflammation—heat, redness, and swelling, sometimes on a microscopic level. But sometimes this reaction proves more damaging than the injury itself. Johns Hopkins urologist Arthur Burnett believes the key to preserving potency after surgery may be to protect the nerves *during* it—to quell this inflammation almost as soon as it starts.

"We have excellent rates of potency here at Hopkins," he says. "But it's not 100 percent, and it can take months to recover. What accounts for that discrepancy? It may be that the nerves are inadvertently injured with traction, or even that the dissection adjacent to them somehow exposes them to injury—something causes the nerves to sustain an inflammatory setback." Indeed, some nerves are sluggish after surgery because they've been traumatized, a condition known as "neurapraxia." It takes time for them to recover. If this is the case, Burnett adds, then what's needed is a way to "preserve, recover, regenerate, or otherwise just regain nerve function that is critical for erection."

These nerves need extra protection; they need the time and necessary ingredients to heal. They also need to be shielded from their own immune response, says Burnett, a surgeon who has also spent the last decade doing research in collaboration with neuroscientist Sol Snyder. For the last few years, Burnett has been working with special proteins called neuro-immunophilins, which are being studied in a host of ailments—stroke, Huntington's disease, and even in organ transplants—for their ability to reduce inflammation and shield nerves from injury. He has found that in rats with nerve injury and erectile dysfunction similar to that found in men after radical prostatectomy, using neuro-immunophilin solutions to "bathe" the nerves provides "greater preservation of erectile function, despite the injury." It is likely that, someday, using such approaches will allow us to shorten the time it takes for men to recover erectile function.

What about Viagra? Although the "nerve-sparing" procedure has been performed successfully for nearly two decades, it's not performed—or, not performed optimally—by every urologist. Drugs such as Viagra will play a role in improving the results of surgery worldwide. Why? Because Viagra *only works if the nerves are preserved*. Over the last few years, many men who were told by their urologists that they had undergone a "nerve-sparing" radical prostatectomy took Viagra, waited for the drug to work and—when nothing happened—returned to their urologists with some tough questions about why their nerves weren't spared. This "wonder drug," which has helped so many men, may increase physicians' interest in preserving the nerves. (For more on Viagra, see Chapter 11.)

Continence and Potency: Quality of Life after Radical Prostatectomy

It used to be, as we discussed early in this chapter, that the long-term quality of life for men undergoing radical prostatectomy was pretty dismal. Every man was impotent, and as many as 25 percent had severe incontinence. The results were so bad that many men felt they'd be better off taking their chances with prostate cancer than submitting themselves to this operation.

Now, of course, the picture has changed. Skilled surgeons at three high-volume hospitals (where hundreds of radical prostatectomies are performed each year) reported almost identical results—92 percent of their patients were continent, and 70 percent were potent. Recently, scientists at Merck Research Laboratories examined Medicare claims filed between 1991 and 1994 by more than 100,000 radical prostatectomy patients. They compared the volume of prostatectomy patients at various hospitals with the patients' length of stay, surgical complications, readmission rate, and number of patient deaths in the thirty days after surgery. Their results, published in the *Journal of the National Cancer Institute*, showed that institutions that perform a large number of radical prostatectomies have lower readmission rates, lower risks of serious complications, lower risks of death, and shorter hospital stays. Again, men do better if they have this operation done at a hospital where it's performed often.

And yet, as surgical procedures go, radical prostatectomy remains one of the most delicate, intricate, and flat-out difficult to perform correctly. Proof of this can be found in the widely varying rates of success of surgeons at hospitals throughout the world—not simply in controlling cancer, but in preserving a man's quality of life in two major areas: urinary continence and sexual potency. The unfortunate fact is that when less experienced or less skillful surgeons attempt this procedure, the results can be disastrous. It has taken more than a decade for the results—the good, the bad, and the ugly, if you will—to surface.

Part of this is that it's hard to know exactly what happens after a man leaves the hospital, particularly in areas where men feel so vulnerable. Nobody wants to talk about it. It's different when we look at something as black and white as, say, a man's cancer status. All we have to do is follow his PSA tests, and bingo—we have all the information we need, a definitive means of knowing whether all of the tumor has been removed. But there aren't such objective ways to tell how a man's doing in the other important areas. At many centers, it's up to the patient to report his success in continence and potency—and again, very often these are the last things men want to discuss, even with their doctors.

Recently, before they underwent radical prostatectomy at Johns Hopkins, sixty-four men agreed to participate in a health-related quality-of-life survey, to be sent to an independent third party, a data analyst who had no access to their patient records. (All of the men reported that they were potent and that they had a sexual partner before the surgery.)

By one year after surgery, 93 percent of the men reported that they were dry—that during the previous four weeks, they had not needed a pad or adult diaper to control urinary leakage. When the men were asked to say how much their urinary continence bothered them, 98 percent said they had either a small bother, or none at all. In terms of potency, at eighteen months after surgery, 86 percent of the men were able to have intercourse. When asked about difficulty with erections, 84 percent of the men said they had either a small bother, or none at all. Looking at the potency rates by age, at eighteen months after surgery, 100 percent of men in their thirties were potent; 88 percent of men in their forties, 90 percent of men in their fifties, and 75 percent of men in their sixties were potent.

We were not surprised at the success with urinary continence; we have reported the same results for many years. In the long run, only about 2 percent of our patients have significant long-term problems with urinary control, defined as needing to change a pad more than once a day. And, as mentioned above, we're currently trying to eliminate that 2 percent. (See "Perfecting the Radical Prostatectomy," above.) The men's results with sexual potency, however, are better than we've ever reported. They are also the highest potency rates reported at any academic medical center. We attribute this to several factors: One is that men today are being identified with smaller tumors, which permits us to preserve both neurovascular bundles. Also, over time, the surgical technique has gradually improved. And finally, there's Viagra. In this study, at eighteen months after surgery, one third of the men said they were using Viagra, although only two patients said they could not have intercourse without it.

The good news is that there are many excellent surgeons, at large referral hospitals and academic medical centers, who have obtained similar rates for urinary continence, and potency rates as high as 70 percent. For example, surgeons at the Washington University School of Medicine in St. Louis recently reported on a series of 1,870 men who underwent radical prostatectomy. Their results, published in the *Journal of Urology*, showed that 92 percent of men recovered urinary continence, and this was associated with "younger age, but not with tumor stage or nerve-sparing surgery." They concluded that "better results are achieved in young men with organ-confined cancer. Other complications can be reduced with increasing surgeon experience."

Unfortunately, however, the success of radical prostatectomy is not uniform; patients at some centers report much greater trouble with side effects. For example, researchers at the Fred Hutchinson Cancer Research Center in Seattle looked at changes in urinary and sexual function in men at six different communities in the United States. Although there were some flaws in their study design—at six months after treatment, they were asking men to recall how potent they were before surgery (the authors admitted that their data indicated that the men had overestimated the frequency of intercourse and quality of erections before surgery)—the message they got loud and clear was that most men who undergo radical prostatectomy are impotent. Worse, they may even have underestimated the true extent of incontinence in these men. The authors said that at twenty-four months after surgery, 8.4 percent of the men were incontinent—and by this they meant men who had "frequent leakage" (6.8 percent) or "no control" (1.6 percent). If they had used the definition we use at Johns Hopkins—needing a pad at all—then 42 percent of these patients would have been considered incontinent. It's not as easy to ascertain the results of their impotence study, because the authors did not specify if impotence meant unassisted erections firm enough for intercourse, or whether they included patients who were using injection therapy or who had penile prostheses. The authors did not hint at the possibility that these results could be much better—and, in fact, are remarkably better at many major medical centers—if the surgical technique were improved. Most troubling here is that until urologists believe these results *can* be better—until they're not willing to accept these devastating side effects as routine—they may not understand the need to improve.

One of the worst series of results is reminiscent of the awful situation in the "before" category—before the operation was improved. A study from Boston recently reported in the *Journal of the National Cancer Institute* that only 50 percent of their patients were continent, and fewer than 20 percent were potent after radical prostatectomy. These authors suggested with some bravado that the poor results were not because the surgery by urologists in Boston was faulty, but because their outcome studies were—as opposed to those of other centers—"truly objective." They concluded that nerve-sparing surgery doesn't work, dismissing the far better results achieved at Hopkins and at other centers as unreliable, suggesting that because patients were reluctant to disappoint their surgeons, they were not truthful in discussing their side effects.

Now, there is always a concern that patients may try to minimize their problems to their physicians or—something we must always look out for—alternatively, that there may be an unconscious bias on the part of the surgeon toward minimizing adverse outcomes. But it's difficult to swallow the idea that patients would rather spare their surgeons' feelings than regain urinary continence and sexual potency. I believe that most men who are incontinent or impotent following surgery want help. If the urologist poses these questions with the intention of helping the men overcome these problems and get their lives back to normal, I believe men will tell the truth.

The Hopkins study shows that when radical prostatectomies are performed by experienced surgeons, major side effects are infrequent. We hope these findings will encourage urologists to work on improving their technique. The study from Boston led many urologists who had poor outcomes to believe that *no one* had good results. But the study at Johns Hopkins, along with the good results at other medical centers, shows that the results of surgery can be excellent, with proper surgical technique.

The take-home message here is this: Any man who wants a radical prostatectomy, and believes it's the best form of treatment for him, should seek out centers where experienced surgeons perform many of these procedures, and where the results can be documented through validated, independent outcome studies.

About the men in the Hopkins study: The average age was fifty-seven. Most of the men, nearly 59 percent, had a clinical stage of T1 (a tumor that is not palpable in a physical exam); 40 percent had T2 disease (palpable, but confined to the prostate); and 1.5 percent had stage T3 cancer (palpable with extension beyond the prostate). Most of the men (83 percent) had a Gleason score of 6; 4.5 percent had Gleason 5 cancer, 11 percent had Gleason 7, and 1.5 percent had Gleason 8. I performed the surgery in all of the men, and preserved both neurovascular bundles (the nerves responsible for erection) in 89 percent of them. After surgery, pathologists determined that the tumor was organ-confined in 81 percent of the men; there was capsular penetration with negative surgical margins in 11 percent, capsular penetration with positive surgical margins (at the bladder neck) in 1.5 percent, positive seminal vesicles in 1.5 percent, and positive lymph nodes in 5 percent.

Finally, the Johns Hopkins study revealed some interesting things about men in general. It turns out that some men exaggerated their sexual activity before surgery, and on careful questioning acknowledged that they really weren't potent, or had difficulty with erections, before they had the operation. But after surgery, men did just the opposite: Many of them said they were not potent, but their wives disagreed. In separate questionnaires of the patients' wives, 78 percent reported that their husbands were potent at the same time the husbands said they were. But 20 percent of the wives said potency occurred earlier than their husbands thought it did, and 2 percent thought it occurred later. What accounts for this discrepancy? Often, the women sense that their husbands are doing better than the men think they are. This is because the men feel that their erection may not be as strong as it was before surgery—and until they have a very strong erection, many men feel any intercourse that occurs "doesn't count."

At many top medical centers, the rates of potency after radical prostatectomy are quite good. But there are still men at those centers, and many men elsewhere, who experience problems. The important thing to remember is that sexual function—potency—can be restored to all men after radical prostatectomy. The main problem for these men is the ability to obtain an erection. But sensation, and the ability to achieve orgasm, are intact. Many men don't understand this. They think that they can't have an orgasm if they can't have an erection. They forget that half of the people in the world have orgasms without erections—women. This is because *orgasms occur in the brain.* There are many ways to restore sexual function, and these are discussed in detail in Chapter 11.

URINARY CONTINENCE AND SEXUAL FUNCTION AFTER RADICAL PROSTATECTOMY AT JOHNS HOPKINS

	3 months	6 months	12 months	18 months
Continence				
No pads	54 percent	80 percent	93 percent	93 percent
No/small bother	96 percent	93 percent	98 percent	95 percent
Sexual Function				
Potent	38 percent	54 percent	73 percent	86 percent
No/small bother	49 percent	64 percent	76 percent	84 percent
Used Viagra	7 percent	13 percent	33 percent	33 percent*

*Only two men cannot have intercourse without Viagra.

Long-Term Issues

In this chapter, we've covered everything about radical prostatectomy and the complications that can occur in the months after the operation. But what about the long-term outlook, and the biggest question of all—has your cancer been controlled? For a detailed discussion of the results of all forms of treatment for localized disease—surgery, radiation, and cryotherapy—see Chapter 10.

9

RADIATION AND CRYOABLATION

Read This First

Radiation therapy is an excellent treatment option for many men with prostate cancer. First and foremost, it requires no surgery—this is a key advantage for older men, as well as for men with other health problems that might preclude major surgery. Also, it can be used in men with prostate tumors that are too far advanced to be cured by surgery.

The two standard approaches are: Sending radiation into the tumor from the outside, with external-beam radiation therapy, and implanting radioactive seeds directly into the tumor; this is called interstitial radiotherapy (doctors also describe it as brachytherapy, or simply, seed implantation).

Cryotherapy—killing prostate cells by freezing them—has also been put forth as a less invasive form of treatment for localized prostate cancer. The idea is not new, and many years ago, the freezing was accomplished through the urethra. Today, using ultrasound to guide them, doctors circulate the freezing argon gas through six to eight metallic probes, which are placed in the prostate gland through the perineum. The freezing continues until the ultrasound shows an "iceball" has been created. The procedure can take longer than an hour, and the hospital stay is generally one or two days.

In the future, there are certain to be other, less invasive forms of treatment to deliver tissue-destroying energy to the prostate, in hopes of killing the cancer. At present, on the drawing board, are:

- Transurethral laser treatment, using laser energy to kill prostate tissue.
- Interstitial seeds, activated by radio frequency to heat surrounding tissue.
- High-intensity focused ultrasound, delivered through a probe in the rectum.

In this chapter, we cover everything about radiation and cryotherapy and the complications that can occur in the months after the procedure. But what about the long-term outlook, and the biggest question of all—has your cancer been controlled? For a detailed discussion of the results of all forms of treatment for localized disease—surgery, radiation, and cryotherapy—see Chapter 10.

Radiation Therapy for Prostate Cancer

Like radical prostatectomy, radiation treatment for prostate cancer is not a new idea. In fact, it wasn't too long after urologist Hugh Hampton Young did that first radical prostatectomy (see Chapter 8) that he and another colleague at Johns Hopkins were among the first to pioneer radiation therapy in this country (it had been developed a few years earlier in Europe). The treatment was primitive by today's standards, involving special radium applicators placed in tissue surrounding the prostate—the urethra, bladder, and rectum.

But the next few decades laid the groundwork for some of today's radiation therapies. X-ray treatments were introduced, followed by radium "seeds" that could be inserted in the prostate tumor. These fledgling attempts at curing prostate cancer, however, were not distinguished by astounding success. Compared to today's high-powered technology, the low-energy X-ray beams produced throughout the 1930s were lackluster, and their ability to penetrate the prostate was mediocre and imprecise. Radiation treatment, therefore, was only palliative; it could relieve pain and symptoms, but it did not eradicate the cancer.

In the 1940s, the impact of hormones on the prostate was discovered (see Chapter 12), and radiation was all but abandoned in favor of castration and hormonal drugs. But radiation's exile was not long, thanks largely to scientists who revolutionized the field using an exciting new machine called a "linear accelerator." They produced penetrating, high-powered beams that could target radiation doses to a specific site without harming surrounding tissue. And suddenly, radiation was off the bench and back in the ball game as a major player—a treatment that actually could cure localized cancer, not just relieve the symptoms of advanced disease.

In the decades since then, radiation therapy has been refined and made even more powerful. There are two standard approaches— sending radiation into the tumor from the outside, with external-beam therapy, and implanting radioactive seeds directly into the tumor (this is called "interstitial radiotherapy," brachytherapy, or simply seed implantation). The 1990s saw a mini-revolution in external-beam therapy, thanks to a new technique called "three-dimensional conformal therapy."

Conformal Radiation Therapy

How does an X-ray machine work? The simplest way to think of it is to imagine yourself getting a suntan. The difference here is that you can't feel or see the X-ray energy hitting your body, and the "sunburn" occurs internally. (Actually, what happens is that the radiation particles destroy DNA, causing targeted cells to die.) The best way to get a good, even tan is in increments, not all at once. That's why the radiation doses are spread out over several weeks—usually five days a week, leaving weekends free, for about eight weeks. Each treatment lasts just a few minutes at a time—maybe five minutes, tops. That's it. Then you go home, and come back the next day.

The conformal approach allows for great precision—allowing doctors to maximize the dose of radiation to the prostate tumor and thus sharpen the treatment's cancer-fighting ability, while reducing the damage to nearby tissue. This approach developed because scientists looked at what was *not* happening with radiation treatment: Conventional approaches, studies found, weren't precise enough. For one thing, they weren't accurately estimating the volume of their target; and because of this, they often didn't supply enough radiation to kill the whole tumor. What was happening in some men, researchers have learned, was like what happens when a speaker with an inadequate sound system tries to make himself understood to an audience of 100,000 people in a vast amphitheater—some, maybe even most, of the crowd can hear him, but that still leaves hundreds or even thousands who aren't getting his message. In traditional radiation treatment for prostate cancer, this inadequate coverage meant that many men who suffered local relapses of prostate cancer did so because they were underdosed. Once PSA testing became available and began to be used as a way to track the success of cancer treatment, scientists realized that only 20 percent of men with T1 and T2 disease who had been treated with external-beam radiation had low PSAs after ten years. A devastating study from Toronto, using multiple biopsies, found that even at four years after treatment, 38 percent of men who were believed to be cured turned out to have active prostate cancer. It became all too clear to the radiation oncology field that conventional external-beam radiation therapy wasn't doing the job; in a large and substantial number of men, it failed to eradicate all of the tumor.

This made it imperative for radiation oncologists to achieve better local control of prostate cancer. Research in recent years has found that *the dose of radiation received has a lot to do with who gets cured and who doesn't*. In other words, men who receive *higher* doses of radiation have lower relapse rates than men who receive less radiation. However, in traditional radiation treatment, higher dosage almost always meant more, and worse, side effects, particularly to the bladder and rectum.

Enter the high-tech advances, all of which fall under the umbrella header of "conformal" radiation therapy: Intricate software and imaging systems that allow 3-D treatment planning and computer-controlled radiation delivery systems. Elaborate computer programs that can zip through sophisticated mathematical calculations of prostate volume and radiation dose per millimeter (or even smaller) of tissue. Amazing technological advances that make it possible for doctors to custom-design a three-dimensional model and treatment plan, so each patient's prostate tumor can get the most precise and thorough radiation coverage possible. Refined radiation machines that deliver intense, precise levels of radiation to the prostate, but do as little harm as possible to the surrounding tissue—the rectum, bowel, bladder, bone and bone marrow, and skin.

There are three basic approaches to conformal therapy, all of which rely on intensive planning and intricate treatment maps, made with the help of multiple CT scans:

- *Three-dimensional (3-D) conformal radiation:* In this approach, many X-ray beams—shaped to fit the target area—are focused on the prostate, delivering a homogenous, high dose of radiation. It is slightly more expensive and time-consuming than traditional radiation.
- *Intensity-modulated radiation therapy:* Here, too, many shaped radiation beams converge on the target. But the intensity can be turned up, to blast the cancer, or down, to spare normal tissue. This is more expensive and time-consuming than the 3-D approach.
- *Proton beam radiation:* This uses charged particles, instead of electromagnetic waves. The difference here is that the proton beam shoots in a straight line, but it can be stopped abruptly—for example, at the delicate rectal wall, just on the other side of the prostate, so the fragile tissue in the rectum can be spared.

Because the prostate generally has an irregular shape to start with, and because, like a snowflake, each man's prostate is unique, these new machines are customizing the radiation beams. The intensity-modulated approach relies on as many as sixty pairs of movable tungsten "leaves"—slim, rectangular-shaped plates that open and close like little shutters. These allow the machine to "sculpt" the radiation beam, molding it to fit the individual contours of each man's prostate and pelvic region. The versatile tungsten leaves, a breakthrough in radiation technology, also block the radiation—much like the lead drape you wear in the dentist's office when you get an X-ray—from areas that aren't supposed to receive it.

In all conformal approaches, preparation is key. Like generals masterminding a strategic attack, the radiation oncologist who designs your treatment begins by studying the terrain. This is called "treatment planning," and it begins several weeks ahead of time, with a series of CT images that give enough cross-section views of the prostate, seminal vesicles, and surrounding terrain (including the bladder wall, rectal wall, small bowel, bony structures, and skin) to create a detailed, three-dimensional map of your pelvic region. Unlike an X-ray—which, basically, is a photograph of your insides—these CT scans can be made to appear on the computer screen in several different ways. One manifestation is called a "wire-frame projection"—a gridlike 3-D configuration that can be rotated in any direction.

Dosage, and the area over which it will be distributed, can be calculated and varied plane by plane, millimeter by millimeter. Each radiation beam—the conformal approach allows more segments of treatment than traditional external-beam therapy—is automatically shaped by the computer so the energy focuses on the tumor alone (in the prostate as well as tissue outside the gland where cancer has spread), rather than its entire neighborhood. This is important, because again, when it comes to dosage, more is definitely better. It takes high doses of radiation to kill prostate cancer—higher doses than used to be possible in the years before these 3-D techniques evolved. But more radiation usually means more side effects, and a greater challenge to achieve the right balance—to kill the cancer, but *not* kill healthy tissue right next to it, and thereby keep side effects to a minimum. Here's where the tungsten leaves (or, used in some hospitals, blocks of lead) come in with the intensity-modulated approach, allowing higher than ever levels of radiation to be delivered *safely* to targeted areas, while sparing as much of the surrounding territory as possible. The advanced technology has allowed doctors to increase the standard dose of radiation, measured in units called Gy (pronounced "gray," and named in honor of Louis Harold Gray, an English radiobiologist), from between 65 and 70 Gy to about 81 Gy. After-the-fact or instantaneous dose checks then verify that the radiation went to the right spot for the right length of time, to help guarantee the most successful treatment possible.

Note: The precision of conformal radiation would be wasted, however, if the patient couldn't keep perfectly still—and frankly, nobody can keep *that* still. Imagine the potential for disaster here— one good sneeze, for instance, or a coughing fit, or even a case of nervous fidgets and oops! The bladder gets a full blast of radiation, while the prostate is unscathed. To prevent this, you will be fitted for your own custom-built body cast, which will keep your pelvis immobilized on the table for the few minutes it takes to receive your daily dose of radiation. The cast also makes sure that your exact position can be reproduced every time.

At your treatment-planning session, the radiation therapists will make some temporary marks on your skin. Don't wash them off! When your treatment starts, these marks will help your doctors position the radiation. When the precise alignment is fixed, some of the marks will become permanent—with small tattoos placed at their center. Laser lights may also be used to fine-tune the alignment. Then, at least once a week during your treatment, you'll probably have special X-rays, called *port films*, made to keep the radiation as accurate as possible.

As another quality-control step, a diode (a small electrical device) will be placed on your skin before treatment to measure the radiation dose you're getting.

WHAT IF I'VE HAD A TURP PROCEDURE FOR BPH?

Your predicament is just the same as that of men who are going to have a radical prostatectomy—you've got to wait for the swelling and inflammation to go down, generally about eight to twelve weeks, before you can undergo any new treatment. This waiting period, though it may seem agonizingly slow, is critical. It helps minimize your risk of becoming incontinent or developing scar tissue around the urethra from radiation damage to not yet healed tissue.

Complications

For the first few days or even the first couple of weeks of external-beam radiation therapy, you may feel nothing out of the ordinary; it takes a while for the cumulative effect of radiation to manifest itself. You can continue all of your normal activities—drive, work, exercise, and be sexually active. (Unlike seed implantation, discussed below, this form of radiation therapy does not make you radioactive.) But by the third to fifth week, many men react with symptoms that can range from mild to severe; in most cases, these generally go away within days to weeks after the course of treatment is over. Sometimes, men develop these symptoms six months or more after treatment.

The most common complications are bowel problems (diarrhea, rectal itching or burning, urgency to have a bowel movement, painful cramps) and urinary trouble (feelings of urgency, painful or difficult urination, stress incontinence, and the need to urinate frequently, especially at night). In 25 to 30 percent of men, these symptoms of bladder irritation become acute enough to require medication (such as Hytrin, Cardura, or Flomax). With increasingly better technology, rectal bleeding now develops in fewer than 8 percent of men who undergo three-dimensional conformal radiation therapy. Diarrhea and increased frequency of bowel movements may be treated with dietary changes (adding more fiber to the diet), or with medications such as Imodium or Lomotil.

In one analysis of 1,020 men, about 7 percent of men needed to go to the hospital for treatment of more severe urinary problems. These included blood in the urine, bladder inflammation, and urethral stricture or bladder neck contracture. Urethral strictures accounted for more than half of these problems, and they seemed to develop mostly in men who had previously undergone a TURP procedure for BPH. Fewer than 1 percent of the men needed surgery to fix these problems. A bladder neck contracture can be reopened in an easy, outpatient procedure as a urologist, using a cystoscope, makes a few tiny cuts to relax the tight scar tissue. Most urethral strictures respond well to dilation—stretching the urethra, in one or two sessions—but stubborn strictures also may be treated with tiny incisions, like those done to ease bladder neck contractures. Just a little over 3 percent of the men experienced chronic intestinal problems, including rectal inflammation, diarrhea, rectal bleeding, an intestinal ulcer, or development of an anal stricture (tight scar tissue that can interfere with bowel movement); fewer than 1 percent experienced bowel obstruction or perforation. And complications that proved fatal were extremely rare—0.2 percent. Severe bleeding from radiation cystitis may require treatment with hyperbaric oxygen therapy to encourage the growth of new blood vessels. This provides prolonged relief in 75 percent of men.

In another analysis, researchers at Fox Chase Cancer Center in Philadelphia administered quality-of-life questionnaires to 120 patients, three to six years after treatment. They found that 2 percent of the men were wearing a daily pad because of stress incontinence, and that 2 percent considered their "urinary bother" to be a big problem. No man, however, was totally incontinent. Thirty-three percent of the men reported that they had rectal urgency (the sudden need to have a bowel movement, and difficulty making it to the bathroom in time); 22 percent felt that their "bowel bother" was moderate, and none of the men considered their bowel bother to be a big problem.

Sexual function: Radiation often takes a gradual toll on the small blood vessels that control erection, causing them to shrink, or to become scarred over time. In one Harvard study of men who received standard external-beam therapy, 171 men said they were potent before radiation, but only 38 percent said they were potent afterward. In the Fox Chase study cited above, in men younger than sixty-five, 73 percent were potent at three years, and 59 percent were potent at five years. Sexual potency is difficult to measure: Age, stage of disease, and a man's sex life before treatment all play a role in his ability to have an erection afterward. Men younger than sixty who are sexually active and who are treated when the cancer is in the earlier stages (confined to the prostate) are most likely to remain potent after radiation treatment. However, many men treated with radiation are older, and more likely to have problems with impotence anyway—either because they're taking medications that can interfere with sexual function, or simply because of their age. (This is discussed in detail in Chapter 11.)

One fact you should know about radiation therapy is that its effect on potency is slower and much more incremental than radical prostatectomy's more immediate impact. Radiation seems to cause a man's ability to have an erection to diminish over time (months to years); about half the men who receive it are impotent at seven years after radiation treatment. This is probably because of radiation's effect on the blood vessels, resulting in an eventual decrease in blood flow to the penis. One Australian study found that 62 percent of 146 men who were potent before they began radiation therapy were potent one year afterward; but by two years after treatment, this number had dropped to 41 percent. (Note: This doesn't mean a man who undergoes radiation therapy can't still have a normal sex life. The drug Viagra can improve sexual function in men after radiation therapy, particularly in men who can achieve partial erections. See Chapter 11.)

Adding Hormone Therapy to Radiation

It used to be that doctors would give a man a full radiation treatment, and then—only if the treatment was not successful, months or years down the road—start hormone therapy (shutting off his supply of the male hormone testosterone; this is discussed in detail in Chapter 12). But what if a man takes a temporary course of hormones—two or three months—and *then* begins radiation? This idea, called "neoadjuvant hormonal therapy," has been shown to be beneficial in several studies, although the details are still being worked out. For example, how much hormone therapy, also called "androgen ablation," does a man need—how long should he take the hormones before starting the radiation? Does hormone therapy somehow make the cancer more responsive to the radiation? And will the short-term promise hold out in long-term studies? The answers are not yet clear.

What is it about hormones that makes radiation more effective? For one thing, they *shrink the volume of the prostate,* which means that radiation has *less ground to cover*—and this, in turn, can mean less toxicity (and risk of side effects) to nearby normal tissue in the rectum and bladder. For another, hormones seem *to make radiation more efficient.* Experimental studies have shown that with hormone treatment, a *lower dose of radiation* (fewer Gy) is needed to kill the cancer. In part—with the prostate made smaller by hormones—there are fewer cancer cells that need to be killed. But together, hormones and radiation seem to encourage a process called apoptosis—basically, suicide of cells, in this case, cancer cells (this process is discussed further in Chapter 12). This combination of hormones and radiation also shifts cells from an active to a resting phase—making them much more like "sitting ducks," and easier to kill.

In brachytherapy (radiation seeds), when hormones reduce the size of the prostate, it's easier to place the seeds accurately, and to make sure they're reaching the entire gland. (This is not always an easy task in some men, when the prostate is so large that it extends under the pubic arch.) A three-month course of hormones before brachytherapy also may reduce the likelihood of complications such as urinary retention or incontinence in men with large prostates.

The first study that provided encouragement was reported in the *New England Journal of Medicine;* researchers found that men with locally advanced prostate cancer who received conformal radiation therapy plus hormone therapy were more likely to be disease-free at five years than men who received radiation alone. The men received monthly hormone-suppressing injections for three years. In this study, 85 percent of the men in the combined-treatment group were free of disease at five years, compared to 48 percent of the men in the radiation-only group—impressive results, although once again the researchers' definition of failure was not as stringent as it could have been. Here, PSA failure was defined as a PSA level greater than 1.5, and increasing on two consecutive measurements. Most important, this study showed an improvement in survival rates. However, it's difficult to know whether *hormones alone* would have provided the same effect. In a study now under way, scientists are looking at hormone therapy alone compared to radiation, versus radiation plus hormones. Until we know the results of that study, it will be impossible to distinguish whether hormones are actually augmenting the effect of radiation—or whether the hormones by themselves are prolonging life.

Other recent studies have investigated the influence of hormones plus radiation. Although no study has shown across the board that all patients benefit, with most studies, there have been subsets of men who seemed to do better—particularly, men with positive lymph nodes and high Gleason scores. Thus, it is now generally believed that if a man with advanced disease (for example, a bulky T3 tumor), a high Gleason score, or positive lymph nodes is going to be treated with external-beam radiation therapy, he should also receive hormonal therapy for at least two or three years. There is also some evidence that short-course hormonal therapy, given just around the time of radiation therapy, may benefit men with smaller tumors. As with every other aspect of prostate cancer research, we won't know for sure until there are long-term results, including studies comparing men who receive hormones alone.

Should you receive hormone therapy? Before you make any decision, you should consider another very important issue—quality of life. There are some definite downsides to long-term use of hormone-suppressing drugs. In some men, testosterone production doesn't always return promptly after these drugs are stopped. The side effects of hormone therapy can be profound. Even with short courses (two or three months), men experience the loss of libido and potency, plus "hot flashes" and weight gain. With long-term treatment, there are the additional risks of osteoporosis (and fractures that result from this bone degeneration); anemia; fatigue; loss of muscle mass; and depression. Depending on the particular kind of hormone-suppressors used, this treatment can also be very expensive. (A detailed discussion of hormone therapy can be found in Chapter 12.)

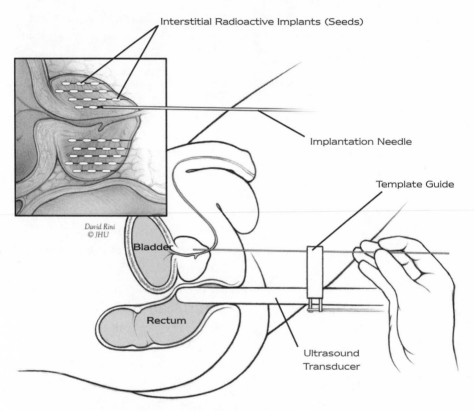

FIG. 9.1   Implanting Radioactive Seeds (Brachytherapy)

Radiation oncologists use advanced-guidance ultrasound systems, three-dimensional treatment planning, and templates to ensure precise placement of seeds, and help guarantee an even distribution of radiation throughout the prostate.

Interstitial Brachytherapy (Implanting Radioactive Seeds)

Brachytherapy is basically hand-to-hand combat, instead of missiles launched from far away, implanting tiny sources of radiation directly in the cancerous tissue. (The term "brachy" comes from the

Greek word for "short," as in a short distance away from the malignancy. Confusingly, doctors often use the terms "brachytherapy," "interstitial radiotherapy," and "seeds" interchangeably.) The concept is not new. Pierre Curie thought of it nearly a century ago—even before external-beam radiation treatment came on the scene—and doctors in New York tried it several years later; they inserted thin glass tubes with a radioactive substance called radon directly into tumors. The treatment killed tissue, but the results were uneven; some of the targeted tissue was devastated while other tissue remained unscathed. In the next decades, scientists improved the technique, but its popularity waned as hormonal treatment developed and as external-beam radiation therapy got better (see above). In the 1950s and 1960s, however, improvements in dosages and radioactive materials helped foster a comeback for brachytherapy: Doctors implanted radioactive gold "seeds," or tiny chunks of radioactive material, in men with prostate cancer; this also was combined with external-beam radiation therapy. A few years later, doctors began using radioactive iodine seeds to fight prostate cancer.

Over the years, several other radioactive materials including palladium have been tested, and the means of implanting them have evolved from a subjective, free-hand technique (which requires surgery to give the doctor access to the prostate) to state-of-the-art, ultrasound- and CT-guided systems involving templates. Doctors have become highly sophisticated in targeting and placing these tiny—2.5 millimeters long, the size of a poppy seed—radioactive pellets, and monitoring the dosage.

Who should get this treatment? Brachytherapy alone (the use of seeds without something else, such as external-beam radiation therapy) is not ideally suited for men with a large, bulky tumor, a high-grade (Gleason score 7 or above) tumor, or lymph node metastases. Most implantation regimens don't include the seminal vesicles or tissue outside the prostate—so if there's the slightest risk that cancer has spread to these areas, implanting radiation seeds *within* the prostate won't do anything to fight the cancer *outside* it. (Although, because the radiation dose can extend a few millimeters beyond the wall of the prostate, some men with "extracapsular penetration" may be candidates for brachytherapy.) *If there is a risk that cancer has spread beyond the prostate, men are also treated with supplemental external-beam radiation therapy.*

The clinical research committee of the American Brachytherapy Society and the Prostate Brachytherapy Quality Assurance Group recently published recommendations for selecting patients who are best suited to brachytherapy alone, brachytherapy plus external-beam radiation therapy, and brachytherapy in conjunction with hormonal therapy. Radiation seeds are not recommended for men who have had a previous TURP procedure; for one thing, because they've had significant amounts of tissue around the urethra removed to alleviate their BPH symptoms, there's not a lot left to hold the seeds in place. Men who have had a TURP are also much more likely to develop urinary problems such as urethral stricture and incontinence from this therapy. Men with urinary problems (who score higher than a 14 on a symptom score questionnaire such as the one in Chapter 2) are not ideal candidates for brachytherapy. Also, men who are in otherwise poor health, men who have a life expectancy of less than five years, and men with distant metastases should not undergo this procedure.

The American Brachytherapy Society also cautions that some men who are not ideal candidates for brachytherapy can be implanted successfully, if the procedure is performed by a physician with expertise in handling cases that present "technical difficulties." The problem here is the risk that the radiation coverage may be inadequate, or uneven. Men in this group include men with prominent median lobes of the prostate (detected by ultrasound), men with severe diabetes, men who have had previous pelvic surgery or radiation treatment, and men with obstructive urinary problems resulting from BPH. Men with a very large prostate (greater than 60 cubic centimeters) are not ideal candidates for brachytherapy. This is because the larger the prostate, the more seeds it takes to kill the cancer, and the greater the likelihood of complications; also, the prostate may intrude on anatomical structures, such as the pubic bone, which may interfere with seed placement. But as we discussed above, some men with large prostates may be able to have this treatment if they have a course of hormone therapy first (lasting about three to six months), to "downsize" the prostate.

The ideal patient for brachytherapy alone is a man with localized disease, who again, is also ideally suited for external-beam radiation therapy and radical prostatectomy—early-stage cancer (T1 to T2a), low-grade Gleason scores of 2 to 6, and a PSA less than 10. Men with stage T2c and higher, men with Gleason scores of 7 or higher, or a PSA greater than 10 will likely be given external-beam radiation therapy, too, as a "boost" to brachytherapy.

As with conformal external-beam therapy, the technology here is continually improving. Before the development of sophisticated guidance systems, major problems arose from seeds being either too far apart or too close together, resulting in an uneven distribution of radiation throughout the prostate; some cancer cells were killed, but some weren't. In many cases, the cancer returned, or never completely went away in the first place. Better placement, thanks to three-dimensional scans like those used to design conformal therapy, may change this picture.

Doctors who sing the praises of brachytherapy—and there are many—are quick to point out its many attractive features. For one thing, there's no hospitalization; it's a simple outpatient procedure; there's hardly any recovery time, and no lengthy time away from work or normal activities. Very high doses of radiation can be concentrated within the prostate, with hardly any damage to surrounding tissue.

Before beginning interstitial brachytherapy, you should undergo an extensive physical examination and a cystoscopy (in which a tiny, lighted tube is inserted through the anesthetized penis and threaded through the prostate and into the bladder, to check for abnormalities) to evaluate your particular anatomy (especially to see whether your prostate has a large middle lobe that protrudes into the bladder) and make sure the cancer is contained within the prostate. Next is the treatment-planning session, which is usually performed several weeks before the procedure (but it can also be done during the procedure; this is called intraoperative treatment planning). With the help of transrectal ultrasound, CT scans, and a computerized guidance system, doctors can establish the volume of your prostate, create a template that marks exactly where the seeds should go, plus determine how many you need, how deeply they should be inserted, and how strong their radiation should be. You may need other tests to make sure your body can tolerate anesthesia; these may include blood tests (to check for bleeding problems), an electrocardiogram (EKG), or a chest X-ray.

To prepare: Starting two days before the procedure, eat a low-fiber diet (fiber is found in fruits and vegetables, and in whole grains such as oatmeal and most cereals). The night before the procedure, you will be asked to drink a bowel-cleansing preparation, such as magnesium citrate (8 ounces). After midnight, drink clear liquids only, and try not to drink anything for six hours before the procedure. Note: If you are on medications that must be taken regularly, or with food, or if you have other dietary needs, don't worry; this is very common. Plan ahead, by discussing this problem with your doctor. Do *not* simply stop taking any medication, just because you're not supposed to eat or drink anything. Because it's essential that the bowels are clear (so that nothing blocks or interferes with the ultrasound image of your prostate), you will be asked to give yourself an enema the morning of the procedure.

During the procedure: A broad-spectrum antibiotic such as ciprofloxacin, levofloxacin, or cefotetan (to minimize the risk of infection), will be administered intravenously. Anesthesia varies; you may be given general or regional anesthesia. In *spinal anesthesia,* a tiny needle is used to inject a local anesthetic into the small of your back through the dura, the membrane lining the spinal cord, and into the spinal fluid. Within minutes, you'll feel numb, relaxed and heavy from your waist to your toes. Afterward, you'll be asked to lie flat in bed until the numbness goes away and you can move your legs again. *This is important; sitting up too soon can cause a severe headache. Epidural anesthesia* is like having an IV tube hooked up to your back, instead of to a vein in your arm. A local anesthetic enters the body through a tiny plastic tube, inserted between the vertebrae of your spine near the small of your back. The epidural anesthetic bathes the area outside the membrane lining the spinal cord, temporarily numbing the nerves in your lower body. Unlike spinal anesthesia, which comes in one dose, epidural anesthesia can be given continuously. The area of numbness can be adjusted; so can the degree of pain relief.

The procedure is performed with the patient on his back in the "lithotomy" position—which gives the best access to the perineum, the area between the rectum and scrotum—with his legs raised in knee stirrups, hips elevated, and buttocks at the end of the table.

Your doctor will probably use transrectal ultrasound during the procedure to guide seed placement, and stabilizing needles to help keep the prostate as still as possible (Fig. 9.1). Depending on the size of your prostate and the radioactive material your doctor is using, you will probably receive between fifty and eighty seeds. At some centers, the needles are inserted under CT or MRI guidance; some centers also use fluoroscopy (an X-ray image that appears live on a TV screen instead of as a still photograph), if the ultrasound does not provide a clear enough picture. The choice of radioactive isotopes (seed material) also varies; some doctors prefer iodine, others palladium. One problem with this still-evolving technology is that nobody has yet figured out the ideal radiation dose needed to eradicate prostate cancer. Palladium has a shorter duration of effect, but puts out a higher initial dose of radiation. Its half-life is seventeen days; the half-life of iodine is fifty-nine days. Because these isotopes emit energy in different ways, the spacing of seeds is less critical with iodine than with palladium (palladium seeds should be implanted less than 1.7 centimeters apart).

The innovations in imaging have helped doctors do a better job of spacing both kinds of seeds, to avoid creating "hot spots"—areas receiving too much radiation, particularly around the urethra, and "cold spots," where cancer or normal tissue are not treated. A refined technique, called a "modified peripheral loading method," also helps keep dosage even. The American Brachytherapy Society looks forward to the development of "real-time, online" dosimetry—which would provide immediate feedback during the procedure—in the near future.

Afterward: You will be taken to a recovery room for about two hours; an ice bag will be placed between your legs to help keep swelling down in the perineal area. When you have regained feeling in your legs (and are able to walk to the bathroom), the urinary catheter will probably be removed. (In some men, the catheter may be left overnight.)

You will probably be given a round of antibiotics, to take for about five days, and some form of pain medication and anti-inflammatory medication. For most men, an over-the-counter medication, such as ibuprofen (Motrin, Advil) or acetaminophen (Tylenol), works well; however, if you are in severe discomfort, your doctor may prescribe a stronger medication (containing codeine or morphine).

Although brachytherapy is an outpatient procedure, you will feel weak and fatigued afterward. Plan on having someone drive you home, and don't try to drive for at least twelve hours afterward. Note:

Most doctors will refuse to perform the procedure, or may want you to stay in the hospital overnight, if you do not have a ride home.

There are no dietary restrictions; after you are out of the recovery room, you can eat and drink whatever you wish. For the first two days, avoid heavy lifting or strenuous exercise. To minimize the risk of blood clots, avoid sitting or standing in the same position for a prolonged period. Drink plenty of fluids (at least six to eight large glasses' worth) to keep your urine clear; eat extra servings of fruits and vegetables (to help prevent constipation), and take it easy; rest often, and apply an ice pack to the perineal area four times a day. Because men are basically radioactive after brachytherapy, you will probably be advised to avoid close contact with children (letting them sit on your lap, or come within two feet of you) and pregnant women for a few weeks after the implantation.

Although your bodily wastes are not radioactive, you may be asked to urinate through a strainer (placed over the toilet) for the first seven days after receiving the seeds. This is because some seeds may become dislodged, and may make their way into the urinary stream. Your doctor will probably give you a small lead container to hold any stray seeds you may find. Don't pick up the seeds with your fingers; use tweezers or a spoon, and return the container to your doctor for proper disposal. (If you can't retrieve a seed that falls into the toilet, don't worry; you won't contaminate the town's water supply by flushing it.)

Guidelines vary, but you will probably be told that it's okay to sleep in the same bed as your wife. There has never been a published account of a man ejaculating a seed into his partner—and the risk of radiation damage from a single seed is minimal—but to be on the safe side, some doctors advise men to abstain from intercourse for as long as two months, and to wear condoms for six months after brachytherapy. There is also a minimal risk that a seed might migrate to the lung. Although this does not cause any symptoms or seem to harm the lung, you may be scheduled to have a chest X-ray at your first follow-up visit. Some doctors perform cystoscopy after surgery, to remove any blood clots and stray seeds from the bladder or urethra.

Call your doctor immediately if:

- You pass blood clots larger than a dime, either through your penis or rectum.
- You are unable to urinate within four hours of drinking two large glasses of liquid.
- You have a temperature greater than 100.5° F or shaking chills.
- You are in pain, and pain medication doesn't help.
- Your Foley catheter falls out of your bladder.

Complications

Evaluating the complications of interstitial brachytherapy is confusing for doctors as well as patients—mainly because there are many studies whose results and criteria vary widely. Some reasons for this are that different surgeons have different techniques and, frankly, levels of expertise; that some doctors implant seeds in patients who would be ruled out for this treatment by other doctors; and that some doctors leading various studies may not specify, may lump in different categories, or may not even be aware of all the complications their patients have had. Anytime you see gaping holes in percentages (like, "From 5 to 85 percent of men had . . ."), it's probably safe to assume that truly accurate results are hard to come by.

The side effects of surgery have been studied in detail. But at the writing of this book, there has not been a critical, long-term analysis of side effects and quality of life after brachytherapy. Because brachytherapy combined with external-beam radiotherapy delivers more radiation than brachytherapy alone, there should be a similar analysis of side effects and quality of life after this combined treatment as well. Also, any form of radiation—or any treatment, for that matter—is "operator-dependent." In other words, it's only as effective as the doctor performing it. It is possible that some doctors today are minimizing the dose of brachytherapy, in an effort to minimize side effects. This used to happen with external-beam radiation therapy. At first, everything is fine—the patient feels great, and maybe three or four years go by before anyone realizes there's a problem, and the PSA keeps going up. The other side of this coin is that some doctors are treating prostate cancer very aggressively, and as a result their patients have more side effects than usual. Again, there needs to be a long-term study comparing aggressiveness of treatment and side effects.

Here are some of the complications you can expect from implantation of radioactive seeds: The incidence of death from any of the procedures is extremely rare, much less than 1 percent. There is a huge fluctuation in the incidence of late (not immediately after surgery) complications—ranging from zero to 72 percent—depending on which study one chooses to quote; the most common range is from 10 to 25 percent.

Urinary retention: The major acute (immediate) complication of brachytherapy is urinary retention, inability to empty the bladder completely. This happens when the tissue surrounding the implants begins to react—with bleeding, swelling, and inflammation—to the trauma of having a needle stuck in it repeatedly (just as, on a smaller scale, the prostate swells after a biopsy). Between 10 and 20 percent of men experience urinary retention during the first few days after seed implantation; this usually gets better after a week to ten days, as the swelling goes down. Urinary retention may have a delayed onset as well, peaking between two and four weeks after brachytherapy. The symptom is the same, but the cause is different—irritation in the urethra and prostate, which develops as the radiation's effects begin to be felt. This, too, is only temporary; it gradually improves and usually goes away within about two months. Some men may need an indwelling Foley catheter for a few weeks, or may need to insert a catheter several times a day to drain the bladder. If the bladder obstruction is severe, some men may need to be treated with a TUIP (transurethral incision of the prostate, a surgical procedure used to treat BPH, in which a surgeon makes a few tiny cuts in the prostate tissue that's choking the urethra; this gives the urethra "breathing room," and improves the flow of urine from the bladder). If surgery is necessary, it should be delayed until three half-lives of radiation have been delivered to the gland—fifty-one days for palladium, and 180 days for iodine. But here, a TUIP may result in long-term incontinence. Thus, the best way to avoid this complication is a proactive approach, beginning well ahead of seed implantation. Some radiation oncologists start all of their patients with enlarged prostates or obstructive symptoms on an alpha-1-blocker, such as Cardura, Hytrin, or Flomax, several weeks before the seeds are implanted. They continue the medication for two or three months after the procedure, and taper it gradually, as the symptoms resolve.

Bowel problems: Several studies report that from 20 to 25 percent of men suffered rectal complications such as diarrhea, cramps, or bleeding; most of these problems were not severe. In one Harvard study, 12 percent of brachytherapy patients had significant gastrointestinal complications—particularly, rectal ulceration, with two men requiring a colostomy, because a hole (called a fistula) developed between the prostate and the rectal wall. In other studies, rectal bleeding has been reported in between 5 and 20 percent of men. Men who were treated more aggressively (for example, men with larger, stage T3 or T4 tumors who also got external-beam radiation) or men who had larger tumors (and therefore got more seeds or a higher dose of radiation) tended to develop more severe rectal problems such as an ulcer. Stool softeners, steroid enemas, and anti-inflammatory drugs may help mild rectal ulcers go away, but more serious ulcers that destroy tissue may require reconstructive surgery. In one study from Memorial Sloan-Kettering Cancer Center, nineteen of 109 men developed "persistent, bright red rectal bleeding from one to 28 months after [iodine seed] implantation." The bleeding eventually resolved in six of these men, "from nine to 48 months from the time of onset." Nine men were treated with steroid enemas, and three men underwent laser treatment to stop the bleeding. Note: If you have rectal bleeding after brachytherapy, there is the chance that it is caused by something else—perhaps colorectal cancer. See your doctor; you may also need to be examined by a gastroenterologist, to rule out other causes.

Prostatitis: In one study of 115 patients who had radioactive iodine seeds implanted, five men developed prostatitis (for more on prostatitis, see Chapter 2) and reported severe irritative urinary symptoms. The investigators suspected that in these men the seeds became infected.

Urinary problems: From 10 to 37 percent of men in several studies had urinary problems including urethral stricture, bladder neck contracture, and damage to the urethra that caused irritative urinary symptoms. Most of these occurred in men who had already experienced such problems (from BPH, for example) or who had undergone a TURP procedure. For example, incontinence, which occurred in 5 percent of men, was not a problem for men who had not had the TURP. As many as half of men who have had a TURP who undergo brachytherapy develop incontinence, sometimes months after the procedure. Another factor in the development of urinary problems seems to be placement of the seeds—in the past, trouble has been much more likely to develop when seeds were planted too close to the urethra. Some doctors now are hoping to avoid this problem by leaving a larger cushion of seed-free tissue around the urethra. Severe prolonged bleeding may also occur, requiring treatment with hyperbaric oxygen (see above).

At the 1999 meeting of the American Urological Association, there were two patient-reported studies comparing urinary function after radical prostatectomy and after brachytherapy. In one study from the University of Virginia, at six months after treatment, there was no significant difference between the two groups on the issues of "bothersomeness," or impact on quality of life. In a study from the University of California–Los Angeles, at one year after treatment brachytherapy patients had worse obstructive symptoms, and were more bothered by urinary and bowel problems, while prostatectomy patients had worse urinary leakage.

Sexual problems: These can include impotence, ejaculatory pain, pain in the testicles, and blood in the semen. In several studies, impotence affects at least 40 percent of men—although not immediately after implantation. A man's ability to have an erection appears to diminish over time, just as it does in men who get external-beam radiation treatment, probably because of gradual damage to small blood vessels. (This can be helped by the drug Viagra, discussed in Chapter 11.)

Much of the information on the recovery of sexual function after brachytherapy is anecdotal. However, a recent study from the University of Pennsylvania used a validated quality-of-life questionnaire in men who underwent seed implantation between 1992 and 1998. In general, the patients were older than men undergoing radical prostatectomy; the average age was sixty-nine. Before treatment, eighty-one men said that they had erections sufficient for intercourse. Two years after treatment, 49 percent of these men remained potent. As with every form of treatment for prostate cancer, younger men fared better: 52 percent of men younger than seventy remained potent, compared with only 45 percent of men over age seventy. The study also found that short-term (for three to six months) treatment with hormones before brachytherapy did not increase the likelihood of erectile dysfunction. More favorable results have been reported by others who claim that at three and six years, 80 and 60 percent, respectively, are potent. The major factors that influenced this were a high implant dose and whether sexual function was normal or marginal before treatment.

Temporary Seeds: High-Dose-Rate Brachytherapy

A variant of brachytherapy, usually given *along with external-beam radiation*, is high-dose-rate (HDR), or "temporary," brachytherapy. As its name suggests, the seeds don't stay in; they're removed at the end of each treatment session. These seeds, used at a few centers in the United States, are made up of high-activity iridium-192. They are inserted (and then removed) with the help of a robotic arm through plastic tubes, or catheters, inserted at precise locations throughout the prostate. Temporary brachytherapy is designed for men with more aggressive cancer, or with cancer that extends slightly beyond the prostate. Although it's too new for its effects to be well studied, one study cites "difficulty achieving optimal catheter stabilization," and trouble getting the seeds placed exactly.

Cryoablation (Freezing the Prostate)

This technique sounds great: For starters, it involves no surgery. Instead, extremely cold liquid nitrogen is used to freeze the entire prostate, causing cancer cells within the gland to rupture as they begin to thaw.

The idea itself is not new. Many years ago, when the technique was first introduced, the freezing was accomplished through the urethra. Today, using ultrasound to guide them, doctors circulate freezing argon gas through six to eight metallic probes, which are placed in the prostate gland through the perineum. The freezing continues until the ultrasound shows that an "iceball" has been created. The procedure can take longer than an hour, and the hospital stay is generally one or two days.

Doctors who perform cryoablation (also called cryotherapy) must be well acquainted with transrectal ultrasound, so they can be sure that the prostate is frozen completely. During the procedure, the tissue around the urethra should be heated so it won't be destroyed along with the rest of the prostate.

The big advantages of cryoablation are its short hospital stay and the absence of an abdominal incision. Proponents of this procedure emphasize cryoablation's ease of treatment and freedom from early side effects. In one study, of sixty-six men with cancers ranging from stages T1c to T3c, Austrian physicians reported that only 10 percent of men had stress incontinence, only 10 percent had impotence, and 8 percent had a temporary rectoperineal fistula (a hole that develops in the rectal tissue). But in other studies, impotence is higher—ranging from about 30 percent to as high as 85 percent. This may be because, in an attempt to destroy all the cancer, many doctors who perform this procedure deliberately attempt to freeze the nerve bundles that are essential for erection (see Chapter 8 for more on these neurovascular bundles).

Incontinence is a serious risk as well. In a large U.S. study of cryotherapy patients, between 40 and 80 percent of men had erectile dysfunction; as many as 27 percent had incontinence; between 3 and 29 percent had bladder outlet obstruction that required prolonged catheterization; about 2 percent developed a fistula between the prostate and rectum; as many as 19 percent experienced sloughing of the urethra (during urination); and as many as 10 percent reported pain or numbness in the penis.

The big unknown is whether cryoablation actually cures prostate cancer. Prostate cancer is a multifocal disease; the average cancerous prostate has seven separate tumors growing in it. *So to cure it, it's necessary to eliminate the entire prostate.* But that doesn't happen with cryoablation. During the procedure, the tissue around the urethra is protected by heat. Does the heat that preserves the urethra also spare a few scattered cancer cells? (For more on cancer control, see Chapter 10.)

Other Forms of Treatment

In addition to cryotherapy, there are other forms of energy—all of them involving the principle of heat—being studied for their potential to destroy the prostate. The list will almost certainly grow longer, but for now, some of these include:

- Transurethral laser treatment, using laser energy to kill prostate tissue.
- Interstitial seeds, activated by radio frequency to heat surrounding tissue.
- High-intensity focused ultrasound, delivered through a probe in the rectum.

In theory, all of these modalities—although promising, and effective in treating benign prostate enlargement—suffer from the same problem as cryotherapy. In an effort to preserve the urethra, the central core of the prostate must be cooled. But sparing even some prostate tissue means that some cancer cells may be spared as well. Also, the nature of the prostate—its irregular shape, and its extreme proximity to vulnerable structures just a few millimeters away—provides further challenges. How to eliminate the prostate's peripheral zone, where cancer often grows, without injuring the rectum, the neurovascular bundles, or other important organs? None of these procedures has been tested widely, or evaluated with long-term PSA follow-up.

But what about the long-term outlook, and the biggest question of all—has your cancer been controlled? For a detailed discussion of the results of all forms of treatment for localized disease—surgery, radiation, and cryotherapy—see Chapter 10.

10

HOW SUCCESSFUL IS TREATMENT OF LOCALIZED PROSTATE CANCER?

Read This First

Will my cancer be cured forever? Out of a massive amount of information about a complicated, confusing, infuriating disease, we have only two incontrovertible facts about cure. If you are going to be cured of prostate cancer, your disease must be diagnosed at a stage when it is curable, before the cancer has escaped to a distant site. And, the treatment has to work.

What's the best form of treatment for localized disease? This is a major dilemma, because it's a moving target: There are multiple options: radical prostatectomy, retropubic, perineal, and laparoscopic; many forms of radiation therapy—3-D conformal, intensity-modulated, proton beam, plus brachytherapy, with or without external-beam radiation; cryotherapy; and all of these with or without hormone therapy. Worse, there are many definitions of success, and study results that can vary widely, depending on the stage of disease at which a patient is treated. Is it possible that the improved techniques for radiation therapy will be able to eliminate all prostate tissue, and approach the "gold standard" achieved by total surgical removal?

Surgeons will tell you that up to now, every time radiation therapy has been used to treat localized prostate cancer, and every time an improved form of treatment has supplanted another, eventually the failure rates were higher than everyone hoped. This is true. However, it's possible that this time it will be different—that with state-of-the-art imaging and high-dose delivery techniques, it may be possible for radiation therapy to kill all prostate cancer. Time will tell.

Curing Localized Prostate Cancer

Will my cancer be cured forever? This question is the bedrock of the book, what everyone wants to know, and what every man with localized prostate cancer has the right to expect.

There are two rules here, two home truths that—like proverbs—sound so simple that, on face value, they seem superfluous. And yet, out of a massive amount of information about a complicated, confusing, infuriating disease, these are the only incontrovertible facts. If you are going to be cured of prostate cancer:

- Your disease must be *diagnosed at a stage when it is curable*, before the cancer has escaped the prostate.
- And, *the treatment has to work.*

Remember what we've said throughout this book—*prostate cancer is multifocal.* It's not like an isolated dandelion that springs up and (if the seeds haven't blown elsewhere in the yard) can be dug up and eliminated. It's more like clover, which crops up in more than one spot at the same time. Prostate cancer starts in many places throughout the entire prostate, simultaneously. The same factors that cause cancer in one site of tissue cause it to develop a few millimeters away, and a few millimeters away from that. *The average number of separate tumors in prostates removed in surgery is seven. Thus, to get rid of the cancer, we must eliminate the entire prostate.* Theoretically, leaving even a handful of prostate cells behind, even if they're actually free of cancer (which they may not be), is a serious gamble. Those instigating factors that started cancer once may—if the same type of tissue is still there—cause it to grow again. Thus, *total eradication of prostate tissue* should be the goal of all forms of treatment for localized cancer.

Now, how do we know when we've scored a bull's-eye? Which forms of treatment mark a direct hit in the target, and which land shy of the middle, leaving room for uncertainty (and for cancer to return)? Our greatest judge of the success of treatment is PSA. Thanks to PSA, we have a better idea, first of all, whether a man is curable (by factoring PSA with the clinical stage and Gleason score, in the Partin Tables). PSA also tells us whether cure has been accomplished. *An undetectable level of PSA is the gold standard of cure.*

As we discussed earlier in the book, the advent of widespread PSA testing in the 1990s has enabled prostate cancer to be diagnosed, on average, five years earlier than it used to be. If your cancer was diagnosed by a change in PSA, be grateful. You've been given a gift of five years over the unfortunate men who used to be diagnosed only when cancer had gotten large enough to feel in a rectal exam—or worse, when it caused symptoms such as urinary retention, because it had grown big enough to interfere with the urethra, or back pain, because it had already spread to the bone. For men with prostate cancer, PSA has been a godsend. This five-year lead time has dramatically shifted the window of curability for most men. Twenty years ago, 75 percent of men diagnosed with prostate cancer clearly had tumors that had extended beyond the prostate. And sadly, of the 25 percent of men we thought were curable back then, fewer than half truly were.

Until PSA, the possibility of being cured of prostate cancer was unlikely, because for most men, even at the point of diagnosis it was already too late. Now, thank goodness, *most men who are diagnosed with prostate cancer have potentially curable disease*—all the more reason why it's so important to identify the best way to cure them. Because the disease can be cured, if the treatment works.

So, what works best? Researchers have been trying to nail this down for decades. Initially, scientists tried to compare overall survival rates of one form of treatment versus another. This didn't work very well. Because most men were older (average age seventy-two) at diagnosis, by the time ten or fifteen years had gone by, most of these men had died from some other cause. Thus, overall survival didn't turn out to be a good measure of treatment success. Next, researchers looked at "cancer-specific" survival—that is, the number of men who lived fifteen years and died of prostate cancer. This proved a better, more specific approach, because it asked the question everyone wanted asked: Of the men healthy enough to live ten or fifteen years, how many died of prostate cancer? In how many of these men did cancer progress to the point where it killed them?

Next, taking this one step further, researchers asked, what percent of men who lived ten or fifteen years had no signs of cancer? That is, they weren't just alive after treatment, but they had *never had a recurrence of cancer that required further treatment.* Why is this important? It's more than just a technicality. Which would you prefer? To be alive ten years after treatment, even if it meant that your cancer had come back, and you then needed additional treatment, such as radiation or hormones, and you were subjected to further side effects? Or to be alive, healthy, with an undetectable PSA, with the prostate cancer as a significant but temporary "blip" on the horizon of your life, only thinking about it once a year when you get your follow-up PSA test? Although both men count on the "plus" side as far as statistics go, because they are alive, it's a "no-brainer"—option B is light-years away from option A in terms of *quality* of life.

But it took ten to fifteen years to reach these answers. During this time, progress in the treatment of prostate cancer dragged on and on, with no one knowing for sure whether any man was really cured, and whether any particular form of treatment was better. In the mid-1980s, with PSA, we had a new way to tell whether any prostate cells existed in men who had undergone treatment for cancer. PSA as a follow-up marker proved very sensitive; after the first elevation of PSA after treatment, we've learned, it can take two, five, or even ten years for a man to develop symptoms of metastatic disease, or signs of cancer on a bone scan.

PSA also provided a rude awakening in the late 1980s, when we learned that only 10 or 20 percent of men who received radiation therapy had a low PSA ten years after treatment. In large part, this was because the men who underwent radiation therapy at that time had been "adversely selected"—they were not considered good candidates for surgery, because it was unlikely that all of the cancer could be cut out of them. But radiation oncologists also realized that there was much room for improvement in the way they were delivering radiation, and they have been trying ever since to do a better job of killing cancer. Since the late 1980s, the field of radiation therapy for prostate cancer has been revolutionized by the techniques (described in Chapter 9) aimed at delivering better treatment to the prostate: 3-D conformal therapy, intensity-modulated therapy, proton beam therapy, brachytherapy (alone, or with external-beam therapy)—and all of these with or without hormone therapy.

The other major development in this field over the last twenty years has been the ability to know the extent of prostate cancer, and to use this finding to predict the probability of cure. Before 1980, only 7 percent of men with localized prostate cancer underwent radical prostatectomy. Thus, for the vast majority of men treated during those years, we never knew whether the cancer was confined to the prostate, or whether it had spread outside the prostate into the seminal vesicles or adjacent lymph nodes. (The only way to know this for sure is for a pathologist to examine the actual prostate and surrounding tissue, and the only way this is possible is for it to be surgically removed and sent to the lab.) For years, we were dealing with a black box: 93 percent of men with what we thought to be localized prostate cancer were all scrambled together—some really were curable, some weren't—and we were using crude end points that took a long time to determine whether or not these men truly were cured.

Then, in 1982, the anatomic approach to radical prostatectomy was developed. Surgeons and patients found this technique more acceptable, because it was safer, and was associated with fewer side effects. Over the next decade, 35 percent of men with localized prostate cancer chose this form of treatment. As a result, we had a lot more prostates to examine, and in many more men we were able to determine conclusively whether the cancer was confined to the prostate, or whether it was more extensive.

These pathologic findings, available only from men who chose surgery, were then correlated with the three things that could be measured in *every man* diagnosed with prostate cancer—the clinical stage, Gleason score, and PSA—the Partin Tables. And then, we could begin to predict which men were really curable. These findings, initially collected at Johns Hopkins, have been expanded to include more than five thousand men, have proven reliable, and now can tell men and their doctors the one most important fact necessary in choosing a form of treatment—the probability of cure.

That's the background. Now, let's examine the success of surgery, radiation, and cryotherapy in curing prostate cancer.

Cancer Control after Radical Prostatectomy

There is no better way to cure cancer that is confined to the prostate than total surgical removal. This is the "gold standard" of treatment, what all other forms of treatment attempt to accomplish. Thus, it's important that you understand the results of radical prostatectomy—just what it can and cannot do—and the fine points in interpreting these results, before you can make an informed evaluation of other treatment approaches.

Start with the facts: The first indisputable fact here is that *for any form of treatment to cure prostate cancer, it must be curable in the first place.* Is your disease curable? We can learn almost everything we need to know about where you stand before surgery from the Partin Tables—the next best thing to a crystal ball—using your clinical stage, PSA, and Gleason score. After surgery, other information fine-tunes this picture. The pathologist can determine the facts of your cancer—the Gleason score of the *entire prostate*, for example (as opposed to the educated guess made by examining just a few cores of tissue). From the pathologist, we can learn whether the cancer was organ-confined, whether there was capsular penetration with negative *surgical margins* (also called "specimen-confined" disease), whether the margins were positive, and whether the seminal vesicles or lymph nodes were involved. All of these factors have a profound impact on the success of treatment.

What are surgical margins, anyway? This is a confusing point for many men. When the prostate is removed, it should be covered by several layers of tissue. It may help to think of the cancerous prostate as a gift box (although it's not much of a present), and the tissue surrounding it as wrapping paper. After radical prostatectomy, your prostate goes to the pathologist, who immediately coats the outside of the entire specimen—the wrapping paper—with India ink. The prostate is then put in fixative for twenty-four hours before it is sectioned, stained, and examined under the microscope. The India ink creates a landmark, so the pathologist can figure out exactly how far the cancer has spread. Is it contained inside the wrapping paper? If the cancer is all contained within the box, we call it *organ-confined*. Even if cancer penetrates the box (this is capsular penetration), it can still be completely covered with wrapping paper. We call this *specimen-confined*. This is an important concept. For example, in men with a Gleason score of 6 or below, the long-term outcome is just as good in men with cancer that's confined inside the prostate (inside the box) as it is in men who have capsular penetration, but negative surgical margins. If the cancer has penetrated the box and the wrapping paper as well, this is called a *positive surgical margin*. The pathologist can see cancer cells at the edge of the India ink, and this suggests that there *may be* cancer beyond the outermost edge where the surgeon removed the prostate.

When surgical margins are positive, or too close to call: In an ideal world, the pathologist would immediately send a triumphant report to the surgeon: "I've looked at the prostate tissue you removed from Mr. Jones, and all of the edges are clear. Congratulations! You've removed all the cancer!"

Fortunately, it often happens that way. At Johns Hopkins, fewer than 10 percent of the patients are found to have cancer at the margins—the edges of the removed tumor. Sometimes, however, the pathologist's report is more ambiguous. The report states that the margins are "close," meaning that cancer is just a hairbreadth away from the edge of the specimen.

Expert pathologist Jonathan Epstein, of Johns Hopkins, has good news about these margins:

Close margins are almost always negative. Epstein recently finished a study of men whose tumors were particularly close—less than two tenths of a millimeter—from the surgical margin. Even though there wasn't a comfortable cushion of tissue between the tumor and the edge of the prostate, "those patients do just as well as if there's more separation between the tumor and the margin."

Even if the surgical margins are positive, this does not necessarily mean that cancer is left behind. How can this be? "There are several different explanations why, when the margins are positive, the tumor may still be cured," says Epstein. "One is that literally, you cut across the last few tumor cells"—that what appears to be remaining cancer is actually a cross section of the perimeter of the tumor. "And even though it looks like it's a positive margin, there's really no cancer left in the patient."

Another explanation is that the act of surgery itself finishes the job, killing any remaining cells. No cut or injury to tissue happens in a vacuum; the area around the cut is affected, too. (Think of lightning striking a tree; the tree dies, but so does a ring of grass around it.) "When the surgeon cuts across tissue, the blood supply is cut off, there's dead tissue, and that can kill off the last few tumor cells that might have been left behind," Epstein says.

There's also the potential, "and this probably accounts for a lot of cases," that it's an "artifact"—basically, a false positive margin. Sometimes, "since there's so little tissue next to the prostate, when the surgeon tries to dissect it from the body, and hands it to the nurse, and then the nurse hands it to the pathologist, everyone's touching the gland. If you're talking about two tenths of a millimeter of tissue, that tissue can be disrupted very easily. It can appear that the tumor is at the margin—but in fact, there was some additional tissue there that just got disrupted during all the handling." In other words, a few good "buffer" cells got rubbed off.

And then there's the sticky cell phenomenon. When cancer reaches beyond the prostate to invade nearby tissue, it produces a dense scar tissue that acts like super-glue. As a surgeon removes the prostate, this thick scar tissue sticks to the surrounding cancer cells—picking them up like a lint brush. So in some cases, although the pathologist may see cancer cells at the margin—and make a judgment of "positive surgical margins"—there are no cancer cells left inside the patient. The sticky scar tissue took them all away.

Epstein recently studied such instances, where the surgeon removed the prostate, looked at it, suspected that some cancer cells were present, went back and cut out more of the surrounding tissue. "So in pathology, we got two separate specimens," says Epstein. "One was the prostate, one was this extra tissue, the neurovascular bundle that the surgeon was thinking of leaving in the patient, but decided to remove." Even when there appeared to be a positive surgical margin at the edge of the prostate, in 40 percent of these patients, there turned out to be *no cancer left behind* in that adjacent tissue.

"So when pathologists call a positive margin, or for that matter, a close margin, it doesn't necessarily mean that these patients need some other form of therapy, like radiation—and also that they need not necessarily be tremendously worried."

PSA after Radical Prostatectomy

The best way to determine whether all the cancer has been removed in a radical prostatectomy is to check for the presence of PSA. Many men are surprised by this; they reason—and rightly so— that if the prostate has been removed, there should be no PSA. Indeed, after a radical prostatectomy, the PSA level should be undetectable. If it is not, this suggests that some prostate cancer cells managed to escape the prostate before it was removed.

But don't have your PSA tested too soon. PSA has a lengthy half-life in the bloodstream (two or three days)—which means it takes quite a while for PSA levels to go down after a radical prostatectomy. For example, if your PSA before surgery was 10, it would take seven half-lives before the PSA fell into the undetectable range (less than 0.1). If you had your blood tested the day after surgery, your same level of PSA would pop right up, suggesting that the operation hadn't done any good. This is misleading, of course. But to avoid having to deal with such unnecessary stress, you should not have your PSA tested until about eight to twelve weeks after surgery—when PSA should be at rock-bottom. After this point, PSA should be tested every six months in men with positive margins, seminal vesicles, or lymph nodes. For most other men, a PSA measurement is only necessary once a year.

What kind of PSA measurement do you need? A simple, total PSA. You don't need a free PSA test. Also, we do not advise getting one of the ultra-sensitive tests. (See "PSA Anxiety: The Downside of Ultra-Sensitive Tests," below.)

Do you need any other tests? No. PSA is extremely sensitive—so much so, that if your PSA is undetectable, there is no other test—a bone scan, CT scan, MRI, other blood tests, or a rectal examination—that could find any residual tumor. For many men, this is good news.

If PSA is undetectable after surgery, no need for rectal exam: Men hate the digital rectal examination—so much so, in fact, that the desire to avoid it may lead men to put off follow-up visits to the doctor after radical prostatectomy. From a medical standpoint, in turn, the rectal exam is only as good as the physician performing it. Similarly, another test often used in follow-up monitoring of prostate cancer patients after surgery, the radionuclide bone scan, is expensive and also may lead to further tests if the findings are inconclusive.

Is there a better way? A Johns Hopkins study led by urologist Charles R. Pound found that PSA is such a sensitive marker of prostate cancer that if the PSA is undetectable, men don't need a digital rectal examination or further imaging studies *at that time.* In other words, they're off the hook. (However, men with a low PSA still need careful follow-up with a PSA test every year, because it is possible for PSA to go up in the future.)

In the investigation, published in the *Journal of Urology*, scientists studied the medical histories of nearly two thousand men who underwent radical prostatectomy at Johns Hopkins over a fifteen-year period—a study of more than ten thousand patient-years of follow-up. Of these men, fifty-six developed a local recurrence of cancer, and 118 developed distant metastases. For some of these men, it took several years for cancer to return—which is why men need to keep getting regular PSA tests, even several years after surgery—but *no man with an undetectable PSA had evidence of local recurrence or distant metastasis.*

For how long do I have to keep getting my PSA tested? When the first PSA test comes back "undetectable," many men feel that they are "home free" from prostate cancer for good. Unfortunately, that is not the case. With some cancers, the magic number is five years; if the cancer hasn't come back by then, it never will. Prostate cancer, as always, is a bit more difficult. If some cancer cells escaped the prostate before it was surgically removed, these tiny offshoots of cancer can exist at very low levels, growing very slowly for years before they reach a size that will produce enough PSA to be detected in the blood. The good news is that almost all men who develop a recurrence of PSA have it within ten years of surgery. Almost. For a very few men, however, prostate cancer can rear its ugly head again between ten and fifteen years after surgery (the good news here being that the longer it takes for PSA to return after treatment, the better the likelihood that it will respond to a second go-round of treatment; see below).

We have carefully followed nearly 2,500 men who underwent radical prostatectomy at Johns Hopkins, some of them for more than fifteen years. Of four hundred men who developed an elevated PSA, it went up in the first five years in 72 percent; between five and ten years in 23 percent, and beyond ten years in 5 percent. Thus, although the likelihood is very rare, the safest bet is for you to keep having a yearly PSA test for the rest of your life.

Results of Radical Prostatectomy at Johns Hopkins, Including Patients in the Pre-PSA Era

How successful is radical prostatectomy? Base your information on facts, and take any scary news reports (and there is always at least one circulating out there somewhere) with a large grain of salt. For example, one "retread" we see every now and then says something like this: "One third of men who undergo radical prostatectomy will have a recurrence requiring treatment within five years." This is misleading, and it terrifies many men who rightly believe they have been cured. In fact, this statistic refers to men who are either not curable at the time of surgery, or who underwent surgery that did not completely remove their prostate. It does not refer to men with specimen-confined prostate cancer, the ideal men who should be having this procedure, and the men selected for this procedure by the Partin Tables. Some men can still benefit from surgery, such as younger men with cancer in their lymph nodes (although surgery can't cure prostate cancer in these men, it reduces many complications of advanced disease and may prolong survival; see below). But the overwhelming majority of men who undergo radical prostatectomy today have curable disease. Thanks to PSA, cancer is being caught earlier than ever before. When did the "one third of men who have a recurrence" undergo surgery? If it was in the 1980s, as we discussed above, many men weren't even diagnosed until the disease was difficult to cure. Because of this, their long-term probability of having an undetectable PSA is far worse than that of men who were treated in the 1990s.

So, how do we measure the success of radical prostatectomy? What is failure? Surgeons like their evidence in black and white. *Therefore, we have a strict cutoff: After radical prostatectomy, we believe that the PSA level should be undetectable—lower than 0.1 nanogram per milliliter.* (Avoid the ultra-sensitive PSA tests; they're often more trouble than they're worth—see "PSA Anxiety: The Downside of Ultra-Sensitive Tests," below.)

At last, we have truly long-term results on a large number of men who have been followed for more than fifteen years. In all of these patients, the probability of maintaining an undetectable PSA at five, ten, and fifteen years was 84 percent, 74 percent, and 66 percent. Furthermore, at ten years, only 6 percent of the men developed a recurrence of cancer at the surgical site; at fifteen years, no one else had a similar local recurrence. Thus, radical prostatectomy was very effective at controlling the local disease, and the reason the other men had a recurrence was that the cancer had spread to distant sites (like the bone) before surgery, in the form of invisible, impossible-to-detect, distant metastases.

These results represent the best long-term cancer control rates of any surgical series for the treatment of localized prostate cancer, and they may well be used as the gold standard, by which all other forms of treatment are compared. *And yet, these results are not the final answer, and ultimately, they won't even turn out to be the gold standard. Better results are on the way.* How can this be? Because five hundred men in this study were diagnosed in the pre-PSA era (before 1989), when cancer was not usually detected early. In these men, it was much more likely that microscopic flecks of cancer had already left the main tumor, even before diagnosis, casting themselves into the bloodstream like dandelion seeds in the wind, taking root elsewhere in the body. In 1980, only 30 percent of men who underwent a radical prostatectomy at Johns Hopkins had specimen-confined disease. But today, 80 percent of the men who undergo radical prostatectomy at Johns Hopkins have specimen-confined cancer. It stands to reason, then, that in men diagnosed today, the fifteen-year probability of an undetectable PSA would be better than 66 percent. And indeed, it is.

We have recently completed a study comparing five hundred pre-PSA era men, who underwent surgery between 1982 and 1988, to men who underwent surgery between 1989 and 1998. The picture keeps getting better: At ten years, the likelihood of having an undetectable PSA for men who underwent surgery between 1982 and 1988, in the pre-PSA era, was 67 percent. But in men who underwent surgery between 1989 and 1992, the result skyrocketed to 80 percent. And once we have ten-year data on men who underwent surgery in the mid- and late 1990s, we expect the results to be even better. Why? Because in the early 1990s, only 40 percent of men had organ-confined disease. But by 1998, this number had increased to 80 percent. Someday, as more men undergo regular PSA screening, and diagnosis comes even earlier, we may be able to declare that virtually everyone who undergoes radical prostatectomy can be cured.

So What Have We Learned about the Probability of Cure?

With the improved outcome of men diagnosed in the PSA era (1989–98), it is possible to divide them into four risk groups based on their pathologic stage:

- *Group I.* These men have an excellent chance of having an undetectable PSA at ten years. They have a Gleason score of 6 or lower, organ- or specimen-confined disease, with or without capsular penetration (there is no difference), and negative surgical margins. At ten years, the likelihood of having an undetectable PSA is 95 percent.
- *Group II.* These men have a good probability of having an undetectable PSA at ten years. They have a Gleason score of 6, with positive surgical margins, or a Gleason 7 with organ- or specimen-confined disease. At ten years, the likelihood of having an undetectable PSA is 72 percent.
- *Group III.* These men have a moderate probability of having an undetectable PSA at ten years. They have a Gleason score of 7 with capsular penetration and positive margins, or Gleason 8–10 disease or positive seminal vesicles. The probability of an undetectable PSA at ten years is 41 percent.
- *Group IV.* These men have a low probability of having an undetectable PSA at ten years. They have cancer in the lymph nodes. Yet, at ten years without any treatment other than surgery, 13 percent have an undetectable PSA.

Of the men who underwent radical prostatectomy at Johns Hopkins in 2000, 70 percent were in Group I, 20 percent were in Group II, 5 percent were in Group III, and fewer than 1 percent were in Group IV.

What will be the long-term results of prostatectomy in the PSA era? These results will keep getting better. Already, in just a few years, we have seen a dramatic shift in the final pathological stage (based on the actual removed prostate, not the educated guess made using the Partin Tables). Remember how only 30 percent of men in 1980 were diagnosed with organ-confined cancer? Even as early as 1993, after just a few years of using PSA as a screening tool, the number had increased to 55 percent, and then, by 1998 it was 80 percent.

To repeat a very important, reassuring point: Today, because so many men are being screened with yearly PSA tests and rectal exams, early detection means that *most men diagnosed with prostate cancer can be cured with surgery.*

Making sense of studies in medical journals: There are hundreds of articles on results of radical prostatectomy and radiation therapy in the medical journals. The results can be confusing, even contradictory. Here are a few tips to help you make sense of what you read:

- First, check the years in which the patients were studied. As the Johns Hopkins studies above illustrate, men who underwent surgery in the pre-PSA era between 1984 and 1988 were much more likely to have advanced disease than men who underwent the same operation in the 1990s.
- Does the analysis include all patients, even the high-risk ones (such as the men in the Johns Hopkins study above, with a high PSA or Gleason score, and advanced pathologic stage)? Some investigators exclude their patients with positive lymph nodes, and "stack the deck," by choosing for their studies only men with low Gleason grades, low PSA scores and pathologic stages.
- What's the end point of the study? How do the investigators define a recurrence of cancer? Is it any detectable level of PSA, or is there a cutoff—some low-level PSA score that's considered acceptable? (In some literature, particularly studies involving radiation, it's permissible for the PSA to go up three times before the treatment is officially considered a failure. This makes it extremely difficult to compare results of various treatments.)

RADICAL PROSTATECTOMY IN MEN YOUNGER THAN FIFTY

Very few men—only around 1 percent—diagnosed with prostate cancer are younger than fifty. So, mainly because of sheer lack of numbers, men younger than fifty have been something of a little known and poorly studied quantity in the world of prostate cancer research. How do these men fare after radical prostatectomy?

Recently, several investigators set out to answer this question in a study of 543 radical prostatectomy patients at the Johns Hopkins Hospital. There were eighty-five men younger than fifty (three of them younger than forty), and 458 men aged fifty or above (the oldest was seventy-six years old). By far the largest study ever done of men in this age group, this analysis, published in *Urologic Oncology,* was also the most thorough: The researchers took into account each man's clinical stage, Gleason score, and surgical margins (in other words, they examined the edges of the tissue that was removed during surgery, and looked for the presence of cancer there); they also checked for capsular penetration, seminal vesicle and lymph node involvement, and followed PSA tests for at least three years.

Their findings: Younger men who are candidates for radical prostatectomy have a better prognosis after surgery than older men. The operation is more successful because these men have smaller prostates. There is more tissue surrounding the prostate, so the margins of resection are wider. Also, the neurovascular bundles are located further away from the prostate, and are easier to preserve. This provides a "win-win"—an excellent chance for cure, with improved quality of life.

The Pathology Report Suggests My Cancer Might Return: What Happens Next?

One of the major advantages of radical prostatectomy is that it gives the patient some early, definitive answers. In contrast, when men undergo radiation therapy, there is no pathologic specimen to evaluate, and many patients find this unnerving. They ask: "You mean I just have to sit around and wait and see what happens?" Well, yes. But for men who undergo radical prostatectomy, the removed prostate is a walnut-sized crystal ball that packs a lot of information about the future. If the cancer is organ-confined, then you know there was no better way to completely eliminate the local cancer. If there is capsular penetration with negative margins, again, the surgery did the best job any form of treatment could do.

But what if the margins are positive, or cancer was found in your seminal vesicles or pelvic lymph nodes? What should you do? Will any other form of treatment help right now?

Let's say, for example, that you've had your first PSA after surgery, and it was undetectable. But from studying the pathology report, you can see that the probability that your PSA will stay undetectable is not that high. Is it possible that you can act now and get rid of any remaining cancer cells? Should you have radiation therapy to the prostate bed, the area where the prostate used to be? What about hormone therapy? Should you consider chemotherapy—or maybe one of the nonhormonal forms of treatment being tested at your medical center? We'll discuss all of these options in Chapter 12. But let's not jump the gun. The major question we need answered right now is, if PSA is going to rise, where are the PSA-making prostate cancer cells? Are they still in the "old neighborhood," the prostate bed—and if so, is it possible now to eliminate them once and for all?

There are two possibilities here. One is that some cancer cells have indeed escaped the prostate locally, but are still in the prostate bed—and that radiation to this area could kill them forever. The other possibility is that these cells have escaped and are hiding, incognito, at a distant site. In this case, radiation to the prostate bed won't do a thing, except cause new complications by needlessly treating an area already free of cancer. Eliminating these stray bits of cancer calls for a more systemic approach—that is, a medical treatment that affects the whole body, not just an isolated section of it. The most common systemic approach used today is hormone therapy, but the big question is, when should it be started? This is covered in detail in Chapter 12.

New options on the horizon. Some of the most exciting advances in the area of systemic therapy are discussed in Chapter 12, but briefly: There are many exciting new strategies for managing a rising PSA after surgery or radiation. They include tumor vaccines, targeted "smart bombs" using viruses or monoclonal antibodies, gene therapy, angiogenesis inhibitors, antimetastatic compounds, cytotoxic chemotherapy, differentiation therapy, inhibition of cell transduction, and cell-to-cell interaction mechanisms. These new treatments hold great promise that someday we will be able to control prostate cancer forever, as a chronic disease like diabetes—or even to cure it, once it has escaped the prostate.

Recently at Johns Hopkins, to determine whether cancer cells are present locally and might be helped by radiation, we carried out a study of fifty-one men who had rising PSA levels after radical prostatectomy. These men were followed until it became clear where these cells were located—the cancer either recurred locally, or showed up as distant metastases. We found that local recurrence was rare in men who had Gleason scores of 8 or higher, or who had cancer found in their seminal vesicles or lymph nodes during surgery. (This study is discussed further, below.) Thus, the men who were at highest risk for developing a recurrence of cancer were those least likely to benefit from radiation to the prostate bed—and we don't recommend postoperative radiation in these men.

What about men with positive surgical margins? Should they have immediate radiation therapy? There is no good answer to this question now, and the definitive study, in which men with positive surgical margins are randomly assigned either radiation or observation, will take years to answer. From the discussion above, we can see that just because a man's surgical margins are positive does not mean that cancer cells were definitely left behind.

But what if a positive margin does mean that there's still cancer in the area? Positive margins are most likely to occur when a man has cancer that has extended outside the prostate, beyond the point where a surgeon could remove further tissue—for example, on top of the rectum. In situations like this, it is also quite possible that the tumor may have escaped through the bloodstream or lymph nodes to a distant site—beyond the reach of *any* form of localized treatment. This is a very important point, especially when a man is considering further treatment—radiation—to the local area.

If you are considering radiation therapy, you must ask: Is there really any tumor left there? And if there is, is this the only tumor you've got, or is there a chance that it's spread to a distant site? Why not just go for it—get radiation anyway? What have you got to lose? Because radiation after prostatectomy is nothing to enter lightly. It is a double assault to very fragile territory, and the side effects are always worse than in men who get either treatment alone. Side effects range from acute, transient problems during radiation therapy itself—fatigue, bladder and bowel irritation—to the long-term problems of impotence, incontinence, and rectal irritation and bleeding.

But how can we possibly know if cancer is lurking somewhere, invisible for now, ready to set up shop in the bone or lymph system? Once again, the massive data collected by Johns Hopkins urologists comes into play. In an attempt to answer this question, and to help patients make the most informed decision possible about further treatment, we recently analyzed the group of men with positive surgical margins who have the highest likelihood of having an elevated PSA ten years after surgery—men with Gleason 7 disease. There were 112 men in this group, who underwent surgery between 1982 and 1987, and who have been followed carefully ever since with further treatment (radiation or hormones). We studied their data to find out the likelihood that the cancer would show up locally alone—only in the prostate bed, and not at distant sites. (If we could figure this out, then we could have informed recommendations as to which men would benefit from radiation therapy.) This study showed that only 6 percent of the men developed a local recurrence—a finding consistent with all of our other results, suggesting that an isolated local recurrence after radical prostatectomy is rare even in men with Gleason 7 disease who had positive surgical margins, and that surgery usually takes care of all cancer in the localized area.

But this finding had another important implication: It suggested that it is unlikely that immediate radiation therapy to the prostate bed would have a major impact on the cure of cancer in these men—because in most of the men who develop a recurrence of cancer, the problem is that there were distant metastases at the time of surgery. And ultimately, if we are going to cure everyone who undergoes surgery, we are going to need better systemic therapy. (See Chapter 12 for some exciting advances in this area.)

What should I do if my surgical margins are positive? First, talk to your surgeon, and find out what his or her experience has been with radiation therapy in cases like yours. At Johns Hopkins, radical prostatectomy patients do not benefit very much from radiation to the prostate bed. We believe this is because our surgeons have done everything they can to remove the cancer locally. However, there are other centers in the country that report better results with radiation therapy. It is possible that some of these men are being helped by radiation because there wasn't a "complete local removal"—in other words, the surgery didn't get all the cancer. Thus, the important question of whether you should receive radiation therapy needs to be answered based on your surgeon's experience with patients like you in the same situation.

What Should I Do if My PSA Comes Back after Surgery?

PSA is a very sensitive marker for the recurrence of prostate cancer—in fact, it's probably the most sensitive marker there is, for *any* cancer. Because PSA is made only by prostate cells, when PSA becomes elevated after a radical prostatectomy, this suggests that some cancer cells are still present (although in a rare case, it is possible that some benign tissue was left behind, which is causing the PSA to show up in the blood).

But before we talk about this, let's make sure you're not having it tested too soon (see above). You should not have your PSA tested until about two or three months after surgery. Next, if your PSA is up more than three months after surgery, the first thing to do is have it checked again. PSA measurements are tricky, and some laboratories are not able to measure PSA at its lowest ranges. (See "PSA Anxiety: The Downside of Ultra-Sensitive Tests," below.) For most men, an elevated PSA means that cancer is present. If you repeat the test and it, too, is elevated, the next question is: Where is the cancer? Is it still localized to the prostate area, or has it spread elsewhere? Were there some cancer cells that slipped outside the prostate—which are still hanging around the old neighborhood, the prostate bed—that were not removed at the time of surgery? Or have the cells escaped to a distant site?

PSA ANXIETY: THE DOWNSIDE OF ULTRA-SENSITIVE TESTS

You've had the radical prostatectomy, but deep down, you're terrified that it didn't work. So here you are, a grown man, living in fear of a simple blood test, scared to death that the PSA—an enzyme made only by prostate cells, but all of your prostate cells are supposed to be gone—will come back. Six months ago, the number was 0.01. This time, it was 0.02.

You have PSA anxiety. You are not alone.

This is the bane of the hypersensitive PSA test: *Sometimes, there is such a thing as too much information.* Daniel W. Chan, Ph.D., is professor of pathology, oncology, urology, and radiology, and director of Clinical Chemistry at Johns Hopkins. He is also an internationally recognized authority on biochemical tumor markers such as PSA, and on immunoassay tests such as the PSA test. This is some of what he has to say on the subject of PSA anxiety:

The only thing that really matters, he says, is, "At what PSA levels does the concentration indicate that the patient has had a recurrence of cancer?" For Chan, and the scientists and physicians at Hopkins, the number to take seriously is 0.2 nanogram/milliliter. "That's something we call biochemical recurrence. But even this doesn't mean that a man has symptoms yet. People need to understand that it might take months or even years before there is any clinical, physical evidence."

On a technical level, in the laboratory, Chan trusts the sensitivity of assays down to 0.1, or slightly less than that. "You cannot reliably detect such a small amount as 0.01," he explains. "From day to day, the results could vary—it could be 0.03, or maybe even 0.05"—and these "analytical" variations may not mean a thing. "It's important that we don't assume anything or take action on a very low level of PSA. In routine practice, *because of these analytical variations from day to day,* if it's less than 0.1, we assume it's the same as nondetectable, or zero."

My PSA Is Back: Should I Get Radiation?

Could radiation therapy eradicate any remaining prostate cancer cells—or would it just cause new complications by needlessly treating an area already free of cancer? This is not an easy dilemma to solve—in part because PSA is so very sensitive, and when so few cancer cells are present, they can't be seen by any of the usual imaging studies, such as MRI or CT. Two studies by Johns Hopkins researchers have shed much light on these troubling questions. The first, led by urologist Alan Partin, studied rising PSA levels in fifty-one men after radical prostatectomy. In 30 percent of these men, cancer returned locally; in 70 percent, the cancer showed up as distant metastases. Based on this study, the scientists found they can estimate which course the cancer will take using the combination of *Gleason score*, *pathologic stage* (the definitive extent of a man's cancer, determined after surgery, when a pathologist looks at the actual prostate specimen and dissected lymph nodes, if any), and *timing*—when the PSA starts to rise, and by how much.

Men most prone to distant metastases, they found, will have one or more of these conditions: Gleason scores of 8 or higher, cancer found in their seminal vesicles and lymph nodes during surgery, or a rise in PSA within a year after their surgery. On the other hand, men with Gleason scores of 7 or lower, no cancer found in their seminal vesicles and lymph nodes, and increases in PSA several years after surgery were more likely to have a local recurrence of cancer—which means their cancer may still be cured with external-beam radiation treatment to the prostate bed, where some residual cancer cells may yet be hiding.

The next study, published in the *Journal of Urology*, confirmed these findings, and took them one step further. It actually followed men who had an elevated PSA after surgery who went on to receive radiation therapy. "We found that no man with a Gleason score of 8–10, positive lymph nodes, or positive seminal vesicles responded favorably to radiation therapy," says urologist Jeffrey Cadeddu. "So in those patients, we do not recommend radiation therapy." In this study, there were sixteen men who experienced a rise in PSA within the first year. One of those men had an undetectable PSA for three years after radiation therapy; then it began to rise again.

But even if radiation couldn't reach a distant metastasis—a bit of cancer that has broken off from the main tumor and established itself elsewhere—couldn't it do some further good to the prostate bed? For a man with metastatic disease, irradiating the pelvis—ironically, an area where the cancer probably is *not*—"does not change survival," Cadeddu says. In addition, radiation therapy to the pelvis in a man who has undergone a radical prostatectomy may cause incontinence and diminish sexual function.

Conversely, for men with a Gleason score of 7 or less, and negative seminal vesicles and lymph nodes, the longer the period before PSA starts to rise, the better the odds that radiation therapy will be worthwhile.

This study also had an unexpected finding: If radiation therapy in men with elevated PSA levels was delayed until the local recurrence was palpable (big enough for a doctor to feel), these men appeared to do just about as well as those who received radiation earlier. If this finding is confirmed in other studies, it might simplify at least one immediate treatment decision in men with elevated PSA levels. The best course may be for doctors to follow these men closely; and then, if they develop local recurrence of cancer, to treat them with radiation therapy, or to begin hormone therapy if distant metastases are found. (Hormone therapy, and promising new approaches for treating advanced cancer, are discussed in Chapter 12.)

Before you undergo radiation after radical prostatectomy: Your doctor may want you to undergo some further tests. If there is a slight chance that the cancer may have spread beyond the local area, your doctor may suggest a bone scan, chest X-ray, and pelvic CT scan (all of these are discussed in Chapter 6). The main reason for these tests is *not* because your doctor expects them to be positive, but to establish a baseline of information. (For example, if you have bone pain in years to come, your doctor can look at the bone scan and say, "Oh, that's the old football injury; see—it hasn't changed in five years.") You probably do not need a biopsy of the prostate bed. If you are going to have radiation therapy after prostatectomy, it's because all signs point to a *local recurrence* of cancer. It might be tiny—so tiny, in fact, that a biopsy might be falsely negative. If local recurrence is likely (based on the criteria described above), even if the biopsy is negative, radiation would still be your best course of action. So why have a biopsy you don't need? Similarly, if all evidence suggests that the PSA is coming from distant metastases, a biopsy is not necessary—because even if it were positive, radiation therapy to the prostate bed will not cure you, and it can cause severe side effects. Another test, called a ProstaScint scan (described in Chapter 6) is often difficult for physicians to interpret, and currently may not be worth the time and money.

If you are a candidate for radiation, your doctor may want you to take a short course of hormone therapy. This has been shown to make radiation after prostatectomy more effective. A study by researchers at Stanford University Medical Center, published in the *International Journal of Radiation Oncology-Biology-Physics*, found that men who underwent hormone therapy for two months before receiving radiation therapy after radical prostatectomy were nearly twice as likely to be free of cancer in five years as men who did not receive the hormones. At Johns Hopkins, we usually treat men with presumed local recurrence of cancer with hormones for three months before radiation therapy. We tell them—and your doctor should discuss this with you—that if they have any urinary incontinence before radiation, the radiation therapy is likely to make this worse. However, the good news is that in most men, the short course of hormones and the radiation do not adversely affect sexual function. (You should know that while you are on the hormones, you will lose your libido—your sexual drive. You may also feel "different," or notice a slight personality change, and this is also because of the hormones. This effect will wear off when the hormones are gone from your system, and you will feel like your old self again within a few weeks.)

IN MEN WITH A RISING PSA AFTER RADICAL PROSTATECTOMY

Men most likely to benefit from radiation after prostatectomy:

- Gleason score of 7 or lower, *and*
- Negative seminal vesicles and lymph nodes, *and*
- Recurrence of PSA more than four years after surgery.

Men most likely not to benefit:

- Gleason score of 8 or higher, *or*
- Positive seminal vesicles or lymph nodes, *or*
- PSA recurrence within a year after surgery.

What Happens if PSA Comes Back Again, or if I Have Distant Metastases?

The return of PSA is a possibility that strikes terror in the heart of every radical prostatectomy patient; in fact, for many men, the dreaded follow-up PSA tests after surgery can be almost worse than having the operation itself. Although radical prostatectomy provides excellent cancer control in most men with clinically localized disease, in the past about 20 to 30 percent of men have experienced a detectable PSA level within ten years of surgery. This number is getting better, and will continue to do so as more men have their cancer detected early. But still, the worry is there: What will you do if your PSA is no longer undetectable? The good news is, *you may not need to do anything for years.*

In a landmark paper, the largest, most complete study of the return of PSA after radical prostatectomy, Johns Hopkins doctors have developed guidelines to help patients and doctors know what to do if PSA comes back. They have produced a simple chart that accurately predicts a man's risk of developing metastatic cancer; it's the postoperative equivalent of the Partin Tables and, like those tables, this chart has the potential to be of great help as doctors and patients make decisions about what to do next.

As we've discussed above, PSA is very sensitive in detecting any recurrence of cancer. That's because only prostate cells make PSA—so if it goes up after a radical prostatectomy, it means prostate cells are still present somewhere. For all intents and purposes, it means the cancer has come back. And that is extremely frightening. The first thing many patients want to know is, "How long am I going to live?" And the first thing many doctors want to know is, "When should we begin treatment, and how should we treat this man?" Does the man have a local recurrence of cancer that would respond to radiation, or does this represent micrometastases to lymph nodes and bone?

Until now, there has been no way to tell. The study, published in the *Journal of the American Medical Association,* is based on ten thousand patient-years of follow-up data. Between 1982 and 1997, nearly two thousand men underwent a radical prostatectomy at Johns Hopkins. Of these, 315 men developed an elevated PSA (defined as being higher than 0.2 nanogram/milliliter). Eleven of these men opted for early hormone therapy, and were not included in the study. The remaining 304 men were followed carefully. This study included eighty-three men in whom radiation therapy—given at the time PSA increased—failed to control the disease.

We set out to answer a few basic questions: Could we predict how long it would take for patients who had metastases to show them on a bone scan, and then once that happened, how long they would live? *The news is actually quite good: Most patients do very well for a long period of time.* On average, it took eight years from the time a man's PSA first went up until he developed metastatic disease—which suggests that *there is no need to panic* at the first sign of a rise in PSA. And at fifteen years after surgery, a projected 82 percent of men will still be free from metastatic disease. Even after developing metastatic cancer (detected by bone scans and other imaging techniques), men still lived an average of five years—and if the metastases showed up more than seven years after surgery, men had a 70 percent chance of being alive seven years later.

"When men see their PSA levels rise again, they think that means the cancer is back and they need to get treated right away," says oncologist Mario Eisenberger, M.D., a co-author of the study. "But men often live for years without having the cancer spread. This information will better equip doctors and their patients to decide what treatment—if any—is most appropriate."

This interval between the reappearance of PSA and the first sign of advanced disease can be predicted, we found, using three pieces of information:

- The Gleason score of the pathologic specimen (the removed prostate, evaluated by a pathologist after surgery). Is it Gleason 7 or lower, or Gleason 8 or greater? *And,*
- The time it takes for PSA to come back. Is it less than two years after surgery, or greater? *And,*
- How rapidly is the PSA level doubling? Is it greater or less than ten months?

Using these criteria, men and their doctors can pinpoint the likelihood of developing metastatic disease. For example: If a man has Gleason 7 disease, has his first PSA recurrence more than two years after surgery, and has a PSA doubling time longer than ten months, his likelihood of being free of metastasis seven years after the first PSA elevation without any treatment is 82 percent. Conversely, if a man has Gleason 7 disease, but his PSA goes up within two years of surgery, and the time it takes PSA to double is less than ten months, his likelihood of being metastasis-free seven years after his first PSA elevation is 15 percent.

So the first thing these tables can do is reassure the many patients who are going to have a long-term, symptom-free, metastasis-free interval, that close observation is all that's really necessary. On the other hand, says urologist Alan Partin, another co-author of the study: "If their chances of progressing rapidly are high, they may wish to start hormonal therapy earlier or get involved in an experimental trial" of more aggressive treatment. "These tables are going to help men who are at low risk and help men at high risk make a more educated decision. We hope it will also decrease the anxiety for some of them." The tables will also provide invaluable baseline data for future drug research, adds Partin. "Until now, it's been difficult to know if a drug was helping someone, because you couldn't be sure what the disease would have done on its own. Now, researchers can compare their treatment groups with our study group and tell if their treatment is improving survival."

WHAT THE NUMBERS MEAN

If you have a Gleason score of 5–7

And your time to first PSA recurrence was greater than two years:

- If your PSA doubling time was greater than ten months:

Your chance of *not developing metastasis* (having a positive bone scan) in:

> Three years: 95 percent
> Five years: 86 percent
> Seven years: 82 percent

- If your PSA doubling time was less than ten months:

Your chance of *not developing metastasis* in:

> Three years: 82 percent
> Five years: 69 percent
> Seven years: 60 percent

If you have a Gleason score of 5–7

And your time to first PSA recurrence was less than two years:

- If your PSA doubling time was greater than ten months:

Your chance of *not developing metastasis* in:

> Three years: 79 percent
> Five years: 76 percent
> Seven years: 59 percent

- If your PSA doubling time was less than ten months:

Your chance of *not developing metastasis* in:

> Three years: 81 percent
> Five years: 35 percent
> Seven years: 15 percent

If you have a Gleason score of 8–10:

- *And* your time to first PSA recurrence was greater than two years:

Your chance of *not developing metastasis* in:

> Three years: 77 percent
> Five years: 60 percent
> Seven years: 47 percent

- *Or* your time to first PSA recurrence was less than two years:

Your chance of *not developing metastasis* in:

    Three years: 53 percent
    Five years: 31 percent
    Seven years: 21 percent

Where do I go from here? The above information can help you and your doctor decide whether you would benefit from immediate treatment, if your PSA comes back after radical prostatectomy. In Chapter 12, we talk about all the options that men in this situation should consider.

Cancer Control after Radiation Therapy

Understanding the results of radiation therapy is complicated. How many meters in a mile, or yards in a kilometer? Comparing the cancer control results of radical prostatectomy and radiation often requires similar deciphering and calculation, as we attempt to convert one system to another and find a common denominator. For surgeons, the definition for success after radical prostatectomy is simple: A PSA level of 0.1 nanogram per milliliter or lower is considered "undetectable." A PSA of 0.2 or higher signals a recurrence of cancer.

But with radiation, many studies have no standardized, definitive PSA cutoff point between success and failure. For most studies, the key concept is *PSA nadir*—the lowest point PSA reaches after treatment. Because radiation's effect is gradual, it generally takes two or three years for PSA to hit rock bottom. Some men reach this nadir much more quickly—as soon as three months—and some men take much longer, almost ten years. Ideally, once PSA has reached its lowest level, it should stay put.

We know that if treatment is going to eliminate the entire prostate, *PSA must be driven to a very low level—less than 0.5, or better yet, 0.2.* In other words, PSA should fall to the undetectable range after radiation, just as it ought to after surgery. Why is this low PSA number so important? Again, prostate cancer is a multifocal disease. In other words, there's usually no single "ground zero," an absolute bull's-eye where cancer starts. Instead, it's more complicated. In most men, as we've discussed earlier, there are usually about *seven separate tumors* within the prostate. *Thus, any treatment that only kills "most" of the prostate may not be good enough in the long run—because if there's any prostate tissue left, it's possible that cancer could develop there, too.* For radiation treatment to cure cancer as well as surgery does, it must accomplish what radical prostatectomy does—eliminate the entire prostate. When PSA levels are undetectable, less than 0.5, it is safe to assume that there is no surviving prostate tissue.

In a study from the DeKalb Medical Center in Atlanta, of men who achieved a PSA nadir of less than 0.5, 95 percent were cancer-free at five years, and 84 percent at ten years. But in men whose PSA didn't fall quite so far—between 0.6 and 1.0—only 29 percent were cancer-free at five years.

Some doctors consider a patient cured if he has a higher PSA—between 1.0 and 1.5. (For that matter, some even assume everything's okay if a man's PSA after radiation is in the "normal" range—lower than 4.0.) But a PSA of 1.0 to 1.5 means that 10 to 15 grams or more of viable prostate tissue could still be there in the body (because the PSA level in the blood is about 10 percent of the weight of the prostate). Even if there is no cancer in this tissue—even if it's perfectly normal tissue—theoretically it could still become cancerous in the future.

With radiation therapy, the standard definition of relapse, or "biochemical failure" (this means that PSA levels start creeping back up), is unique as well. The American Society for Therapeutic Radiology and Oncology (ASTRO) defines biochemical failure as *three consecutive rises in PSA after it reaches its nadir.* The problem with this is that the PSA increases are not always consecutive. A man's rise in PSA with one test might be followed by a transient decrease in the next, followed by another increase. Although there's clearly something not right here, under these guidelines, this man's treatment would still be considered a success—even though it's just a technicality. The ASTRO guidelines suggest that a man should have a PSA test every three or four months during the first two years after treatment, and then every six months after that. But it can take a couple of years for PSA to fall to its lowest point, and then—if the treatment didn't work—several more years before failure is declared. Thus, experts state that the ASTRO criteria are only accurate for patients who have been followed for longer than five years.

Also, if you received an LHRH agonist (a form of hormone

therapy—see Chapter 12) before radiation, this can have a profound effect on PSA. For men who have received an LHRH agonist, the average time to normalization of testosterone is about six months. Also, the time it takes to recover testosterone levels in the blood is shorter in men who have received hormone therapy for less than four months than it is for men who have received hormone therapy for more than two years. Thus, in men who received hormone therapy, the low PSA may be the result of low testosterone levels, rather than the effect of the radiation.

Finally, in a Mayo Clinic study that analyzed outcomes following radical prostatectomy, the ASTRO criteria overestimated the chance of cure at 10 years by more than 20 percent. Be careful when making comparisons between surgery and radiation.

Cancer Control after External-Beam Therapy

As we've just seen, one problem for doctors and patients wrestling with statistics and results is simply figuring out how success and failure are measured by the authors of a particular study. Another is that *we probably need to throw out the longest, most mature data we have on the older, standard external-beam approach, and start all over.* The old picture of radiation is no longer accurate, and it's unfair to compare the results from even a decade ago with those achievable today. For one thing, it has become clear that in the past many men didn't get enough radiation to do the job of killing all the prostate cancer. For another, many men who received radiation were what doctors call "adversely selected" for this approach, because their cancer was too extensive for them to be cured by surgery. Unfortunately, this means that many men who received radiation in the past probably did not have curable disease to start with. Plus, the technology today is markedly better than it was a few years ago. And finally, one of our best markers for determining the extent of disease, PSA, was not available when most of these men were treated.

The bottom line is that the standard radiation therapy administered in the pre-PSA era before the 1990s did not always eradicate prostate cancer, and in many men, PSA levels have risen over time. In the past, most studies of radiation therapy relied on prostate biopsies to monitor the progress (or lack of it) of cancer. Depending on how many biopsies were taken, anywhere from 30 to 90 percent of men who received standard external-beam radiation therapy had a positive biopsy two years or more after treatment. This does not mean that *all* of these men have treatment failure, that their cancer has come back. But long-term follow-up studies have found that in many men cancer has returned. At five years after treatment, only 25 percent of patients who underwent standard external-beam therapy had low or undetectable levels of PSA. At ten years, only 10 percent did. However, despite the fact that PSA may be measurable, in many of these men it takes *several years* before any clinical signs of treatment failure (urinary tract obstruction, for example) appear. *These findings suggest that radiation therapy can effectively control local symptoms from prostate cancer in many men.* (And frankly, for many older men, it isn't going to matter too much if PSA rises slightly ten years from the time they received treatment, if the therapy has controlled the cancer.)

The conformal techniques have brought great promise to radiation therapy. Still, because these techniques have only been in widespread use for about a decade, there can be some uncertainty in understanding the results. The clearest short-term yardstick may be the PSA nadir, the lowest point PSA reaches after treatment. One study, of 743 patients at Memorial Sloan-Kettering Cancer Center in New York, confirmed that higher-intensity radiation does a better job in achieving a rock-bottom PSA. Of the men who received higher doses—76 to 81 Gy—90 percent achieved a PSA nadir of 1.0 or less; 76 percent of men who received 70 Gy, and 56 percent of men who received 64.8 Gy, achieved those low PSA levels. But there was a tradeoff—the men who received higher doses of radiation also had a significantly higher rate of gastrointestinal side effects, urinary tract complications, and impotence. To overcome these side effects at high doses, intensity-modulated radiation therapy (IMRT) may have an advantage.

In a study of proton therapy, scientists at Loma Linda University Medical Center in California looked at men with early-stage (T1 to T2b) prostate cancer. They found that 65 percent of the men achieved a PSA nadir of 0.5 or lower.

Because all of the new, high-dose, conformally directed, external-beam techniques for radiation therapy have been in widespread use for such a short time, it is difficult applying the ASTRO criteria. However, at five years, in favorable patients (men with low-grade, early-stage cancer), cancer control rates of 91 percent have been reported.

If you study the medical literature, you will find many studies using the ASTRO criteria to evaluate short-term results of all of the forms of radiation therapy. But again, for now it remains unclear—for all the reasons mentioned above—just how durable these results will turn out to be over the long run. The good news is that (as outlined in the surgical section above) men are being diagnosed sooner than ever. This means that more curable patients are being treated with all forms of therapy—and thus, the results of all forms of therapy should be getting better. The real question is, what will be the gold standard ten years from now? Time will give us the answer.

Cancer Control after Brachytherapy

How effective is brachytherapy by itself, without the boost of external-beam radiation, at controlling localized cancer? This is one of the most heated controversies in the field of prostate cancer treatment and research.

Interstitial radiation seeds are like little grenades, inserted directly into a prostate tumor. In theory, each radioactive seed blasts a targeted area of tissue, ultimately destroying the prostate. In practice, however, it hasn't been that simple: In the 1960s and 1970s, brachytherapy was very popular, because it appeared to have fewer side effects than surgery. Back then, doctors used a free-hand technique—crude by today's standards—and placed the seeds somewhat randomly, during open surgery. Basically, they "eyeballed" it, estimating where the seeds should go. The coverage was uneven—some of the target tissue was obliterated, but other tissue was left unscathed—and the procedure's ability to control cancer ranked a distant third behind radical prostatectomy and external-beam radiation. It took more than a decade—as it always does, when we evaluate any new procedure—for doctors to realize that this form of treatment was not effective. At ten years after seed implantation, overall about 90 percent of men had a detectable PSA level. Even in the most favorable subset of patients, men with the smallest tumors, the PSA level remained low in only 60 percent of patients. The procedure wasn't well suited for men with large or high-grade tumors; also, because most implantation regimens focused only on the tissue within the prostate and ignored the seminal vesicles and tissue outside it, the seeds were unable to reach cancer that had spread locally. Unfortunately, many of these patients eventually died from prostate cancer.

The ideal patient for radioactive seeds was (and still is) a man who is also an ideal candidate for radical prostatectomy and external-beam radiation therapy. Is interstitial brachytherapy as good as, or better than, either of those treatments? The answer twenty years ago was a definite no, and this procedure was abandoned.

Today, brachytherapy—now billed as an "easy outpatient procedure"—is once again gaining great popularity. Instead of the old freehand approach, doctors now use sophisticated, high-tech guidance systems, working with ultrasound or CT, and crafting a custom-designed template, for each patient. Now that the seeds can be placed more accurately and closer together, there are fewer "cold spots" that do not receive radiation. This has led many doctors and their patients to assume that brachytherapy is now effective in curing prostate cancer. Let's examine the evidence.

How do the results of seeds compare with radical prostatectomy? The most widely quoted results on brachytherapy come from the Pacific Northwest Cancer Foundation, a small hospital in Seattle. Radiation oncologists at the Seattle hospital have carefully analyzed their results, and to their credit have reported both the probability of having a low PSA nadir (less than 0.5) and the probability of cure using ASTRO criteria. These doctors are often quoted as saying that their results with brachytherapy alone are as good as the results of surgery at Johns Hopkins. We mention this claim here, not to discredit these doctors, but to illustrate how complicated it is to compare one series of patients to another.

As we discussed earlier in this chapter, a long-term study of radical prostatectomy at Johns Hopkins, dating back to 1982, found that at ten years, 66 percent of men had an undetectable PSA. In the series of patients who underwent interstitial brachytherapy at the Pacific Northwest Cancer Foundation, at ten years, 60 percent of men had a PSA less than 0.5. On the surface, these results do sound very similar. However, the results reported from Johns Hopkins included five hundred men who underwent surgery in the pre-PSA era (before 1989)— when, unfortunately, many men were diagnosed when the cancer was not curable. Furthermore, the results at Johns Hopkins included everybody—men with all grades and stages of cancer—as opposed to the men in the Seattle study, who were selected for brachytherapy alone because they were "best-case" patients; all had Gleason scores less than 7, and most had small tumors with relatively low PSA levels.

How would these men have fared if they had undergone surgery instead? At Johns Hopkins, we decided to make a true comparison, looking at a group of men who—following the selection criteria used by the doctors in Seattle—had comparable Gleason scores, PSAs, and clinical stages. In that group, *at ten years after surgery, 98.6 percent of the Johns Hopkins patients who underwent surgery continued to have an undetectable PSA, of less than 0.2 nanogram per milliliter.*

It is difficult to compare two different treatments at two different institutions. But these findings, and the way they are presented to patients, give us concern as to whether brachytherapy alone, in the long run, will prove to be an effective means for controlling cancer. These Seattle results are the same as those achieved with the old, free-hand approach—the handheld technique for implanting iodine seeds in open surgery—which is now nearly universally considered to have been unsuccessful. The same group of Seattle radiotherapists used external-beam radiation plus seeds to treat men with larger tumors, with Gleason scores of 7 or higher. At ten years, 75 percent of these men had a PSA of less than 0.5. Why weren't the men who received seeds alone, who had less aggressive cancer to begin with, faring as well as the men with larger, more aggressive cancer who received external-beam radiation therapy plus the seeds? This evidence raises further concerns about whether seeds alone are maximally effective.

However, the Seattle doctors counter that the results may be inferior because the men who had a recurrence of cancer were more likely to have palpable disease, higher PSAs, and their Gleason scores may have been undergraded. Men who are contemplating radiation seeds, who have a life expectancy of at least fifteen years, should consider this statement very carefully. This may be true, but there is often more tumor in the prostate than doctors expect. It is difficult to know who may need more than seeds alone.

How does radical prostatectomy compare to combined therapy— radioactive seeds plus external-beam therapy? This combination may prove more successful. Radiation oncologists at the Georgia Center for Prostate Cancer Research have actively studied this approach, using ProstRcision—iodine seeds followed by external-beam radiation. They, too, have been consistent in reporting PSA nadir as the best end point for judging success. In doing so, they also have reported that their ten-year disease-free survival rates were comparable to the ten-year results after radical prostatectomy at Johns Hopkins. However, a closer look at the evidence suggests that when apples are compared to apples, this may not be the case.

Between 1984 and 1993, 90 percent of the men in the Georgia series were treated with open retropubic implantation of radioactive seeds, and all of these men underwent removal of the lymph nodes. But the center only reported its results on the patients who had cancer-free lymph nodes; again, the Johns Hopkins study includes everybody—even men who turned out to have cancer in the lymph nodes (about 7 percent of the men in this study).

At ten years, the Georgia Center reported that about 65 percent of these men had a PSA less than 0.5, and about 57 percent had a PSA of less than 0.2. When we look at the patients with negative lymph nodes who underwent a radical prostatectomy at the Johns Hopkins Hospital during the same time interval, about *77 percent* of patients who underwent radical prostatectomy during the same time period had PSA levels less than 0.2 at ten years. Thus, 20 percent more patients who underwent surgery had undetectable PSAs than patients who received ProstRcision. In a more recent study, the Georgia investigators updated their results by adding 670 men who underwent transperineal implantation of iodine seeds beginning in 1993. However, the average follow-up in this recent group is only two years, which is the average time it takes to develop the PSA nadir, and the longest follow-up is only five years—not enough time to predict long-term outcome. Thus, it's unclear how they claim that at ten years, the disease-free survival rate is 72 percent.

Which Form of Radiation Therapy Is Best?

This is the $64,000 question. And the answer is . . . we don't know. Again, no long-term studies are long-term *enough*, yet, to tell us how men fare with brachytherapy, conformal external-beam radiation therapy, or a combination of the two, with or without the addition of hormonal therapy.

In studies comparing seed implantation's results in controlling cancer to other therapies, the seeds have come in a distinct third to radical prostatectomy and 3-D conformal radiation therapy. One Harvard study, published in the *Journal of the American Medical Association,* concluded that at five years after treatment, there was no real statistical difference in outcome among men at low risk of metastases (T1c or T2a cancer, PSA less than 10, a Gleason score of 6 or lower) who had surgery, external-beam radiation, or brachytherapy (with or without neoadjuvant hormone therapy). However, men at intermediate risk (stage T2b or Gleason score of 7, or PSA between 10 and 20) and high risk (stage T2c, PSA greater than 20, or Gleason score of 8 or higher) treated with radical prostatectomy or external-beam radiation did better than those treated by implant. But that's about it: *The pinnacle achieved by brachytherapy so far is that at five years after treatment, for the men in the "best" category of prostate cancer—those most likely to be cured—it's not any worse than the other two treatments.* In no major study has interstitial brachytherapy ever proved a *better* method than the other two main forms of treatment for prostate cancer. Nor has the combination of seeds plus external-beam radiation been shown to outperform high-dose 3-D conformal treatment.

What will the results of these radiation treatments be after ten or fifteen years? This is a crucial question for healthy men under age seventy-five, who can expect to live long enough to *really need to know* the answer. But nobody knows. Remember that—especially if somebody tries to tell you that a certain form of radiation treatment, or a particular hospital's success rate, has excellent long-term cure rates. People who make these claims should be able to back them up, and prospective patients have the right to know such criteria as:

- What was the preoperative PSA, clinical stage, and Gleason score of the patients they treated? (If they're all in the elite, low-risk group, then the five-year success rate *ought* to be good.)
- What are they using as an end point? Does "success" mean an undetectable PSA? Or is the definition slightly more fuzzy—a low PSA, or a PSA that fluctuates, but hasn't risen a certain number of times?

- In what era were their patients treated? Before or after PSA came into widespread use?
- Are they comparing apples to apples—men treated during the same era?

It is possible that during the next ten years, we'll know for sure which form of radiation therapy is best. But if radiation oncologists keep changing the technique, because they're not yet satisfied with the results, we may not—because when the treatment changes, results achieved with the outdated model of therapy are meaningless.

What about high-dose-rate (HDR) brachytherapy? The results with these high-powered, "temporary" seeds (described in Chapter 9) are just coming in. Using ASTRO definitions of biochemical failure in men with PSAs lower than 10, at five years, 94 percent of men appear to be cancer-free.

The bottom line: Radiation—brachytherapy and external-beam— is a moving target now. The good news is that more patients are curable today, and radiation oncologists are constantly trying to improve their approach to the disease, working to improve curability and reduce side effects. But it's going to take years for the dust to settle, and for results to become clear. These approaches sound good, and look promising. We just don't know yet for sure.

What Happens if My PSA Goes Up after Radiation Treatment?

The purpose of radiation treatment is to disable the prostate, to stop cancer there from continuing to grow. Because the prostate is the source of PSA, it's pretty obvious that something is wrong if PSA is still being made, and there are two possibilities here: either the cancer has reactivated locally, to the prostate or surrounding tissue, or a distant metastasis—a tiny bit of cancer that probably escaped the prostate before treatment began—has started causing trouble.

It is often difficult after radiation therapy for a patient to know where he stands. Many doctors delay making the call that treatment has failed—sometimes even for several years—on a technicality. This is especially true with the ASTRO guidelines, discussed above, which require waiting, first of all, for the PSA to "bottom out," or achieve its nadir, and *then,* for three consecutive rises in PSA. Unfortunately, if the treatment does fail to control the localized cancer, and if time goes by before corrective action is suggested, the window of opportunity may be squandered; it may not be possible to salvage the situation with further treatments to the prostate bed.

But what if a man has been followed closely, and he and his doctor face the possibility that the cancer has not been controlled sooner—when his PSA starts to rise—rather than later?

To determine if you are a candidate for surgery after radiation, you will need to have a prostate biopsy, to confirm that the return of cancer is local, and an evaluation for distant metastases. The guidelines above (see "What Should I Do if My PSA Comes Back after Surgery?") may eventually be adapted for men after radiation, but the overriding principles can be useful here in identifying the probability of metastases. If you have a high Gleason score (8 or greater), or if the PSA begins to rise early after radiation therapy, or if the PSA has a rapid doubling time, it is likely that you have metastases.

If the cancer appears to have stayed put—to still be localized to the prostate—what are the options? "Salvage" radical prostatectomy, "salvage" brachytherapy, and cryotherapy.

In the past, with standard radiation therapy and with less sophisticated brachytherapy, performing a radical prostatectomy on a man who had undergone radiation treatment was a nightmare. The prostate was adherent to everything around it, and very difficult to remove cleanly; in fact, it was often necessary to remove the bladder as well. The side effects were high, particularly the risk of incontinence and of rectal injury. With the advent of 3-D conformal external-beam therapy, it may be easier to perform surgery as a salvage procedure. There is too little information yet about salvage surgery after brachytherapy to make a judgment. Under the best circumstances, in men who appear to have no evidence of distant metastases, the likelihood of being cancer-free following a salvage radical prostatectomy at five and ten years is about 50 percent and 30 percent, respectively. The price for this, in quality of life, is high. About 60 percent of men have persistent urinary leakage requiring two or more pads a day, and about 20 percent eventually undergo placement of an artificial sphincter. Erectile dysfunction is almost inevitable.

Recently cryotherapy—freezing the prostate, discussed below—

has been considered as a plan B for radiation patients with a rising PSA. Although there is little long-term information yet on how this affects the tumor, complications are much more likely here, as with any salvage procedure. One study from researchers at the University of Texas M.D. Anderson Cancer Center and the University of California–Los Angeles found that complications are much worse if the urethra is not warmed (in an attempt to kill the entire prostate) during cryotherapy. In a study of 112 men who underwent salvage cryotherapy between 1992 and 1995, the researchers found that "quality of life may be compromised by urinary incontinence, impotence, tissue sloughing [during urination], problematic voiding symptoms and/or perineal pain [pain between the rectum and scrotum] in a substantial number of patients following salvage cryotherapy. Effective urethral warming is essential in reducing complications and maximizing quality of life. Salvage cryotherapy does not appear to offer any quality of life advantages compared to salvage prostatectomy." In a review of cryotherapy in *Urology Times,* one urologist from the University of Texas M.D. Anderson Cancer Center in Houston cited the rate of side effects for cryotherapy after radiation (as opposed to the side effects of cryoablation as a primary treatment) as "too high."

What about additional radiation? This is a third option—either additional external-beam radiation, or brachytherapy. Long-term results and complications of either treatment as a salvage procedure are not yet known. There is limited experience with salvage brachytherapy, in men whose cancer returns after external-beam radiation therapy. Although preliminary results suggest that it might be effective, about 25 percent of the men who undergo this procedure are incontinent within five years. If you are considering this option, it is essential that the procedure be performed by someone who is skillful in delivering more radiation to an already irradiated area.

Or, your doctor may want you to start long-term hormone therapy. If you are otherwise feeling fine, with no evidence of metastatic disease, this may not be a good idea. Hormone therapy, discussed in detail in Chapter 12, is nothing to enter into lightly. Many men have very slow, gradual elevations in their PSA for years and have no symptoms of cancer. If you're not on hormone therapy, you can enjoy a normal life (including a normal sex life), and simply be followed closely with watchful waiting. Then—only if or when you develop symptoms from local recurrence or metastatic disease—you can consider further treatment.

In "New Options on the Horizon," above, we mention some of the most exciting advances in treating advanced disease. These are discussed in greater detail in Chapter 12.

How Well Does Cryotherapy Work?

Again, the downside of evolving technology: There are no long-term studies to help us evaluate the success of cryotherapy in controlling cancer. The procedure has been refined recently; doctors performing it have switched to argon from liquid nitrogen, and increased the number of probes from five to as many as eight. Have these changes made a difference? We won't know for several years. Whenever any technology is improved, the clock starts all over again for scientists who are evaluating it. As we've discussed earlier in this book, even if a miracle cure comes along tomorrow, it won't be proven to eradicate prostate cancer until the men who have been treated with it have been cancer-free for at least a decade. We do know that results of cryotherapy in the early 1990s were not impressive. At two years after treatment, 20 percent of men treated with the five-probe method had positive biopsies, and 70 percent had detectable levels of PSA. A critical study that used biopsies to determine whether men had any residual prostate tissue found that only 39 percent of men had complete prostate ablation (destruction). With the six- to eight-probe method, the prostate is completely killed in only 53 percent of men. Researchers at the University of California–San Francisco found that only 60 percent of men had a low PSA four years after treatment. The very best results show only 70 percent of men have a low PSA at five years after treatment—the same result seen at ten years after surgery.

Currently, cryoablation is used to treat men with localized prostate cancer as well as men who have undergone unsuccessful radiation treatment. Again, we come back to the critical question: Does it work? As more men opt for this therapy, this question is becoming increasingly important. To answer it, we need thoughtful studies that not only determine the risks of late complications, but that demonstrate cryoablation's long-term success in controlling cancer. Even the pioneers of this treatment do not recommend it for the young, otherwise healthy man who most likely has organ-confined disease. However, reported two researchers from Allegheny University of the Health Sciences in Pittsburgh, in the journal *Contemporary Urology,* there is a role for cryoablation. It is a "very viable option for patients with bulky lesions, high-grade lesions, clinically localized legions with high PSA, radiation failures, and for those patients whose age or comorbidity [other health problems] make them a suboptimal candidate for conventional surgery." For example, the researchers stated, cryoablation may benefit a man with stage T2b, Gleason 8 cancer, who has a PSA of 20: "Even if biochemical 'cure' is not obtained, one can achieve very effective local control with low morbidity," or side effects.

Final Thoughts on Treatment for Localized Prostate Cancer

What's the best form of treatment for localized disease? This is a major dilemma for men and their doctors, because it's a moving target: There are multiple options. Worse, there are many definitions of success, and study results that can vary widely, depending on the stage of disease at which a patient is treated. Is it possible that the improved techniques for radiation therapy will be able to eliminate all prostate tissue, and approach the "gold standard" achieved by total surgical removal?

Surgeons will tell you that up to now, every time radiation therapy has been used to treat localized prostate cancer and every time an improved form of treatment has supplanted another, eventually the failure rates were higher than everyone had hoped. This is true. However, it is possible that this time it will be different—that with state-of-the-art imaging and high-dose delivery techniques, it may be possible for radiation therapy to kill all prostate cancer. Unfortunately, we have—at best—only five- and ten-year data on which to make this decision. Many men who can expect to live for fifteen, twenty, or more years may be unwilling to take this gamble—especially when they know that with a time-tested technique such as radical prostatectomy, their quality of life after treatment can be excellent if they find the right person to perform the surgery. There are other, equally thoughtful, people who will be willing to take this chance, because they don't want to be subjected to the risk of side effects associated with surgery.

In addition to this uncertainty about outcomes, you must take into consideration some of the external factors that can sway someone's decision. The news media are constantly reporting "what's new." That's their job; but it's not always clear from the newspapers and TV that "new" doesn't always equal "best." Prostate cancer is a publicized disease these days (unlike the bad old days, when men didn't speak of the disease, and either didn't know to get tested for it, or were afraid of what they'd find out). At least once a month, we hear about some celebrity or political figure who is diagnosed with prostate cancer, and what form of treatment he has chosen. It's easy to think, "That guy is a multimillionaire; he must have the best doctors in the world, and if this is what he's chosen, it must be the best treatment there is." Well, sometimes it is, sometimes it isn't. Also, in today's world of instantaneous everything, many patients have the idea that they should be able to receive effective treatment without any complications—that they should be cured today, and be able to play golf tomorrow.

There are more subtle factors at work here, too. In today's health care economy, many physicians are being strongly affected by reimbursement patterns. Insurance companies and HMOs are paying less for traditional surgery. Frankly, many urologists have found that they can make more money during the same period of time it would take to perform one very difficult operation by performing two outpatient procedures that require no postoperative care. Finally, the companies that make devices, and the pharmaceutical companies that make drugs, are in a high-stakes business, where marketing their wares to patients (through advertisements, and carefully placed stories in the media) and physicians can bring in astronomical profits. So when you sit down and talk to your doctor about what you should do, take into consideration these outside influences.

What's the best form of treatment? The traditional way to determine this, for any disease, is "randomized" clinical trials, in which men are randomly assigned to undergo one form of treatment or another, and the long-term results are eventually collected. If this route is taken in prostate cancer, it will take many years for mature results to become available. This will be a very good thing to do. But what do we do in the meantime? One problem is that men choose specific medical centers for a reason—namely, that center's expertise in a particular form of treatment. It is unlikely that a man who goes to a center known for one particular treatment strength would choose another form of treatment in the interests of impartiality and the betterment of science.

I believe the quickest, most reliable results will come from non-randomized comparisons of treatment by a blue-ribbon registry. Experts in all the fields here—urology, oncology, radiation, and radiation oncology—should name their most respected, impartial colleagues to a registry that can compare treatments performed at different centers. This registry should agree on the characteristics of the candidates for treatment—their age, any other illnesses they may have—and should develop a stratification of risk to determine, in groups, who is curable and needs to be cured, using standard, easily available criteria such as PSA, Gleason score, and clinical stage.

Furthermore, they need to agree on a standard for cancer control. Should it be an undetectable PSA, a PSA less than 0.5, or should the ASTRO criteria be used across the board? And finally, they should agree on ways to evaluate the quality of life of men before and after treatment. When all of this is in place, they should enlist medical centers of excellence—centers where the side effects are the lowest, and cure rates highest—to participate, so that comparable patients given different forms of treatment at separate institutions can be compared. With a powerful resource such as this, over the next decade we can know with confidence which form of treatment is truly better.

11

ERECTILE DYSFUNCTION AFTER TREATMENT FOR LOCALIZED PROSTATE CANCER

Read This First

Men who have trouble with erections after surgery or radiation therapy have normal sensation, normal sex drive, and can achieve a normal orgasm. Their only trouble may be in achieving or maintaining an erection—that's the bad news. The good news is that this problem, called erectile dysfunction (ED), can always be treated.

Why does ED occur? There are many reasons in addition to the fact that a man has had prostate treatment. Aging is one reason for ED. But ED can also result from medical conditions such as diabetes or hypertension, from certain medications, from overuse of alcohol, cigarettes, or other drugs, even from emotional or psychological problems.

The bottom line is that for most men, ED does not have to be a permanent situation. If there's a will, there's generally a way.

The important message here is that after treatment for prostate disease (except for men treated with hormone therapy), recovery of sexual function is almost certain. Take heart!

What Is Erectile Dysfunction?

As its name suggests, erectile dysfunction (ED) means trouble having or maintaining an erection. There's no minimum age requirement for ED; it can happen to *any* man, at any time. It's especially common after treatment for prostate cancer with prostatectomy or radiation therapy. Having ED does not mean your sex life is over—far from it. In fact, a man with ED has *normal sensation, normal sex drive, and can achieve a normal orgasm.* He may just need a little help with erections. And this is a problem that can be fixed.

The purpose of this chapter is to let you know two things: First, that *you're not alone.* By age sixty-five, about 25 percent of all men—those who have been treated for prostate cancer, as well as men who have never had it—experience at least some trouble with ED. In the United States alone, ED affects an estimated *10 to 30 million men.* (Note: ED is different from the loss of libido, or sex drive, that results from hormone therapy—discussed in Chapter 12.) A recent report from the Massachusetts Male Aging Study suggests that the incidence of ED triples from 5 to 15 percent between ages forty and seventy. Aging (and the general nerve loss that goes along with it; see below) is one reason for ED. But ED also can result from medical conditions such as diabetes, hypertension, or multiple sclerosis, from certain medications, from overuse of alcohol, cigarettes, or other drugs, even from emotional or psychological problems.

The second point here is that *help is available.* For most men, ED does not have to be a life sentence. If there's a will, there's generally a way.

AFTER RADICAL PROSTATECTOMY, TESTOSTERONE GOES UP

Some men experience a loss of libido—sex drive—after radical prostatectomy. This is different from impotence or difficulty with erections. It's not about having trouble with sex—it's about not wanting to have it at all. Some scientists have theorized that perhaps after surgery, there is a decrease in male hormones (particularly, testosterone), and maybe this accounts for the diminished libido in some men.

But a recent Johns Hopkins study has found that this is not the case; in fact, it's the opposite of what we suspected. Before we go any further, let's take a quick look at testosterone: The story begins in the brain—in the pituitary gland, which makes a hormone called LH (luteinizing hormone). In the chemical chain of events involved in the production of testosterone, the pituitary is the thermostat, a regulator that controls the testes—the "furnace," in effect. The furnace cranks out heat—testosterone—which, in turn, stimulates the prostate. The level of testosterone in the blood is constantly monitored by the brain, which regulates how much LH is needed.

This study showed that when the prostate is removed, LH goes *up*—and so, then, does testosterone—suggesting that the prostate somehow produces a substance that controls LH secretion. The investigators were studying the effect of radical prostatectomy on these hormones in sixty-three men, wondering whether some change in hormonal makeup might explain a loss of libido experienced by some men after surgery. In normal men, the major factors that influence sexual function are blood flow, nerve supply, and hormones. A great deal of attention has been placed on studying how to avoid disrupting the nerve supply and blood supply during surgery—but up to this point, there has been little attention as to what happens to the hormones.

The newly discovered information, that the pituitary gland makes more LH after radical prostatectomy, suggests that the prostate is also making an inhibitor that regulates the release of LH from the pituitary, raising the fascinating hypothesis that the prostate itself may influence hormone levels in an effort to modulate its own growth.

The increase in testosterone is not noticeable, but it certainly dispels the idea that a loss of male hormones contributes to a loss of the sex drive. Instead, a more likely cause of this diminished libido after surgery is depression. In many cases, treating the depression restores the sex drive back to normal.

What Happens in Normal Sexual Function?

Normal erection in men can be reduced in medical terms to a "vascular event," but this seems too simple a description for the delicate, complex interplay between blood vessels (veins and arteries) and nerves. The penis itself is a remarkable structure, made up of nerves, smooth muscle tissue, and blood vessels. It has three cylindrical, spongy chambers that are essential to erection; one of these is called the *corpus spongiosum*, and the other two are called the *corpora cavernosa*.

When sexual function is normal, this is what happens: A man becomes sexually aroused. A substance called *nitric oxide* is released by the nerve endings, and the smooth muscle tissue in the penis begins to relax. The spongy chambers (also called sinousoids) within this smooth muscle tissue begin to dilate. Meanwhile, arteries continue to pump blood, as usual, into these spongy chambers of the penis. As the penis elongates, the veins are stretched; they clamp down against the thick tissue that surrounds the corpora cavernosa—shutting themselves off so the blood can't leave the penis. The chambers become engorged, and this keeps the penis "inflated" during sexual activity. An erection is born.

After ejaculation, nitric oxide stops being released; the smooth muscle tissue contracts and the blood flow to the penis is reduced—the veins ease their viselike grip. Once again, blood is allowed to leave the penis, and the erection goes away.

What Can Go Wrong?

There are four components to normal sexual function in men—*libido* (sex drive), *erection, emission of fluid* (ejaculation), and *orgasm*. All of these elements are regulated separately; there is no centralized "sex control center."

Libido: The sex drive is controlled by two things—by male hormones, and by psychological and environmental factors. The major male hormone that affects libido, testosterone, is made in the testicles. When this hormone supply is shut off—as it is in hormonal therapy (actually, hormone *deprivation* therapy) for advanced prostate cancer—testosterone levels fall considerably, to extremely low levels. When this happens, most men on hormonal therapy lose all interest in sexual activity. Men who have undergone a radical prostatectomy or radiation therapy may also experience a loss of libido, but it's not caused by the loss of testosterone, and it's not usually as severe. There is some evidence that radiation therapy may cause a slight decrease in the production of male hormones, although this is unlikely to be significant enough to reduce sexual function. Surprisingly, after radical prostatectomy, testosterone levels actually go *up* (see above). The most likely cause of diminished libido after surgery is depression (one of the body's natural responses to stress, this can happen after any serious medical treatment), and in many men, treating the depression restores the sex life back to normal. (Other pharmacological agents may help with loss of libido, as well; see below.)

Erection: Probably the most common sexual problem for men after prostate treatment is the inability to have an erection sufficient for sexual intercourse. The nerves that lead to and from the penis are extremely important to erection. Particularly essential are nerves in the two bundles that sit on either side of the prostate (see illustrations in Chapter 8). Even if these nerve bundles are not removed during radical prostatectomy, they can still be damaged by the surgery. They also can be injured during radiation treatment, and other procedures including cryotherapy. But remember, these nerves are only necessary for erection—not for sensation, and not for orgasm. The nerves that are responsible for sensation travel outside the pelvis for a long distance. These nerves are not close to the prostate, and should not be damaged. Loss of erection after radical prostatectomy or radiation is what doctors call "multifactorial"—in other words, it's probably not caused by one single problem.

In the most skilled surgeon's hands, if both neurovascular bundles are preserved during a radical prostatectomy, potency should return in at least 80 percent of men in their forties and fifties, and 60 percent of men in their sixties. However, only about 25 percent of men over age seventy are potent after surgery. Why are the numbers so much lower? We think a large part of the problem is something that comes with the territory of aging in general—a gradual loss of all nerves, including those involved in erection. When a younger man undergoes a nerve-sparing radical prostatectomy, it's likely that about 20 percent of the nerves involved in erection are damaged, 60 percent are preserved normally, and 20 percent are temporarily disabled, but eventually recover. This explains why, for most men, sexual potency doesn't just snap back like a coiled spring.

So at best, a younger man after prostatectomy has about 80 percent of these nerves left for erection. But as we age, we constantly lose nerves. By age 60, a man only has about sixty percent of the nerves he was born with—which means that if 20 percent of them are damaged by treatment for prostate cancer, fewer than 50 percent remain. This explains why ED is more common in older men after surgery, and in men in whom it is necessary to remove one neurovascular bundle.

Erection problems also can result from vascular injury—damage to the blood vessels in the penis. For a normal erection to occur, the arteries that supply blood to the penis must be intact. This blood supply can suffer after radiation treatment; in fact, damage to these arteries is believed to be the main cause of ED after radiation treatment, although recent studies suggest that radiation may also injure the neurovascular bundle. In a few men, this blood supply also can be reduced by radical prostatectomy—even though the major arteries that supply the penis do not normally travel next to the prostate. In these men, for some reason the major blood supply to the penis runs *inside* the pelvis—instead of outside, as it does in most men, and these arteries can be damaged inadvertently during radical prostatectomy. At Johns Hopkins, once we recognized this, we modified our surgical technique, and now any major arteries that run on top of the prostate can be saved.

Another major problem with erections in men after radical prostatectomy or radiation therapy results from a problem called "venous leak." What happens here is that, although the blood flows normally into the penis, it doesn't stay there; the small veins that carry blood back to the heart can't keep it trapped inside. The valve that "dams up" this venous blood works passively. The penis must be fully engorged with blood in order for these veins to be shut off. If a man never gets a full erection, then there's a constant leak. Also—yet another consequence of aging—as men get older, the fibrous tissues that surround the penis weaken, and this, too, undermines the ability of the veins to hold back the blood.

Dry ejaculation: In normal ejaculation, several events must take place. Sperm, which are made in the testicles, travel to the epididymis, a "greenhouse," in which they mature. During orgasm, sperm are rocketed from the epididymis through the vas deferens during a series of powerful muscle contractions. They shoot through the ejaculatory ducts and mix with fluid produced by the prostate and seminal vesicles. Simultaneously, a muscular valve in the bladder neck slams shut, forcing this fluid out the only possible exit—through the urethra and penis to the outside world, rather than backward into the bladder.

After radical prostatectomy, there is usually no emission of fluid because the prostate and seminal vesicles, which produce the vast majority of this fluid, are gone and the vas deferens has been shut off. (Thus the term "dry ejaculation." A few men, however, do continue to produce a small amount of ejaculate. This fluid comes from the nearby Cowper's glands; like the prostate and seminal vesicles, these are known as "sex accessory" tissues.)

After radiation therapy, many men also have a loss of ejaculate fluid because the glands responsible for making this fluid are dried up. In any event—no matter what causes dry ejaculation—the lack of fluid should not interfere with orgasm. This is because orgasm doesn't really have much to do with the prostate. Think about it—women don't have prostates, yet they do have orgasms. Here's why:

Orgasm: Orgasm happens primarily in the brain. For orgasm to take place, there must be sensation and stimulation. In men who are impotent after radical prostatectomy or radiation therapy, sensation is not interrupted; therefore, orgasm should always be possible and it should be no different from the way it was before treatment. Many men don't realize that they can have an orgasm without an erection, and they're surprised to hear that half of the people in the world have orgasms without an erection—women. (Again, it's different for men receiving hormonal treatment for prostate cancer; orgasm is not an issue because—although a few can still have erections—the treatment causes a loss of interest in sexual activity.)

What Can You Do about ED?

Talk to your doctor. The first thing you can expect is to have a detailed history and physical taken. The doctor is going to try to pinpoint the exact problem, and figure out what's causing it. Is it trouble with libido, erection, ejaculation, or orgasm? Even though it may seem pretty obvious—your erections were just fine before prostate cancer treatment and inadequate or nonexistent afterward—the doctor needs to rule out the possibility that any other medical or psychological problem is causing this.

You may be asked to fill out a questionnaire so you don't have to discuss details face-to-face, or your doctor may ask you some very specific questions. You'll probably be embarrassed; most men would rather be almost anywhere else, discussing almost any other topic, than in a doctor's office talking about ED. But you shouldn't be embarrassed. This is private, sensitive, confidential information. Everything you discuss in the doctor's office will remain there. Remember: This certainly won't be the first time that your doctor has heard about such problems, and it won't be the last—there are millions of other men in America alone with this same problem. And finally, remind yourself that this discussion is the first step to solving the problem.

Probably one of the first questions your doctor will ask is whether you ever wake up at night with an erection. Most men have several erections while they're asleep; these are usually associated with dreaming, and they happen during a particular phase of sleep called REM, for rapid eye movement sleep. (Because men tend to wake up in the morning with these erections, they often connect them with having a full bladder; this is just coincidence.) The idea behind this question is to make sure there's no mental or emotional problem causing the ED. In other words, if a man can't produce an erection during sexual activity but has several a night while he sleeps, this is a clue that the nature of the problem is not physiological, but psychological. This type of erection problem is called "psychogenic," and it's often treated successfully with counseling.

Your doctor will also ask whether you have a history of cardiovascular disease. Men who have had a heart attack, men who have coronary artery disease, hypertension, elevated blood lipids, or who smoke have a greater chance of having vascular problems. Aside from the obvious health risks, smoking causes arteries to contract. Smoking is an easily reversible cause of ED; if you quit smoking, you could greatly improve your ability to have an erection. One of the first steps in erection is for the arteries to dilate; they fill up the penis with blood. If they're contracted, they won't be able to dilate very well. *The arteries in the penis are the same size as the arteries in the heart.* If you have heart disease, hypertension, atherosclerosis ("hardening" of the arteries), or high cholesterol (which can contribute to heart disease), it is very likely that these arteries in the penis have already been compromised.

A history of neurological disease—diabetes, for example—may be a cause of ED. Also, certain drugs may contribute to sexual problems, and combined with prostate treatment, they may result in ED. Cimetidine, for example, is a drug used to treat ulcer disease; but it's also an antiandrogen; it blocks the action of testosterone. Other medications that can cause ED include drugs to treat high blood pressure such as beta-blockers and thiazides, medications to treat depression such as monoamine oxidase inhibitors and tricyclic antidepressants, antipsychotic drugs, sedatives, drugs to treat anxiety, and drugs of abuse such as opiates. (And don't forget alcohol and cigarettes—they're drugs, too.) Basically, it's a good idea if you're on *any* medication—even herbal or dietary supplements—to check with your doctor and make sure the side effects don't include ED. Switching from one drug to another may make a big difference.

Diagnostic tests: Your doctor may want you to undergo further evaluation, which may include something called a "nocturnal penile tumescence test." This sounds like a form of torture, but all the name means is that it's a test to see whether you have erections during your sleep (see above). If your doctor suspects a problem with penile blood flow, you may need to undergo pulsed Doppler evaluation. This test uses high-resolution ultrasound to evaluate the arteries' blood supply to the penis. Another test involves the injection of smooth muscle relaxants through a small needle directly into the penis; the idea here is to see whether an erection can be produced. If this shot doesn't cause an erection, this is a good hint that there's a vascular problem—trouble with arterial blood flow. Sometimes during this test a man develops an erection but gradually loses it; this usually signifies that there's a problem with the veins—they're not shutting off the blood supply, so the blood is escaping from the penis, and thus the erection is failing. Note: Surprisingly, psychological factors can prevent the penis from becoming erect in spite of this powerful pharmacological stimulation. This shows the true influence of mind over matter, and here again, counseling may provide significant help.

PEYRONIE'S DISEASE AND RADICAL PROSTATECTOMY: IS THERE A LINK?

Peyronie's disease is a disorder of the connective tissue within the penis that can cause curvature during erection. It's fairly rare—diagnosed in only twenty-six out of 100,000 men each year, most of them in their fifties and sixties. But Johns Hopkins urologists have spotted what they believe may be a small yet significant trend: Peyronie's disease seems to be more common in men who have had a radical prostatectomy. Is this just coincidence? The age group is roughly the same. Or does the procedure itself—or a man's recovery from it—somehow contribute to development of the disease?

"Peyronie's disease is like arthritis of the penis," says urologist Jonathan P. Jarow, who specializes in treatment of erectile disorders. "When you get scar tissue deposited in the connective tissue of your joints, you get arthritis. It's a similar problem in the penis." Sometimes this buildup of scar tissue causes a telltale bend, or curvature in the penis (which appears only during erection). It may also manifest itself as palpable or painful lumps—which may be terrifying for a man to discover. "Many men worry that they have penile cancer," says Jarow, "but we can tell just by examining them exactly what it is." He hastens to reassure his patients that although the disorder may be annoying, it is not life-threatening: "Men aren't going to live any longer or shorter because of it."

Although nobody knows what causes Peyronie's disease, scientists believe that it's related to a series of minor injuries—or, as Jarow explains, "wear and tear." One theory "is that it's due to repetitive, minimal trauma to the penis from buckling that occurs when you're attempting sexual relations with an incomplete erection, and that this repetitive trauma leads to buildup of scar tissue." Peyronie's disease appears to be more common among men who have ED, notes Jarow. "It's not clear whether it's secondary to some of the treatments, such as vacuum erection devices, or injection therapy, or whether it's due to having erection problems to begin with, and is independent of the treatment."

In a new study that will include one hundred patients, three out of sixty-four radical prostatectomy patients so far have developed "rapid appearance of new-onset Peyronie's disease" after surgery, says Jarow. "This sounds very low. But if you compare that to the incidence of Peyronie's disease in the general population, it's one-thousand-fold greater."

In some men, there may be an inherited component to Peyronie's disease (as there is with other connective tissue disorders); Jarow is seeking men with a family history of the disease in hopes of finding genetic proof. "What makes us so interested in the radical prostatectomy patients—and we are just beginning to investigate this—is that, hopefully, if we can understand the mechanism behind Peyronie's disease in this setting, we may be able to prevent it in men undergoing radical prostatectomy in the future, as well as in other men."

The good news is that Peyronie's disease does not progress forever. "In some men [fewer than 20 percent], it goes away completely by itself," says Jarow. "For most people, it eventually stabilizes. The pain goes away. The lump becomes less prominent, and the curvature lessens. In just about everybody, the disease process, the deposition of scar tissue, stops with time."

Men who were fully potent when the disease began generally remain so, Jarow notes. "In other words, erection problems—specifically, problems with rigidity—are a rare result of Peyronie's disease in general." But most men who have had a radical prostatectomy have at least some temporary trouble with erection; thus, treatment depends on a man's specific symptoms.

"If a man's problem is curvature—if the penis is bent so he cannot en-
gage in sexual activity, or it's uncomfortable to his partner—then we can
do an outpatient surgical procedure to straighten the penis," says Jarow.
"If, however, he has significant curvature that prevents sexual relations *and*
problems with rigidity, then he's treated with insertion of a penile prosthesis combined with penile straightening," also an outpatient procedure.
If a man simply has erection problems but no serious curvature, he is
"treated like anyone else with an erection problem, starting with pills, then
shots, then the vacuum device, then if necessary, a penile prosthesis."

Recovery of Potency after Radical Prostatectomy

You've had a radical prostatectomy, and one or both bundles were
preserved. Which means that the potential for erection is there. So
what's the problem? Why isn't it happening?

The first bit of advice your doctor will probably give you here is:
"Be patient." Erections return gradually. Maybe better advice is: Be *very*
patient. It can take up to four years for some men to experience full
recovery of potency. Your body has been through a trauma; it needs
time to recover. Now, this doesn't mean you should give up on sexual
relations until the day you wake up with a full erection, or until four
years goes by—whichever comes first. By no means. Also, know that
the erection you have two months after surgery is not the same one
you'll have two years from now. *Most patients experience an improvement in their erections over time; the quality improves month by month.*

Normally, men become sexually aroused, have an erection, and
then pursue sexual activity. But after radical prostatectomy, the
stimuli that cause an erection are different; visual and mental stimulation are not nearly as important as tactile sensation—what the penis
can feel directly. Usually, soon after surgery the only way a man can
achieve an erection is with direct sexual stimulation. This changes the
sequence of events. Before surgery, visual or psychogenic stimuli
would bring on an erection, which led to interest in sexual activity.
Now, men need sexual stimulation to produce an erection sufficient
for intercourse. You will need to be proactive. In other words, you and
your partner need to bypass the brain as an instigator or even a "mid-
dleman," and speak directly to the penis. Thus, don't be afraid to
experiment with sexual activity (although it's best to wait until six
weeks after surgery, to be sure everything is well healed).

If you have a partial erection, go ahead and attempt intercourse—vaginal stimulation is the best stimulation to improve your erection. So don't wait until you have the "perfect erection." (If you do, you could be waiting a long time and missing out on this important aspect of your life.) Use whatever erection you have to attempt vaginal penetration; you will probably find that the erection soon becomes much firmer. Use of lubrications such as Astroglide (available at most drugstores) also will help tremendously. Remember, you can have an orgasm even without an erection (and don't be surprised that it is dry—see above).

Early on, however, erections are often not sufficient for traditional vaginal penetration. One common reason for this is the venous leak described above. Even though the arteries are doing their job and filling the penis with blood, producing a partial erection, the veins aren't keeping the blood trapped inside the penis. To improve this situation, many men find that if they attempt sexual activity standing up, they'll be able to achieve a much firmer erection. (The escaping blood has to travel all the way back up to the heart, and this takes longer if a man is standing up than if he's lying down.) Sexual activity can continue either while a man remains standing, or while he's kneeling. Also, it may help to attempt entry from behind; the vagina opens more easily if a woman is bending forward.

Another way to combat venous leak is for men to place a soft tourniquet at the base of the penis *before* they begin foreplay or sexual stimulation. The purpose of the tourniquet is to *keep blood in the penis,* once the stimulation causes the arteries to dilate and penile blood flow to increase. The tourniquet doesn't impede blood flow *into* the penis; it just keeps it from going back out. You can achieve the same effect with a rubber band, a ponytail holder, or—if you're brave enough to venture into a novelty store—a device called an erection ring.

To sum up: The return of sexual potency is different in every man. Again, for some men, it can take as long as four years for full potency to return. For others, intercourse is possible just a few weeks after surgery. In any case, you don't have to wait for the penis to become erect on its own.

Finally, it's worth repeating that almost all men who can't obtain an erection after radical prostatectomy still have normal penile sensation and are able to achieve a normal orgasm. Therefore, even if you are not having erections—and even if you need some extra help—your recovery of sexual function is almost certain. Take heart. As for the extra help you may need, there are five basic approaches, discussed below.

Loss of Potency after Radiation Therapy

Radiation's effect on potency is much more gradual than surgery's immediate impact. Sexual function may be fine immediately after radiation therapy. However, ED may develop gradually, over the next one or two years. The slow, late progression of ED has been blamed on radiation damage to the arteries that provide blood to the penis. However, there is some recent evidence that radiation also may damage the neurovascular bundles, especially after brachytherapy. In an effort to protect these delicate nerves and reduce the chances of impotence, radiotherapists are developing new ways to estimate the amount of radiation delivered to this area.

Solutions to the Problem of ED

Before we go any further, let's just say right here that some men have very little sexual activity before treatment for prostate cancer, and frankly aren't that interested afterward. That's very common, particularly in older men, and there is absolutely nothing wrong with a man who is not concerned about having an erection.

However, many men who were very sexually active before treatment want this part of their lives to continue. What's next? The first thing that needs to happen is that you need to involve your partner. The worst thing you can do—take it from a doctor who has seen the unnecessarily devastating effect ED can have on patients' relationships—is to clam up, wrap yourself up in shame, self-pity, failure, anger, or any other negative emotion you can think of, retreat to a distant corner of the bed, sulk, agonize, and not talk to your wife about this. Your wife should understand what's going on, and she should be part of the solution. Shutting her out will only make her feel rejected, and will compound the problem in many different ways.

Second, as mentioned above, experiment early (as soon as six weeks after surgery, sooner after radiation treatment). *Anything* you can do to bring new blood into the penis will speed up your recovery of spontaneous erections. Many men don't understand this. They don't want to use a "crutch," because they think it will slow down the body's own efforts to recover potency. This is hogwash. Think of it, if you will, as recovering from any other injury—a broken leg, for example. At first, crutches are necessary. Two of them. Then, as you get stronger, maybe you taper down to one crutch, then a cane. Then you walk, run, and join a marathon, if you wish. The same is true for sexual activity. Experiment early—with a tourniquet or elastic band, if necessary—and if you need more help, we suggest the following "crutches," in this order:

- Phosphodiesterase inhibitors, such as Viagra
- Intraurethral therapy
- Penile injection therapy
- Vacuum erection device
- Penile prosthesis (implant)

We suggest you begin with a pharmacological approach—phosphodiesterase inhibitors such as Viagra; intraurethral therapy; or an injection—because these truly bring new blood flow into the penis, and are most likely to "jump-start" the spontaneous recovery of erections. Some men worry that if they start using some of these approaches, they will always need them—they'll become dependent on them, and spontaneous sexual activity will never return. This couldn't be further from the truth. These approaches will actually *speed up* recovery, by bringing in blood flow to the penis. Remember: Think of them as a crutch. Once spontaneous activity begins to recover, you can throw them away.

Viagra and Similar Drugs

The phosphodiesterase inhibitor Viagra (the chemical name is sildenafil) is a remarkable breakthrough. (Note: Viagra has become the generic name of its class, like "Band-Aid" or "Xerox." But at the writing of this book, several similar drugs are being developed and tested, and one of these agents may turn out to be more effective for you.) It works very well in many men after radiation therapy, and in men after radical prostatectomy, too—but only if the neurovascular bundles have been spared. (Investigators who report that Viagra isn't terribly effective after radical prostatectomy are probably working with men who did not undergo an effective nerve-sparing operation.)

Viagra has been called a wonder drug. What does this mean? Will it put a spring in your step, revitalize your marriage, pay your bills, and generally solve all your problems? No. Is it an "instant erection" pill? No. Contrary to the plots of some recent TV sitcoms, and despite many a comedian's monologue, taking the drug Viagra is not followed by a hearty "boing!" Instead, to understand what happens, we need to take a brief look at the biochemistry of erection.

Several years ago, researchers discovered that the chemical messenger, or neurotransmitter, nitric oxide plays a crucial role in erection. We discussed this briefly above, but here are some of the nitty-gritty details: When a man is sexually stimulated, tiny nerve endings in the penis release nitric oxide, which causes the smooth muscle tissue in the penis to relax and the blood vessels to dilate. If an erection, like every chemical process in the body, is a domino effect, or cascade of events, then nitric oxide is roughly step one. For the next link in the chain, nitric oxide activates another chemical switch, called cyclic GMP—known in scientific terms as the "second messenger"; this is the active agent within the blood vessels and smooth muscles that causes the dilation and relaxation. Here, we might consider cyclic GMP to be the "gasoline" running the engine: How much cyclic GMP you have determines how strong your erection is, and how long it lasts. Obviously, erections aren't meant to last forever, so there is also an "off switch"—another chemical, an enzyme called phosphodiesterase. Now, cyclic GMP is active in many organs of the body, and the "off switch" phosphodiesterase comes in many forms, specifically targeted to various tissues. In the penis, the particular brand of phosphodiesterase needed is called Type 5. Viagra acts by *blocking* the action of Type 5 phosphodiesterase, and in this way, it amplifies the action of whatever cyclic GMP (the "gasoline") is present. This is why, fortunately, Viagra has little effect in any other tissue in the body—except for the retina. One of the minor side effects of Viagra is that it may cause some temporary vision disturbances (in 3 percent of men who take it). Other side effects include headaches (in 16 percent of men), flushing (in 10 percent), and upset stomach (in 7 percent). Future generations of phosphodiesterase inhibitors may do a better job of protecting the retina as well.

How well do phosphodiesterase inhibitors work after radical prostatectomy? In the Johns Hopkins experience of men who are unable to have intercourse more than one year after an operation in which both neurovascular bundles were spared, *80 percent* are able to have successful intercourse after treatment with Viagra. But again, not only is Viagra not an "instant erection" pill—it may not even work very well early on, in the first few months or even the first year after surgery. We think this is because the nerves are temporarily paralyzed. However, as these nerves recover, Viagra works better and better. Thus, if you take Viagra six weeks after surgery and it doesn't work, you should try again every month until it does.

Also, be sure you're taking it right: Viagra works best if it's ingested on an empty stomach. Never take Viagra after a big meal, or a meal heavy in milk or fatty food; these can block absorption of the drug. Then, it takes about an hour for Viagra to reach its peak strength in the blood. At this point, a man needs to have sexual stimulation. (Again, as discussed above, immediately after surgery, just thinking about sex isn't going to be enough. Here, sexual stimulation needs to be tactile.) Soaking in hot water increases blood flow in the pelvis; this might be a good way to spend the hour between the time you take Viagra and when you attempt intercourse. (This has also been reported to improve the effectiveness of MUSE—see below.) Remember, Viagra does not create an erection; it only facilitates one. If you find that an initial dose of 50 milligrams doesn't work, you can increase the dose to 100 milligrams. Do not take more than 100 milligrams of Viagra every twenty-four hours.

Who should not take Viagra? If you have any history of cardiovascular disease, talk to your cardiologist before you take Viagra. Despite the fact that it's mainly targeted to the penis, Viagra is not safe for men with certain medical conditions.

Do not take Viagra if:

- You are taking any form of nitrate, such as nitroglycerin.
- You have had an irregular heartbeat or heart attack in the last six months.
- You have low blood pressure (lower than 90/50).
- You have high blood pressure (greater than 170/110).
- You have congestive heart failure or chest pain.
- You have retinitis pigmentosa.

Some men who have used Viagra to have intercourse have had heart attacks and died. This is probably not a direct effect of the drug, but was probably related to the exercise associated with intercourse. Many men who have heart disease do not exercise, or don't exercise regularly. These are the "weekend warriors" who have heart attacks after exertion they're not accustomed to—playing pickup basketball, perhaps, or shoveling snow or moving heavy furniture. If these men have ED, they may rarely experience intercourse, and the sexual excitement that goes with it. However, if Viagra makes them able to have intercourse, and this causes them to exercise to a point where they shouldn't, then this is probably the reason for the heart attacks. The safest bet for you is to talk to your doctor first. If you can't exercise, or you have any other limitations on your physical activity, do not take this drug.

The "sons of Viagra": The next generation of Viagra is on its way. There is promise that these newest drugs may work faster, in less than half an hour; that they may last longer—for example, that you might be able to take the drug at night, and still have it active in the morning—and that they may cause less of a drop in blood pressure, and thus be safer.

Other pharmacological approaches: New medications, not yet commercially available, may join the market within a few years. One is an oral form of phentolamine. Another is apomorphine, a drug that acts centrally in the brain as a dopamine agonist. Apomorphine has been reported to induce erections in as many as 60 percent of men with ED. However, it has undesirable side effects that are not conducive to romance—mainly, the fact that many men who take it become nauseated or vomit. Also, it appears that a drug called a melanocyte-stimulating hormone (MSH) may have a powerful effect on libido. As we mentioned earlier, many men, for reasons that are unclear, state that their libido is reduced after treatment of prostate cancer. One reason for this is depression, and antidepressants can be of great help here. There is a new super-potent MSH analog, which has been effective in inducing erections in early studies—even in men with psychogenic ED.

In the future: We've talked about why injury to the nerves that control erection can cause ED. A number of experimental studies currently under way are aimed at preserving these nerves. In animals, several studies have shown that growth factors may enhance recovery of nerve function more rapidly. There is also some exciting evidence that gene therapy may one day be used to transfer growth factors directly into the penis, and boost nerve stimulation.

New methods of application are also under study. Scientists are working on a topical approach, salves or gels that contain vasodilators (drugs that cause blood vessels to open up) such as prostaglandin, papaverine (a calcium channel blocker derived from the opium poppy), or nitroglycerin.

Intraurethral Therapy

Another approach to pharmacological treatment is the use of agents that can be placed directly into the urethra. One of these is called MUSE (Medicated Urethral System for Erection), a tiny suppository that contains a vasodilator called prostaglandin E1. The best thing about MUSE is that it's easy to administer. First, urinate (to empty and moisten the urethra). Then, place a suppository into the end of the urethra while you are standing. Then, massage the penis for fifteen minutes while the drug is absorbed; it may help to use a tourniquet at the base of the penis as well. MUSE works in about 40 percent of patients. However—and this is a big "however"—MUSE probably won't be ideal for many men after radical prostatectomy. For some reason, prostaglandin E1 often causes severe pain in men who have undergone a radical prostatectomy. But men who have ED for other reasons (including ED after radiation therapy) do not experience such pain, and for these men, it can be a valuable resource.

Penile Injection Therapy

Injection therapy is one of the best ways to bring new blood flow into the penis, and encourage recovery of sexual function. Again, the ideal situation is that you won't need this forever—consider it a crutch or a "jump-start," as described above, until your body recovers enough to handle erection on its own.

How does it work? The keys to a normal erection are for the arteries to open and fill the penis with blood, and for the veins to close, so the blood can't escape the penis; the smooth muscle tissue also needs to relax. Several drugs can produce erections by making these events happen; most of these are in a class of drugs called alpha-blockers, which are used to treat some forms of hypertension and also to treat BPH. They are vasodilators; they open up blood vessels, making a wider channel for blood to go through. They also cause the smooth muscle tissue to relax and the veins to close. The main advantage here is that these drugs produce an *absolutely normal erection.* Some of these erection-producing drugs include papaverine, phentolamine, and prostaglandin E1.

It usually takes less than five minutes for one of these drugs to work, and the erection can last as long as a couple of hours. It will be important for your doctor to determine the *lowest possible dose* you need to achieve an erection; this will help reduce the risk of side effects. Other ways to help lessen side effects include limiting injections to no more than once a day, and using an insulin syringe (which has a smaller needle than many syringes) to minimize pain and bleeding from the injection. Also, men should compress the site where the needle went in for three minutes after the injection; this also helps reduce bleeding and tissue damage.

Again, a common side effect for men after radical prostatectomy is that prostaglandin E1 is often very painful. These men should ask their physician to prescribe a different blend of injection, called "trimix," which contains papavarine, phentolamine, and smaller amounts of prostaglandin E1. This may reduce the pain considerably.

Penile injection is not for everybody. These erection-producing agents may not help men with vascular problems. However, they do work in most patients. Because of the nature of this therapy—giving the penis a shot—it obviously is not ideal for men who can't see well, men with poor hand-eye coordination, or men who are very overweight. Also, because many erection-producing drugs reduce blood pressure, this can cause problems for some men with heart disease.

One side effect is that if the injection is too strong, it can produce a prolonged erection that may require some medical therapy to relieve it. Some doctors ask patients who opt for penile injections to sign a consent form because of some other side effects—some of them long-term—associated with the injections. These can include tiny blood clots, burning pain after injection, damage to the urethra, or minor infection. But the worst is that in some men, over time, painless, fibrous knots of tissue build up in the corpora cavernosa, and this can cause the penis to become curved. (For more on this condition, also called Peyronie's disease, see above.) Doctors aren't entirely sure why this happens; it may be related to the frequency of injection, strength or dosage of the drug used, and the amount of bleeding resulting from the shots. Some doctors believe compressing the site at the time of injection may be critical to minimizing this risk; also, keeping the dosage to a minimum, or using a blend of several drugs, may help.

Vacuum Erection Devices

The idea here is to create suction using an airtight tube that is placed temporarily around the penis. An attached pump withdraws air, creating reduced atmospheric pressure—a vacuum—around the penis, causing it to become engorged with blood. The penis becomes erect. Then a constricting ring, like a rubber band around the neck of a balloon, keeps the blood trapped in the penis, so the erection can be sustained. (This imitates the clamping action of the veins in normal erection.) It usually takes about five minutes to produce the erection, and it generally lasts for about half an hour. (The erection probably shouldn't last much longer than that; leaving the constricting band on too long can cause distention or swelling due to fluid retention in the penis.)

This erection is not quite the same as a normal erection—it begins only above the constricting band. But it is sufficient for successful intercourse. However, the penis is usually cold, and sometimes numb, and from the man's standpoint, the erection is often less than desirable. Also, because this approach does not bring new blood flow into the penis, it may not do much to facilitate the recovery process. Vacuum devices have few complications; these can include trouble with ejaculation, pain in the penis, and tiny, pinpoint-sized bruises. (Men taking aspirin or other blood-thinning medications may be more likely to experience such complications.) Some men are highly satisfied with the result of vacuum devices; others are not.

Penile Prostheses (Implants)

Penile implants, or prostheses, are available in several varieties; the simplest are bendable, and the more complicated ones are inflatable or mechanical. The implants are not a new idea, but they have improved considerably since they were first introduced about twenty years ago. The bendable prostheses, for example, were exactly the same size *all the time*—whether or not the penis was in the erect position—which, as you can imagine, often proved awkward in social settings. Earlier models of the inflatable prostheses that did allow for a "nonerect" size sometimes failed to work and needed to be replaced.

If these relatively clumsy but functional early designs were the prosthetic equivalent of the typewriter, then the latest models are more like a Macintosh—sleek, sophisticated, and user-friendly. They are more reliable, easier for surgeons to implant, and are designed to look more natural in the "nonerect" phase—even the bendable prostheses, which are more malleable than before. *And they can restore sexual function entirely to normal.*

Now, most prostheses are implanted into the penis through an incision in the scrotum. Some of the more complicated devices involve a pump and a reservoir for fluid, housed in the abdomen or scrotum, and inflatable chambers, which are placed in the corpora cavernosa. (Fluid is pumped into the penis to create an erection and held there by a valve. Afterward, the valve is released, and the fluid returns to the reservoir.)

Penile prostheses used to be offered routinely to most impotent men. Now, with other good treatments available, many urologists have come to regard penile prostheses as a last resort because they do involve surgery—and thus, they carry the risk of complications. These can include infection, scarring, damage within the corpora cavernosa, or a problem with any part of the prosthesis. However, these side effects are relatively rare. Most men who have penile prostheses are satisfied with the result and have a normal sex life.

Prostate cancer is hard on everybody. Wives, partners, and family members feel the stress of prostate cancer and treatment, too. You're all sharing the burden of this disease. Your priorities change, your focus shifts, and your usual best lifeline—each other—may temporarily flag, from the physical and emotional stress. The worst thing you can do during this recovery process is try to "go it alone." The best thing you can do is talk about it—with each other, your doctor, other patients and their wives, a counselor or member of the clergy. And go back and read this chapter over again, as many times as you need to—because it is full of hope. Be patient. You will get your life back.

12

HELP FOR ADVANCED PROSTATE CANCER

<table>
<tr><td>

Help if You're In Pain
    Drugs for Pain
    Complementary Approaches
      to Pain Management
    Drugs for Milder Pain
    Drugs for Moderate to
      Severe Pain
Treating Specific Pain
    Spot Radiation
    Radioactive Strontium
When Additional Treatment
    May Be Needed
    Spinal Cord Compression
    Pathologic Fracture

</td><td>

Other Complications
    Fatigue
    Urinary Tract Obstruction
    Weight Loss
    Constipation
Complementary Medicine
    The Mind-Body Connection
    Faith, Prayer, and Spirituality
    Can Changing Your Diet
      Affect Your Cancer?
Note for Wives, Partners, and
    Caregivers—Take Care of
    Your Own Health, Too

</td></tr>
</table>

Read This First

As you are reading this, scientists are working on the cure. Research into advanced prostate cancer has exploded with whole new classes of innovative, cancer-fighting drugs and treatments targeted at various stages of the disease. Perhaps even more exciting, scientists are rethinking their strategies for giving these drugs—going after prostate cancer when it is still relatively young and vulnerable, hitting it hard, and hoping to change the course of the disease. The bottom line: Even when cancer has escaped the prostate, there is still much hope—more now than ever before.

Hormonal therapy: The mainstay for the management of advanced disease is hormonal therapy—shutting down the hormones that feed the prostate and nourish the cancer. Unfortunately, some prostate cancer cells aren't affected by hormonal therapy at all. These are called hormone-independent (or androgen-independent) cells.

When a man starts hormonal therapy, the early results are successful and highly encouraging: The tumor shrinks, PSA levels drop in the blood, and the patient feels better. When this happens, many men rejoice, believing the cancer cells to be utterly defeated. But only the hormone-*dependent* cancer cells have been affected—and the drop in PSA may be misleading. So when PSA falls, it signals that the cancer is responding to treatment—which is good, but it's no guarantee that the cancer is completely gone. The cancer cells that have nothing to do with hormones are oblivious to all of this.

There are several forms of hormonal therapy; these treatments can be used individually, or in combination. They are all designed to accomplish the same goal: to lower testosterone levels in the blood. The most direct and least expensive way to control testosterone is to surgically remove a man's testicles; this is called an orchiectomy, or surgical castration. The same effect can be accomplished medically, with drugs called LHRH agonists, or anti-androgens. For obvious reasons, this is the most popular approach today.

When should you begin hormonal therapy? First, if you have metastases to bone, or bone pain, or a large mass of cancer that is obstructing your kidneys or bladder, you need to start hormonal therapy now. In this situation, hormone therapy is the right course of action—one that can make a huge, vital difference in the quality of life and can protect your body from the ravages of cancer.

But what if you have no cancer in your bones, no sign that anything is wrong—except a rising PSA after surgery or radiation, or the presence of cancer in your lymph nodes—and you feel fine? Many doctors would advise you to start hormonal therapy as soon as possible. Others—and I'm in this group—believe that there is no evidence that starting hormonal therapy now, as opposed to later, will prolong life. *But doesn't early hormonal therapy delay the progression of cancer?* The answer is, yes and no. It delays your *knowledge* of progression. It doesn't stop the clock. Hormonal therapy does two things: It stops cells from making PSA, and it shrinks the hormone-sensitive cell population. However, hormone-insensitive cells continue to grow, silently.

"Nonhormonal" approaches: These are a far cry from the old chemotherapy drugs, with their "buckshot" approach—killing everything, good and bad, in range, with limited effect in prostate cancer. These new treatments work like a high-powered rifle, with only one target in their sights: prostate cancer cells. They're specifically designed to target the biological mechanisms involved in cancer progression and metastasis. They can be grouped based on their mode of attack. The most promising strategies include immunotherapy, gene therapy, drugs that put roadblocks in the way of cancer's progress and keep it

from invading other tissues, drugs that slow down the cancer growth rate, and drugs that interfere with the way cancer cells communicate.

Complementary medicine: Can changing your diet help slow down prostate cancer? We don't know. It is not reasonable to assume that diet can reverse cancer after the fact—that it can "unring the bell." However, it may help. If you want to change your diet to reduce the intake of fat and increase your intake of soy, you should do it. But be careful not to lose too much weight too quickly. A rapid, ten percent drop in your weight can compromise your immune system—which may be the major self-defense mechanism that is holding your cancer in check.

A final word, for caregivers: Take care of yourself, too. You need your strength—emotional as well as physical—now more than ever. We have some advice for you in this chapter, too.

Revolution in Treating Advanced Prostate Cancer

As you are reading this, scientists are working on the cure. There have never been so many promising drugs being developed for prostate cancer, and never before have doctors been so hopeful about their ability to help men with advanced disease—cancer that either has spread beyond the prostate, or cancer that has returned after surgery or radiation.

Not only has research in advanced prostate cancer exploded with whole new classes of innovative, cancer-fighting drugs and treatments targeted at various stages of the disease—perhaps even more exciting, scientists are rethinking their strategies for giving these drugs. Armed with the guidelines (discussed in Chapter 10) that—for the first time—allow doctors and patients to predict what will happen if a man's PSA returns after treatment, oncologists, radiation oncologists, and urologists are working together to go after prostate cancer when it is still relatively young and vulnerable, hitting it hard, and hoping to change the course of the disease.

What a difference in hope this is from even a few years ago! Traditionally, oncologists have begun chemotherapy in men with advanced prostate cancer only after other treatment—surgery or radiation, followed (sometimes even years afterward, when men developed symptoms of advanced cancer) by hormonal therapy—has failed to control the cancer. But over the last few years—in breast and colon cancer, as well as prostate cancer—there has been a sea change in scientific thinking. As Johns Hopkins oncologist Mario Eisenberger puts it: "Why should we wait until it's a last-ditch effort? Why not go all-out first?"

In the past, oncologists have been unwilling to take a man who is, for all practical purposes, healthy—who has steadily increasing PSA levels, but no other symptoms of disease—and make him sick. Chemotherapy drugs have been notorious for their side effects, which often include vomiting, hair loss, and debilitating fatigue.

But the newest generations of drugs are remarkable for their relative lack of side effects: They're smarter, more specific, and many of them are aimed at containing prostate cancer, rather than eradicating it. Most are relatively nontoxic, outpatient oral medications. There are many new approaches, but the basic ideas are to stabilize the disease and inhibit growth. "So ideally, in men with minimal disease, they may delay further progression of cancer, and thus the development of symptoms. And if they're used in men with more advanced disease who are well, these men may stay well for a longer period of time," says Johns Hopkins oncologist Michael Carducci.

Carducci and Eisenberger, a pioneer in developing and refining drugs to treat prostate cancer, have identified key groups of men with advanced prostate cancer, all of whom have different needs, and who probably respond best to different drugs:

- Men who have undergone surgery, who have been identified as having a high risk of cancer recurrence.
- Men who have undergone surgery and/or radiation, who have a detectable PSA level, but no other evidence that the cancer has spread.
- Men with metastatic disease, in whom hormonal therapy has lost its effectiveness (this is also called "hormone-refractory" cancer).

"Most of the drugs have traditionally been developed and tested in this last group of men," says Carducci. "But increasingly, the drugs are showing few or limited side effects, and laboratory models suggest that they work best in patients who have hardly any disease."

The bottom line, to paraphrase a popular saying, is that *it's not your father's prostate cancer anymore*—at every step of the way. Even when cancer has escaped the prostate, there is still much hope—more now than ever before. We will cover these and other new approaches in this chapter.

Treatment of Advanced Prostate Cancer: An Overview

This is the part of the book we wish we didn't have to write, and that no one would ever have to read. But it's necessary to spell out all the facts about where we stand today—with the understanding, as we said above, that there is great hope for major advances in this area of prostate cancer.

As we will discuss in depth, the mainstay for the management of advanced disease is hormonal therapy. Hormonal therapy means shutting down the hormones that feed the prostate and nourish the cancer. (Androgens are male hormones, and many doctors use these words interchangeably; hormonal therapy is also called hormone or androgen deprivation, or hormonal or androgen ablation.) Prostate cells need male hormones to grow and develop—think of a houseplant that flourishes because it receives a steady supply of fertilizer. If the supply of hormones is shut off, the normal prostate shrinks—but *does not disappear*. If a houseplant doesn't get fertilizer, it doesn't die, either. It might struggle along on nothing but sunlight and water, but it still hangs in there. Normal prostate cells can survive without hormones, and so can cancerous prostate cells. Not having the hormones is a setback—one from which it can take years for prostate cancer to recover—but it's not a lethal blow. In fact, some prostate cancer cells aren't affected by hormonal therapy at all.

Why doesn't hormonal therapy serve as a "knockout punch" for prostate cancer? Because prostate cancer is "heterogeneous"— which means it's a cellular melting pot. It's a bunch of different cells mixed up together. When all of these cells are confined within the prostate, the fact that they're not all alike is not much of an issue. No matter how many different kinds of cells there may be, if they're all in the prostate, bang—they're all equally dead when the prostate is surgically removed or effectively irradiated. But when some cancer cells have escaped to distant sites, this diversity becomes a major challenge. A drug or hormone treatment that targets only one kind of cell won't have any effect against another variety; the "one-size-fits-all" approach doesn't work here. Plus, some of these cells have learned to be resistant—to grow in the absence of male hormones. These are called *androgen-independent* or *androgen-insensitive* cells. (And cancer that seems to defy hormonal therapy is called *hormone-refractory* disease.)

When a man starts hormonal therapy, the early results are successful and highly encouraging: The tumor shrinks, PSA levels drop in the blood, and the patient feels better. When this happens, many men rejoice, believing the cancer cells to be utterly defeated. But in the prostate, only the hormone-*dependent* cancer cells have been affected—and the drop in PSA may be misleading. Guess what controls the production of PSA? Hormones. When male hormones are shut off, the PSA-making process may indeed stop—but this doesn't necessarily mean that the cancer cells are dead, or that they've stopped growing. In animal models, scientists have shown that cancer cells can continue to grow, even when PSA is no longer made. One process has little do to with another; in fact, the nastiest, most malignant cells don't make much PSA anyway. So, when PSA falls, it signals that the cancer is responding to treatment—which is good, but it's no guarantee that the cancer is completely gone.

The cancer cells that have nothing to do with hormones just go on about their merry, proliferative business, oblivious to the hormonal war being fought just cells away. Say you had a weed problem in your garden, and instead of spraying Roundup, you sprayed Raid. What effect would this have on the weeds? Not a lot.

Scientists believe that these androgen-independent cells probably inhabit the prostate for years; they don't just suddenly appear one day after the cancer is diagnosed. Ultimately, the androgen-independent cells manage to dominate through two different means. One of these is *genetic drift.* In this case, each time the cancer cells reproduce, or divide, they accumulate more mutations, and become increasingly malignant. In the process, cells that used to depend on hormones manage to wean themselves; they learn to survive without them. The other mechanism is called *clonal selection.* Here, the most malignant cells (which originally may have been in the minority) grow faster than the better-differentiated, more sedate cells. Over time, they overtake these more normal cells. This may actually be aided, inadvertently, by hormonal therapy: The androgen-dependent cells shrink back, and the androgen-independent cells take their place.

Hormonal Therapy

Specific ways to control hormones: Doctors have long known that hormones play a major role in the life of the prostate. In 1786, an English surgeon named John Hunter became the first to demonstrate in animals that a radical operation—castration—caused the sex accessory tissues, including the prostate, to shrink. But it wasn't until the 1930s that anyone discovered *why* this happened. At the University of Chicago, Charles Huggins discovered that removing the testes *shut down production of testosterone*. And, when shots of testosterone were injected back into castrated animals, these tissues were restored to normal size and function. This Nobel Prize–winning research included another valuable finding—that castration also could shrink prostate cancer.

Huggins also was able to achieve the same effect chemically; he found he could shut down testosterone with doses of female hormones called estrogens. Estrogens blocked a signal, transmitted in the brain by the pituitary gland, called *luteinizing hormone* (LH), which stimulates testosterone. The oral estrogen, called *DES* (diethylstilbestrol), produces what's known as chemical castration; it lowers testosterone levels, just like removal of the testicles.

For now, hormonal therapy means one of two main choices: surgical castration, a "one-shot effect"; or chemical castration, a lifetime of medication. Loss of sexual function is likely with almost every kind of hormonal therapy; 90 percent of men on hormonal therapy lose sexual drive and the ability to have an erection.

What's the best method of stopping these hormones? Think of a car going through a series of checkpoints—Points A, B, C, and D—to cross over a border into another country. You want to stop this car from reaching the other side. At what point do you stop it? Do you set up a roadblock at Point A, the first stop? Or do you simply wall off the border at Point D, so the car can never cross over? Or do you divert the car at some point along the way? The androgens that affect the prostate reach their destination through a multistep process that begins in the brain. Medical roadblocks are now available to stop or detour this process at Point A (the brain), Point D (the prostate), or several spots in between.

How hormonal therapy works: Each therapy targets a different link in the chain of hormonal interactions that affect the prostate. Some of them work better than others, and some are more expensive. The chain of hormonal actions is long and complicated; put together on paper, it's a confusing jumble of letters, mostly consonants, that looks

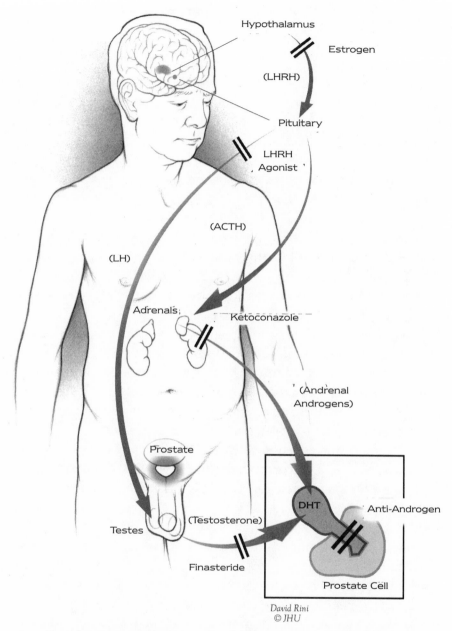

FIG. 12.1   Sources of Male Hormone Production, and Where Hormonal Therapies Actually Work

Different forms of hormonal therapy act in different ways, and break the hormonal chain at different places. Here are drugs that block either the *effect* of testosterone and other androgens (anti-androgens and finasteride), or the *production* of testosterone itself (LHRH agonists, estrogens, ketoconazole).

like alphabet soup. And if you're like most men, just thinking about this muddle will make your eyes glaze over. But, stripped down to its essential steps, this code is not so tough to crack—you can do it! (And you need to master this information, so you can not only understand what your doctor's talking about, but help choose the treatment option that's best for you. See Fig. 12.1.)

To understand this hormonal chain, let's start at the beginning— the brain, where the hypothalamus makes, among other things, a substance called *LHRH* (luteinizing hormone–releasing hormone), which acts as a chemical signal. It's dispatched in pulses, like Morse code or flashes of light, to the nearby pituitary gland. Its message? "Make LH and FSH," it tells the pituitary.

LH (luteinizing hormone) and *FSH* (follicle-stimulating hormone) are other chemical signals, and they bring us to the testicles, or testes, where LH motivates certain cells (called *testicular Leydig cells*) to make *testosterone*. (FSH has its major effect on sperm production.)

And testosterone brings us to the prostate. Testosterone circulates in the blood and enters the prostate by diffusion, like water through a tea bag. Soon it undergoes a metamorphosis: Testosterone is transformed, by an enzyme called 5-alpha reductase, into a hormone called *DHT* (dihydrotestosterone)—which is more than twice as powerful as testosterone. Several studies have shown that the prostate contains less 5-alpha reductase when it is cancerous; therefore, DHT is not believed to be as important in prostate cancer as it is in the normal prostate or in BPH. Both testosterone and DHT can bind to the same receptor in the prostate cell—like two different keys fitting the same lock. (DHT *really* binds to it, with great affinity; testosterone does not cling as strongly to the receptor.) When DHT or testosterone hooks up to the receptor, this complex attaches to DNA, which then activates certain genes.

Testosterone in the blood circulates back to square one, the hypothalamus, which acts as a thermostat. It measures the level of testosterone and decides whether to boost or cut back on its LHRH production, and the cycle begins all over again (scientists call this a "feedback loop").

Also, the adrenal glands, which sit on top of the kidneys, make weak male hormones called "adrenal androgens," including androstenedione, dehydroepiandrosterone (DHEA), and dehydroepiandrosterone sulfate (DHEAS), plus small amounts of testosterone. These are minor players, believed to make up only 5 percent or less of the total androgen stimulation to the prostate. Their total effect on the prostate has been a controversial issue (see below).

So there are several potential checkpoints in this chain of events. Currently, hormonal therapy can target the hypothalamus (LHRH), the pituitary (LH, FSH), the adrenal gland (adrenal androgens), the testes (testosterone), and the prostate (DHT). They can be used individually or in combination.

Surgical Castration

Surgical removal of a man's testicles (also called an orchiectomy) is the most direct and least expensive way to control testosterone. As surgical procedures go, it's simple. The operation can be performed under spinal anesthesia (for a description of spinal anesthesia, see Chapter 8) or, if the patient is not strong enough to tolerate this, even a local anesthetic. This is what happens: A surgeon makes a small incision in the scrotum, and brings out each testicle individually through this opening. Then the surgeon cuts the vas deferens and blood vessels that supply each testicle, and the testicles are removed. Some surgeons perform what's called "subcapsular orchiectomy." In this operation, the surgeon opens the lining to the testicles and empties the contents of each testicle. The lining is closed again, and this empty shell is placed back inside the scrotum—so nothing looks different; in other words, no one can tell from outward appearance that there's nothing inside the scrotum. The basic differences here are cosmetic—and therefore psychological—and for some men, this makes the thought of castration easier to accept.

After surgery, patients usually can go home from the hospital the same day—or, at the very latest, the next day. The only major complication to worry about with surgical castration is bleeding. However, this shouldn't be a problem if the surgeon makes a point of checking that all bleeding is stopped before the scrotum is closed, and that a compression dressing is left in place to control the smaller, harder-to-see blood vessels.

Castration works fast; it reduces the body's amount of testosterone by 95 percent almost immediately, and permanently. Boom; within about three hours after surgery, testosterone levels begin to plummet to a level called the "castrate range." This is considered the gold standard, an important point of comparison in monitoring hormonal therapy—as certain drugs are judged by their ability to reduce testosterone to this range.

Some doctors used to believe that several months after castration, the body began producing more testosterone at other sites—and that this was the reason prostate cancer continued to grow. This is not true. There is no delayed increase in testosterone and, anyway, that's not why prostate tumors keep growing—they continue to spread because of the cancer cells that are *not* affected by hormonal therapy.

What happens to the prostate tumor? It begins to shrink, and men with symptoms of obstruction or pain caused by the cancer begin to feel better right away.

Castration's advantages are that it is effective almost immediately, and that its results are permanent—there's no need to take daily medication. And, because it is a "one-shot" treatment, it's relatively inexpensive.

Specific side effects: Its disadvantages are certainly psychological (this can vary depending on a man's age and stage of illness) and cosmetic. To help alleviate the stigma of castration, some surgeons perform what's called a "subcapsular technique"—see above—in which *only* the testosterone-producing parts of the testicles are removed, and the outer shell remains. (Also, testicular implants—which make the testicles appear normal—are available for some men.) However, castration is irreversible, and for many men this is too final a treatment. (For a discussion of the general side effects of hormonal therapy, see below.)

Medical Castration

Medical castration can be accomplished in three ways: By shutting down the hypothalamic-pituitary connection (see above); by directly blocking the ability of the testicles to make testosterone; or by blocking the effects of testosterone at the target organ—the prostate. (See Fig. 12.1.)

Drugs That Shut Down the Hypothalamic-Pituitary Connection: Estrogens and LHRH Agonists

Estrogens: Many men, for many reasons, don't want to undergo surgical castration, so they opt for chemical castration—taking drugs that accomplish the same result without the cosmetic change.

DES, the main oral estrogen, targets a different checkpoint—the hypothalamus. It works by blocking the release of LHRH; in turn, the pituitary stops making LH, and this virtually shuts down the Leydig cells, the testicles' testosterone-making factories. So testosterone drops to the castrate range.

The effect is not as speedy as with surgical castration; it generally takes ten to fourteen days for testosterone to fall to the castrate range. And, it's not permanent—in most cases, the testicles start making testosterone again soon after a man stops taking DES.

We talk about DES here because it's the most widely used oral estrogen, and it's the gold standard of *estrogen* therapy (but no longer the mainstay of hormonal therapy) for prostate cancer. Other drugs, such as Premarin and ethinyl estradiol (both medications used by women during menopause) and PC-SPES are considered as effective as DES; none is clearly better. Another drug, called chlorotrianisene (Tace), is a synthetic estrogen that lowers testosterone but doesn't completely shut down its production; it also permits the body to make a little bit of LH. (It has proven to be ineffective, and is no longer used in completely lowering testosterone levels.) A drug called polyestradiol phosphate (Estradurin), injected once a month, may be easier to tolerate for men with gastrointestinal problems.

Twenty years ago, oral estrogens—easy to administer, and much cheaper than other forms of treatment—were the foundation of medical treatment of advanced prostate cancer. They aren't today, mainly because of their major, potentially fatal side effect—they raise your risk of having a heart attack or developing a blood clot. Some investigators in Europe believe that polyestradiol phosphate (Estradurin) produces fewer side effects, and may be a preferable form of treatment. However, this drug is not used widely in the United States.

Decades ago, doctors gave high-powered doses of DES—10 to 20 milligrams a day—thinking that it would not only eliminate testosterone, it might also kill cancer cells. This didn't happen; testosterone was lowered, but that was it. Then, studies by the Veterans Administration showed that lower doses could achieve the same results. But even 5 milligrams a day proved to be too much. One study found that, over time, men on 5 milligrams of DES a day died—from heart disease caused by the estrogen, not from prostate cancer! Then doctors tried 3 milligrams, and then 1 milligram a day. *And 1 milligram of DES a day*

proved sufficient to suppress testosterone without endangering the heart.
A large study in Europe found that men on 1 milligram of DES a day
showed no signs of *irreversible* damage to the cardiovascular system.

Other studies have proven that there is no statistical difference in
the life span of men who were castrated or who took 1 milligram of
DES a day. Some doctors argue that it takes 3 milligrams of DES a day
to lower testosterone to the castrate range. This is true. However, if
there's no difference in the length of survival, and the heart-related
side effects are fewer with 1 milligram than with 3 milligrams, what's
to be gained by taking the higher dose? The very interesting aspect of
this finding is that men can live just as long by taking the lower dose—
and not even lowering testosterone to the castrate range. This adds
more fuel to the fire that combined androgen blockade (discussed
below)—eradicating every last iota of male hormones—is not important, or necessary.

Still, because even with 1 milligram a day DES can cause cardiovascular problems, many doctors believe even this slim risk is not
worth the benefits, and prefer other forms of hormonal therapy.

Other specific side effects: The other main side effect is enlargement
of the breasts. This problem can be eliminated, however, with three
low-dose treatments of radiation, given directly to the breast *before*
estrogen is started. Edema (water retention, which causes swelling in
the ankles) is also common, and can be managed effectively with
diuretics. Some physicians also recommend that their patients on
DES take an aspirin every day to avoid other cardiovascular side
effects such as thrombophlebitis (blood clots in the legs) and to lower
the risk of a heart attack. Because of the risk of cardiovascular problems, men with a history of heart disease or thrombophlebitis should
not use estrogen as their main form of treatment. (For general side
effects of hormonal therapy, see below.)

Conclusion: One milligram of DES a day is just as effective as
higher doses, and 1 milligram of DES is just as effective as surgical
castration in prolonging life. However, because even this very low
dose can cause cardiovascular side effects, most doctors believe that
it's just not worth the extra risk.

LHRH agonists: Like oral estrogens, LHRH agonists shut down
production of LH and FSH. Here's how they work: LHRH is a small
protein, built of ten blocks of amino acid. A synthetic substance called

an *LHRH analog,* or *agonist,* made by changing one of the ten blocks, works by blocking LH (the hormone that tells the testicles to make testosterone). The hypothalamus acts like a lighthouse, sending out LHRH in signal pulses—like Morse code in flashes of light—to the pituitary gland. LHRH agonists work by providing prolonged signals—by turning on the light and keeping it on, instead of just sending flashes. So these drugs trick the pituitary; because the pituitary receives no flashes, or pulses, it thinks no signal is being sent—and it doesn't make LH. In turn, the testicles do not produce testosterone.

These drugs don't work right away. In fact, for about a week after a man begins taking an LHRH agonist, his testosterone level kicks into overdrive. This is called a "flare," and it happens because the constant LHRH signal initially stimulates LH production. But by about ten days, testosterone falls into the castrate range. For the first few weeks, doctors often prescribe an antiandrogen—flutamide (Eulexin) or bicalutamide (Casodex) to block this surge. On the horizon are newer LHRH analogs called LHRH antagonists, which do not produce this brief testosterone "flare," and with these drugs, short-term treatment with an antiandrogen is not necessary. (This appears to be the only major advantage of these new drugs.)

The most commonly prescribed LHRH agonists are leuprolide (Lupron) and goserelin (Zoladex). In large studies, researchers have found that these LHRH agonists are equivalent to treatment with DES or surgical castration in their ability to lengthen the time until the cancer progresses, and to prolong survival.

To sum up: LHRH agonists are basically equivalent in testosterone-lowering and life-span-lengthening results to DES, which is basically equivalent to surgical castration. The chief advantages of LHRH agonists are that they avoid the need for surgery, and they don't carry the risk of cardiovascular complications that can accompany estrogen treatment. Also, they don't cause breast swelling as often as treatment with estrogen.

Specific side effects: LHRH analogs require an injection. Long-acting agents need to be injected either monthly, or every three or four months, and a new osmotic pump has been developed that dispenses medication for one year. However, to insert it, a small incision must be made, requiring local anesthesia. Other disadvantages include the tremendous expense—LHRH agonists cost thousands of dollars a year. In 1994, the total Medicare expenditure for the treatment of prostate cancer was a staggering $1.4 billion. Of that total, $478 million was for LHRH agonists. (For general side effects of hormonal therapy, see below.)

Drugs That Block the Effects of Hormones at the Prostate

Antiandrogens: These drugs don't care how much LHRH, LH, testosterone, or DHT you make; it doesn't matter to them. (Actually, antiandrogens cause testosterone levels to go *up* because of an increase in LH.) All they do is make sure testosterone and DHT don't reach their targets—the receptors. In other words, antiandrogens act as dummy keys in the "locks," or receptors. When testosterone and DHT reach the receptors, there's already a key sitting in the lock—so they can't enter the lock and activate the receptors. Therefore, the tumor doesn't get the hormones it needs to nourish its androgen-dependent cells.

Bicalutamide (Casodex) and flutamide (Eulexin) are the most widely used antiandrogens. In Europe, cyproterone acetate is also common. (This drug, however, acts like estrogen, and rather than stimulating testosterone, it actually suppresses the hypothalamic-pituitary connection, so it lowers LH, thus reducing testosterone.)

Originally, antiandrogens were used for specific reasons, in combination with other treatments. For example, their most common use, even today, is to block the surge, or "flare," of testosterone that occurs during the first week or ten days after treatment with an LHRH agonist. (To stop this surge, antiandrogens are usually given for the first month of treatment with an LHRH agnoist.) Antiandrogens also have been given to men who needed more urgent treatment—men who came to the doctor with severe bone pain, for example, or who had large, local cancers that were obstructing urinary flow. Treatment with an antiandrogen immediately blocks the effect of testosterone, and brings relief to men who are awaiting either surgical castration, or for an LHRH agonist to achieve its full effect. They also have been administered chronically in combination with castration or an LHRH agonist—the form of treatment called combined androgen blockade (see below).

More recently, however, doctors have become interested in using antiandrogens, especially bicalutamide, as "monotherapy"—that is, as a single agent, without any other form of treatment. The main goal here is to attempt to preserve sexual function. When bicalutamide is given in doses of 50 milligrams, three times a day, sexual interest is maintained in many men; however, beyond one year, only about 20 percent of men remain potent. This 150 milligram daily dose of bicalutamide has been compared to castration in men with locally advanced and metastatic disease, although it's not entirely certain how well it works. The survival of men who start bicalutamide when they have metastatic disease appears to be less. Thus, men with metastatic disease should not be treated with antiandrogen monotherapy. However, for men who start taking it when they have locally advanced disease, the survival appears to be about the same. Thus, there is great interest in using these drugs in men with advanced cancer that has not yet metastasized to bone. Note: As we will discuss below, no form of early hormonal therapy delays progression of the disease. The only thing it delays is your *knowledge* of this progression.

Specific side effects: In addition to maintaining sexual interest, antiandrogens appear to have a lower risk of osteoporosis than surgical castration or treatment with LHRH agonists, most likely because testosterone levels are maintained. Both bicalutamide and flutamide cause breast enlargement (called gynecomastia) in about 75 percent of the men who take them. Flutamide's major side effect is diarrhea. Also, it can cause significant liver damage in some men; therefore, it's a good idea for men taking flutamide to have their liver function checked after the first few months of treatment.

Conclusion: The fact that men can retain sexual interest makes antiandrogens the focus of intense research—particularly, scientists are investigating combining these drugs with others in hopes of improving quality of life in hormonal therapy.

5-Alpha reductase inhibitors: In prostate cells, testosterone is converted by an enzyme called 5-alpha reductase into a more potent hormone, DHT; 5-alpha reductase inhibitors—drugs such as finasteride (Proscar)—block this enzyme. Finasteride's big advantage is that it preserves potency because testosterone levels in the blood remain unchanged.

Finasteride works well in shrinking benign enlargement of the prostate (BPH), where DHT plays a major role. But in prostate cancer, testosterone is more of a villain than DHT, and finasteride does little to stop it. So, by itself, finasteride is not enough. Some scientists are investigating whether finasteride may prove more effective when combined with an antiandrogen (see above).

Drugs That Inhibit Production of Testosterone

The best known drug in this class, ketoconazole, got its start as an antifungal agent. Then doctors noticed that men taking it developed breast enlargement—clearly, more than fungal problems were being treated here! Doctors learned that ketoconazole blocks production of testosterone by the testicles as well as by the adrenal androgens. It works quickly; taking 400 milligrams of ketoconazole every eight hours reduces testosterone to the castrate range within twenty-four hours. Another drug in this group, aminoglutethimide, has a similar effect. Neither drug is used very commonly today. Before antiandrogens were available, these drugs were the only way to suppress testosterone quickly. However, when antiandrogens were approved, these drugs became more or less obsolete.

Combined Androgen Blockade

This idea is not new. Investigators have been pursuing this concept since the 1930s, when scientists first began to understand the ramifications of shutting down every single hormone that could possibly affect the prostate. Some approaches have been more drastic than others—surgical removal of the adrenal glands or the pituitary, for instance.

The theory here is that even low levels of testosterone and DHT—engendered by the adrenal androgens—can stimulate cancer in the prostate, and they must be stopped. This can be accomplished by combining whatever achieves a castrate level of testosterone—surgical castration, estrogen, or an LHRH agonist—with an antiandrogen.

Combined androgen blockade became a hot concept in the medical community in the 1980s, due largely to the work of one scientist. This scientist reported that combining an LHRH agonist with an antiandrogen was far more successful than using either approach alone. But there are a few things you should know about this research: One is that *no other scientist has ever reproduced this man's original spectacular results.* In his study, 97 percent of men with advanced cancers who were treated with an LHRH agonist plus flutamide were still alive eighteen months later.

The sad truth is that in nearly every other doctor's experience, only half of patients diagnosed with metastatic prostate cancer are alive two or three years later, and no treatment, so far, has made a real difference in those numbers.

Most studies since then have shown either no difference in survival or an overall survival time lengthened by only a few months. (For more on these studies, and an oncologist's view of flutamide, see "The Flutamide Disappointment: An Oncologist's View," below.)

Unfortunately, the idea that the combined therapy can somehow stretch out the time that hormones work—lengthening by several months the time to progression of cancer—just hasn't borne fruit. These findings confirm those of another study of men on the combined treatment: In a huge analysis of about five thousand prostate cancer patients in Europe and America, doctors studied overall survival and found, at five years after treatment, *virtually no difference* between the men on combined androgen blockade and the men who underwent castration or took LHRH agonists alone. Again, unfortunately, not a stunning display of the success of combined androgen blockade.

And, after a certain point, some patients actually benefit from *stopping* antiandrogens. For example, if a man taking an antiandrogen in combined therapy begins to relapse—if his prostate cancer begins growing again, and his PSA level goes up—one step his doctors should take right away is to *stop* the antiandrogen. In from 40 to 75 percent of these men, PSA levels drop when the antiandrogen is stopped. (See "What Happens if Hormonal Therapy Doesn't Seem to Be Working?" below.)

Paradoxically, antiandrogens can make some patients—who initially were helped by them—worse. Exactly why this happens is not clear. In certain prostate cancers, over time, the androgen receptors (the part of the cell responsive to hormones) undergo a mutation—and all of a sudden, the antiandrogen *stimulates* the cancer. Remember, antiandrogens normally act like a dummy key in the "lock" (the receptor), whose purpose is to block testosterone and DHT from activating the receptor. With this mutation, however, the antiandrogen key actually works—it turns in the lock and activates the receptor. Because of this odd twist, some doctors have questioned the long-term value of taking these drugs, and believe they should be used only for a month by men taking LHRH agonists.

What about quality of life? If the addition of an antiandrogen to castration (surgical or chemical) doesn't make life longer, does it make it *better*? In one study, scientists compared the quality of life between castration and a placebo, and castration plus flutamide. Although most patients reported improved quality of life over time, the men in the flutamide group tended to show less improvement in most areas, particularly in the area of emotional functioning. (For more on depression and prostate cancer, see below.) Men in the flutamide group also had more trouble with diarrhea.

There is one crucial concept here that you need to understand: *Ultimately—although it may take years—combined androgen blockade is going to stop working, just as every other kind of hormonal therapy does.* Anyone who leads you to believe otherwise is not doing you a favor. And if hormone treatment stops working, it's not because of the tiny amounts of testosterone and DHT being made by the adrenal androgens—in other words, it's not the fault of some renegade hormones that are sneaking through the hormonal blockade. It's because of the hormonally *independent* portion of the cancer—the cells that couldn't care less what hormones its host is taking, because *hormones have no effect on this portion of the tumor.* Using hormones to fight these cells is (going back to our bug spray analogy) like trying to kill a cockroach with weed killer instead of insecticide. The problem is, we're still looking for the right "Raid," as well.

As Johns Hopkins scientist John Isaacs explains: "Cancer cells are very efficient. And as they keep dividing, they jettison some deadweight. One of the first pieces of unnecessary baggage to go may be the system of controls—the part of the cell that takes orders from hormones. Over time, the deadliest cancer cells survive because they become pure, stripped-down growing machines."

If adrenal androgens really were the key to fighting prostate cancer, antiandrogens should produce a dramatic improvement in men who were castrated, took estrogen or an LHRH agonist, and then had a relapse. This just isn't the case. Sadly, what happens for these men is that beginning combined androgen blockade has little effect—again, suggesting that this approach is not the answer.

Finally, other studies have demonstrated that adrenal androgens have little effect on the prostate. In one investigation at Johns Hopkins, researchers studied the autopsy records of four men who had their pituitary glands removed before they reached puberty—which means that not only did their bodies fail to make LH, they failed to make a hormone that stimulates the adrenal gland, so it was virtually shut down; in other words, they had combined androgen blockade. They also studied three men who had a genetic disorder called Kallmann's syndrome (in which the hypothalamus doesn't make LHRH, and therefore the pituitary glands don't make LH or FSH); and one unfortunate man who had been castrated at age seven, when a dog bit off his testicles. None of these men ever received treatment with testosterone; at autopsy, their average age was about sixty-five. Using age-matched "control" (normal) patients for comparison, the investigators showed that at autopsy there was *no disparity in prostate size* in men with both testosterone and the adrenal hormones out of commission and in men with only testosterone missing. (In all of these men, the prostate was tiny. In all but the castrated man, there were no Leydig cells, the tiny testosterone-making factories in the testicles.) In other words, *combined androgen blockade made no difference.*

THE FLUTAMIDE DISAPPOINTMENT: AN ONCOLOGIST'S VIEW

Kill all androgens! Don't stop at shutting down the testes, the body's main testosterone-making factory: Eliminate every single one, even weak male hormones produced in tiny amounts by the adrenal glands—anything that could possibly affect the prostate. This is the concept of combined androgen blockade, combining surgical or medical castration with LHRH agonist drugs (castration deprives the prostate of its chief hormone, testosterone, causing the prostate cancer cells that are hormone-controlled to die) with an antiandrogen.

The idea was that this one-two punch would be far more successful than either approach alone, and it became a huge issue in prostate cancer treatment in the 1980s. Scientists around the world conducted trials of flutamide; Johns Hopkins oncologist Mario Eisenberger conducted two of them, with about two thousand patients. "The first trial we did was marginally positive, a six-month difference in survival" in favor of the group of men randomly assigned to receive combined androgen blockade (versus the men who took LHRH agonists alone). Eisenberger's results were good enough for the FDA to approve the drug in 1989.

"The problem," Eisenberger says, "is that the issue continued to be controversial. There were two more positive trials, and everybody focused on those three trials," despite the fact that in one of them, the difference in survival was only about three months. "There were twenty-four other trials, all negative. This included my second trial—the largest ever done, with close to 1,400 patients. In the end, close to eight thousand patients were entered in twenty-seven clinical trials, and *only three of the trials were marginally positive.*" Eisenberger estimates that more than $1 billion has been spent in clinical research on combined androgen blockade. The sum could be justified, he adds, "if it generated something that would consistently be shown to improve the survival of our patients." But that didn't happen. The twenty-four negative trials didn't receive nearly as much attention as the three marginally positive ones. Combining LHRH agonists or surgical castration with antiandrogens "became a standard treatment, and added substantially to the cost of prostate cancer treatment." Antiandrogens cost about $300 a month. The negative result of Eisenberger's second trial, reported in the *New England Journal of Medicine*, confirmed what he had suspected: "Men with prostate cancer don't really need an antiandrogen. Anti-androgens provide what we consider a clinically insignificant advantage." Worse, in another trial designed to look at patients' quality of life, Eisenberger found that flutamide caused men to have more hot flashes (side effects of hormonal therapy in general), cramps, diarrhea, nausea, vomiting, and depression.

These results, Eisenberger concludes, show that men with advanced prostate cancer "don't need an antiandrogen together with castration. By not taking it, they're saving money, not affecting their quality of life, and not losing anything." Antiandrogens are best used as a backup to surgical or medical castration, he adds. "For patients treated with one form of castration who demonstrate a rising level of PSA in the blood, antiandrogens represent an option. About 20 percent of patients will get a second response."

General Side Effects of Androgen Deprivation

Testosterone is the hormone that makes men feel "manly." When it is missing, some of the characteristics associated with being male vanish along with it. Side effects of castration—surgical or medical—can include a loss of muscle mass (because male hormones are involved in making men muscular); and osteoporosis ("thinning" of the bones), which eventually can lead to fractures (one study has found that the long-term bone loss is worse for men who undergo surgical castration, instead of medical castration). The loss of bone density—because testosterone helps strengthen bones—may be as much as 7 to 10 percent in the first year; men who smoke may be more susceptible. You can help prevent this bone loss by taking vitamin D supplements (400 IU daily) and boosting your calcium intake to 1,200 milligrams a day. Also, there is some evidence that drugs called bisphosphonates (particularly, pamidronate) may help increase bone density. (Note: Specific risks are discussed with each form of hormonal therapy.)

Other general risks of hormonal therapy include anemia (because male hormones act on the bone marrow to encourage the formation of red blood cells in men), loss of sex drive, and decreased mental acuity. In older men, scientists have learned that testosterone levels are strongly linked to cognitive function—particularly, verbal memory (for example, naming the months of the year backward) and mental control (for example, the ability to recall a name and address after a ten-minute delay). Impotence is not an absolute certainty; 10 percent of men do remain potent. However, they are rare exceptions to the rule. (Impotence here, unlike impotence in other situations, means loss of libido as well as the ability to achieve an erection.) Some men also experience tenderness, pain, or swelling of the breasts (gyneco-mastia). This is not common after castration or treatment with an LHRH agonist, but it occurs in 50 to 70 percent of men treated with antiandrogen monotherapy, and in all men on estrogens. It can be pre-vented by low-dose radiation to the breasts *before* treatment begins.

Hot flashes: The other major side effect is hot flashes, and these are like the hot flashes experienced by women during menopause—a sudden rush of warmth in the face, neck, upper chest, and back, lasting from a few seconds to an hour. Although they aren't harmful to a man's health, they can be bothersome. They probably occur because the change in hormones affects the hypothalamus, the brain's "ther-mostat" for regulating body temperature, and the brain's response to this makes the body feel out of kilter. The blast of heat happens because blood vessels underneath the skin are dilating; this causes sweating, which helps bring the body back to normal.

Hot flashes are unpredictable; no one knows what sets them off, or what makes them go away. Some men don't have any; other men are plagued by them. There is some evidence that outside triggers such as radiant heaters, eating hot food, drinking alcohol, or taking certain medications can bring them on. However, there is help: Hot flashes can be treated with progestational drugs such as medroxy-progesterone (Provera), or megestrol acetate (Megace).

Other changes: Finally, many men on hormonal therapy report that they don't feel "normal"; in addition, they may feel irritable and less aggressive. Weight gain and subtle changes in physical appearance—differences in skin tone and hair growth—also are common. However, contrary to popular belief, there is no change in the pitch of the voice; nor, unfortunately, do balding men regrow a full head of hair.

Note: It is important for you to know that you're not alone, and many men undergoing this same treatment are experiencing the same feelings. Ask your doctor about a local support group. (For more, see "Where to Get Help," at the end of this book.)

LOSS OF SEXUAL FUNCTION: WHAT'S REALLY IMPORTANT HERE?

Loss of sexual function is an awful thought, one that makes most men shudder. This loss of identity is not a pleasant concept; it can be even worse when combined with the fear and uncertainty that are part of having cancer. This is a scary time, but you are not alone. It might help to talk to your doctor, or family, or men and their wives who are going through this, too (see the "Where to Get Help" section at the end of this book).

For many men with prostate cancer, when it comes down to choosing between sexual potency and holding off cancer, the sex life takes a back seat to survival. If hormonal therapy can truly mean the difference between life and death and you're preoccupied with sexual potency, you're missing the bigger point. (On the other hand, *if you have no symptoms of advanced cancer, this is one of the best reasons to wait until you do.* The long-term benefits are the same, but the difference in quality of life can be tremendous—see below.) But if you have cancer in the bones, or other symptoms of advanced disease, the message is clear: Taking hormones now can prolong your life, ease your pain, and make you feel better in countless ways.

One of the greatest challenges with any illness is to find a way past the physical limitations imposed on your body. Even if your sex life has moved to the back burner, you can still be intimate. In fact, intimacy—physical and mental closeness and sharing—is more important now than ever. It's easy, and very tempting, to let yourself become angry at what you *can't* do, and many people fall into this trap as they struggle to come to terms with a serious illness. This kind of frustration ultimately boils down to a control issue—it's human nature; we want to be in charge of our lives. But most of us, throughout our lives, have the point made—repeatedly—that there's remarkably little over which we have direct control. We are at the mercy of—well, God, if you believe in God; infinite other factors, if you don't.

One of the hardest pieces of advice doctors can give to patients—but one of the best things we can do for them—is to tell you to take the hard road: Make it your daily mission to avoid bitterness, which is not only unproductive and time-wasting, it consumes your vital energy and strength like the plague. Don't just ignore negativity; go a step further, and substitute positive thoughts and actions in its place. A rabbi once told his congregation, "We all have the same amount of time—today." With this in mind, treasure every extra, precious moment you get to spend with your loved ones. Now is the perfect time to do some things you've always wanted to do—take that trip you've always dreamed of, for instance. Take your wife out dancing. Learn to sail. Teach your grandchild how to fish. Investigate your family tree, and look up long-lost relatives. Realize there is so much more to living than sexual potency.

How Long Do Hormones Work?

This varies from man to man. In the past—*note; we expect these numbers to change, with the explosion in new strategies for attacking hormone-resistant cancer*—10 percent of men who are started on hormonal therapy when they have metastases to bone have lived less than six months. Ten percent live longer than ten years. The other 80 percent fall somewhere in the middle. Traditionally, statistics have shown that half of these men live three years or less, and 25 percent are alive after five years.

What accounts for the extreme disparity in these numbers? *It all has to do with the ratio of hormone-sensitive cells to hormone-insensitive cells, and how fast the cancer grows.* In some men, nearly every cell is responsive to hormones; in other men, very few cells are hormone-sensitive. Some cancers take hundreds of days to double in size; others double every few weeks.

There is a mathematical model of how these cancer cells grow, called "tumor kinetics." A tumor must double in size thirty times before a doctor can even feel it, before there's a centimeter of cancer. This growth is exponential—two cells, then four, then eight, and so on. Say a tumor is at its tenth doubling; it has 1,024 cells. And say that three fourths of these cells are responsive to hormones. The patient is castrated, and all the hormone-responsive cells drop out of the picture, leaving only 256 cells. What happens? These cells aren't affected by the hormones; they continue to grow. The now smaller tumor doubles. There are 512 cells. It doubles again—1,024 cells. It's back to where it started. And when it doubles again, there will be twice as many cells as before.

Now say only 1 percent of this cancer is not responsive to hormones. It's going to take many more doublings before this tumor becomes dangerous. So how long hormones work depends on two things: the ratio of hormone-resistant cells to hormone-dependent cells, and how long it takes for the cancer to double in size. Relapse will come a lot sooner in a man whose cancer doubles every thirty days, for example, than in a man whose cancer takes one hundred days to double. Unfortunately, today we have no way to predict these two important numbers.

When Should You Begin Hormonal Therapy?
Some Factors to Consider

Of all the issues in the controversial field that is prostate cancer treatment, this remains one of the most controversial. In fact, many well-informed, thoughtful individuals have reached diametrically opposed conclusions—often based on information from the same studies. One group says: Start hormones right now. Time's wasting, and if you start hormones today, you can delay the progression of the androgen-insensitive cell population, and add years to your life. The naysayers believe that there is no evidence that hormonal therapy cures prostate cancer, nor does it have any effect on the androgen-insensitive cell population, which for so many men is the factor that eventually determines life and death. They say that starting hormonal therapy early will only add side effects, and will actually take life out of the years a man has to live, without adding any years to that life. Still another group says: Let's use hormones intermittently. We'll start and stop it, maintain the quality of life, and have the best of both worlds. And finally, there's a new group, using what's called "step-up" treatment. Here, men start with innocuous therapies that have little effect and hardly any side effects, and then increase the intensity of treatment (and the potential for more side effects) as the cancer progresses. We will discuss all of these approaches.

Finally, there's something that might fit in the category of "worldly issues." You should be aware that the medical debate in this area is strongly influenced by factors that don't often get talked about openly. The pharmaceutical industry makes at least a billion dollars a year on hormonal agents for the treatment of prostate cancer. There is no question that they look after their financial interests by stoking the furnace to keep sales (prescriptions) up. This happens in many ways—through direct advertising, distribution of multicolored "scientific summaries," which endorse the widespread use of their products, or surreptitious support for medical meetings at fancy spas, in which "experts" (who receive generous honoraria, frequent-flier miles, and a free trip)—promote the company cause. In addition, at a time when HMOs and Medicare reimburse very little for a return visit and a long conversation with the doctor, it is tempting for a physician to advise a form of treatment for which he or she may receive hundreds of dollars for each visit, in the form of a shot. The massive financial and political clout—and largesse—of the pharmaceutical companies is widespread, and well known among physicians of every specialty, not just urology. Not all physicians are swayed by it; many aren't. But it's out there, it's yet another element in this complicated mix, and something for you to take into consideration.

Now, all that said, let's discuss the timing of hormonal therapy.

First things first: We need to get one thing straight right away: *If you have metastases to bone, or bone pain, or a large mass of cancer that is obstructing your kidneys or bladder, you need to start hormonal therapy now.* In this situation, hormone therapy is the right course of action—one that can make a huge, vital difference in the quality of life, and can protect your body from the ravages of cancer. Also, you should select some form of treatment that will drive your blood testosterone to the lowest level—either an LHRH agonist (accompanied for the first month by an antiandrogen, to block any possible "flare" reaction—described above) or by surgical removal of both testes. This is not the time for treatment with an antiandrogen alone—you need effective, immediate action. Also, if your bone scan is positive for metastatic disease—even if you don't notice any symptoms—you should start hormonal therapy now.

But what if you have no cancer in your bones, no sign that anything is wrong—except a rising PSA after surgery or radiation, or the presence of cancer in your lymph nodes—and you feel fine? Many doctors would advise you to start hormonal therapy as soon as possible. The rationale here, as one oncologist puts it: "Treat the tumor while a greater percentage of cells are responsive to hormones, and the patient should do better." Advocates of this approach also believe that it preserves quality of life, because it delays the onset of symptoms.

Others—and I'm in this group—believe that there is no evidence that starting hormonal therapy now, as opposed to later, will prolong life. (This is discussed in detail below.) However, if a man adopts this philosophy, he must be followed very closely—so that hormonal therapy can be started before any symptoms develop. This means a man should go back to the doctor every six months or less. At each visit, he should: be questioned closely about any signs or symptoms that could be bone pain; undergo a physical exam, to check for any increase in the size of a local tumor; have a bone scan every six or twelve months, or any time a new pain develops; and have blood tests—a PSA, and a serum creatinine test, to measure kidney function. (An elevated creatinine level in the blood may signal that the cancer has silently obstructed the kidneys.)

Does early treatment prolong life? The real issue in debating when to start hormonal therapy does not relate to symptoms and quality of life, because if you choose delayed hormonal therapy and are followed carefully, you will be started on active hormonal therapy at the earliest signs of progression (such as a positive bone scan), before you have any symptoms. Instead, the simple question is: Does early hormonal therapy prolong life? The best evidence to date is based on a study done by the Veterans Administration Cooperative Urological Research Group. (See Fig. 12.2.) When prostate cancer began to progress in the men on the placebos—this eventually happened to 65 percent of the men with locally advanced disease, and all of the men with metastases to distant sites—they began hormonal therapy, too. The study, though not originally intended for this purpose, turned into a comparison of early hormonal therapy versus delayed treatment. *There was no difference in survival between the men who started hormonal therapy late and the men who had been on it all along.*

This study, as your doctor can probably tell you, took place thirty years ago. Why are we quoting something that clearly is old news? Because its results are rock solid, and still hold up today—because, unfortunately, there have been no breakthroughs or improvements in long-term survival with hormonal therapy over the last fifty years.

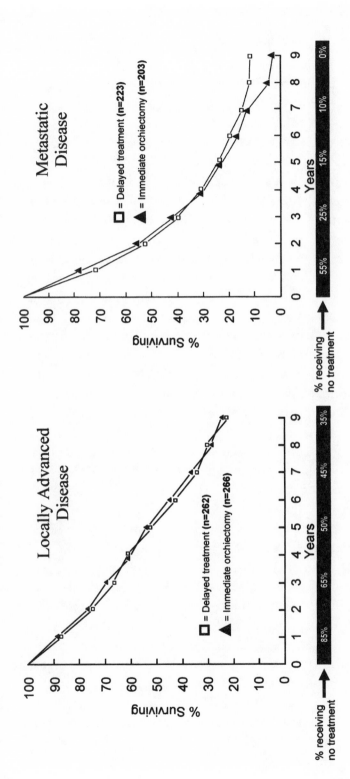

FIG. 12.2 Does Early Hormonal Therapy Prolong Life?

These two graphs show the results from the Veterans Administration Cooperative Urologic Research Study I, of 954 men with prostate cancer. The men were randomly assigned either to immediate surgical castration, or were followed on placebo therapy until their cancer progressed, at which point they underwent definitive hormonal therapy. The percentage of men left untreated is shown in the dark band below the X axis. With follow-up intervals out to nine years, there is no difference in survival in the men who received early versus late treatment. This must be addressed by anyone who tries to argue that early hormonal therapy prolongs life—because if it does, then what's wrong with this carefully executed, long-term study of almost one thousand men? [Modified from Blackard, C. E., D. P. Byar, W. P. Jordan, *Urology* 1:553–560, 1973; reproduced with permission.]

Because, ultimately, hormones aren't the answer for the long haul. Hormonal therapy never cures; at best, it palliates cancer—often for many years. What is the answer? A new plan of attack—many different strategies are being tested today—designed to kill the cancer cells that don't respond to hormones (see below).

But what about the studies that have shown a benefit from early hormonal therapy? One of the most quoted is another study by the Veterans Administration, originally designed to determine the ideal dose of estrogen. What happened was a lot like Goldilocks and the Three Bears: Some men were randomly assigned to receive a very low dose of estrogen—too low, actually, to be effective. Some received a very high dose—so high that it caused cardiovascular toxicity. And some men got an intermediate dose that turned out to be "just right." These three groups of men were then compared to men treated with a placebo. The men treated with the intermediate dose did better; they lived longer. But about half of the men on a placebo, and the men who *might as well have been on a placebo* (those in the "too low" dosage group) *never received hormonal therapy*—so this study didn't really turn out to be a comparison of early versus late treatment with hormones. Instead, it compared early treatment versus no treatment. This happened because many investigators in this study misinterpreted the first Veterans Administration study. They believed that first study showed that hormonal therapy did not prolong life; they missed the fact that the men in the placebo-treated group eventually did receive hormones.

More recently, scientists in Great Britain, in an investigation similar to the first Veterans Administration study, looked at the influence of early versus late hormonal therapy in men with locally advanced and metastatic disease. However, this study was not terribly uniform (for example, bone scans were available for some men, but not all), and there was no defined interval for follow-up. When the scientists first looked at the results, they concluded that men with locally advanced cancer who received early hormonal therapy lived longer. However, the comparison wasn't that fair. For men assigned to the delayed treatment group, treatment was *really* delayed—often until men had irreversible damage from the cancer. For example, some men didn't receive hormones until they had developed a pathologic fracture or spinal cord compression (when the bones had become riddled with cancer). There were fifty-four more deaths in the delayed treatment group than in the patients who received hormonal therapy up front—but of these fifty-four men, twenty-nine *never* received hormonal therapy before they died of prostate cancer. These men were, in effect, hung out to dry—and this study is not a true comparison of early versus late hormonal therapy. Instead, it's a comparison of early treatment versus *no* treatment, or treatment that comes too late to do any good. And several years later, when they looked at the results again, they concluded that there was no overall survival difference in the early and late groups.

A study from the Eastern Cooperative Oncology Group (ECOG), published in the *New England Journal of Medicine,* has received a lot of attention. This study looked at radical prostatectomy patients who turned out to have cancer in the lymph nodes. These men were randomly assigned either to hormonal therapy right away, or to delayed treatment—hormonal therapy given only when these men developed signs or symptoms of metastatic disease. After a relatively short follow-up interval of seven years, the authors found that the men who received early hormonal therapy lived longer. However, these findings have proven somewhat surprising—at least to scientists heading similar studies. One of these is a European study, in which 304 men with cancer in the lymph nodes who did not undergo radical prostatectomy were randomly assigned to early or delayed therapy. In this much larger study, where patients have been followed for an equal length of time, no significant difference in survival has been reported yet. Another study, led by the Mayo Clinic, retrospectively reviewed data of a large group of men with cancer in the lymph nodes, many of whom were treated with hormonal therapy. At seven years after treatment, the Mayo scientists found no overall cancer survival benefit for men receiving early hormonal therapy. Beyond ten years, however, they identified a small subset of men (twelve out of 790) with diploid tumors (which have the normal number of chromosomes—an indication that they are slower-growing), whom they felt did benefit from early treatment.

Why haven't other scientists been able to achieve the same success? One possible reason is that there weren't enough men in the ECOG study. When scientists carry out a randomized study, they need to have comparable patients in each group. This study was designed to evaluate 240 patients; however, the scientists had trouble recruiting men for the study, and ended up with only ninety-eight men. This left a smaller number in each group, and it's possible that unintentional bias might have been introduced. Another problem: The most powerful predictor of outcome is the Gleason score on the radical prostatectomy specimen. Unfortunately, these scientists did not have a central place where all pathologic specimens were analyzed, and they were unable to show that the Gleason scores of men in this study correlated with their response to treatment. If the Gleason scores were not performed evenly, it is possible that there was an unequal distribution of men with more adverse pathologic findings in the delayed group without hormonal therapy. For example, we know that in men with cancer-positive lymph nodes who have Gleason 8–10 disease, 82 percent will have metastatic disease within five years, compared to only 15 percent of men with Gleason 5–7 disease. In this study, 50 percent of the patients in the delayed treatment group had metastatic disease by five years, and 22 percent had died. This is much higher than in three other studies.

But doesn't early hormonal therapy delay the progression of cancer? The answer is, yes and no. It delays your *knowledge* of progression. It doesn't stop the clock. Another way to look at it is, "pay me now, or pay me later." Eventually, the result is the same. Hormonal therapy does two things: It stops cells from making PSA, and it shrinks the hormone-sensitive cell population. Say a man begins hormonal therapy when his PSA is elevated, but the bone scan is negative. His PSA will drop dramatically, and he may feel that his cancer is gone. But it's not; it has just slipped below the radar screen. Those hormone-insensitive cells continue to grow, silently. There is a euphemism for this: It's called a "delay in progression." What it really is, unfortunately, is a "silent progression." Over time (and this may take years), these hormone-insensitive cells will reappear on the medical radar map—the PSA will begin to rise again, the bone scan will become positive, and the tumor will begin to attack bone, producing the signs and symptoms of advanced, hormone-refractory disease.

Actually, this "delay" is just a "time shift." Say the man waited to start hormonal therapy until his bone scan was positive. Right away, his tumor would shrink, the PSA would fall, and the man would experience a remission of indefinite duration—until, just as in the first scenario, his hormone-insensitive cells reached a critical mass. Eventually—whether the man started hormonal therapy early or late—the result would be the same. If the man had begun hormonal therapy early, his cancer would have progressed, but he wouldn't have been aware of it. The trade-off is that he would have endured the side effects of hormonal therapy for a much longer time. If the man had begun hormonal treatment later, he would have had fewer side effects. What about peace of mind? Well, in both cases, the cancer is growing. The man who begins treatment early has a false peace of mind, based on the idea that what he can't see won't hurt him. Unfortunately, as we've discussed at length, hormones are not the long-term answer to controlling prostate cancer. The best hope is in the nonhormonal approaches, discussed below.

What I believe: So far, there has been no convincing scientific evidence to prove that early hormonal therapy prolongs life. In Chapter 10, we talked about the Johns Hopkins study that followed men who had an elevated PSA after radical prostatectomy. We found that, on average, it took eight years until these men developed metastases in the bones. We also developed a means of predicting when metastases may show up, using the Gleason score on the radical prostatectomy specimen (whether it was more or less than 8), the time after radical prostatectomy when the PSA first increased (whether it was more or less than two years), and how long it took for the PSA to double (whether more or less than ten months). Using this information, a man can quickly determine his risk of developing metastatic disease. In one of the most common scenarios, a man with Gleason 7 disease who developed a PSA elevation more than two years after surgery, who had a PSA doubling time longer than ten months, had an 82 percent likelihood of being metastasis-free at seven years. On the other hand, if the PSA had gone up within the first two years, and the PSA doubling time was less than ten months, then the freedom from metastatic disease at seven years would be only 15 percent. This information can tell men how long it will be before they actually need hormones—if they ever do.

If a man is treated with hormonal therapy immediately, as soon as the diagnosis of advanced disease is made, or if his doctor waits until the man has signs of progression and *then* begins treatment, we believe the *survival is exactly the same.* There is no compelling evidence that any kind of hormonal therapy works better earlier than later, when a man begins experiencing symptoms such as urinary obstruction or has a positive bone scan. And yet, it's highly unlikely that a man who is symptom-free (also called "asymptomatic") is going to feel any better once he has been deprived of his normal hormones. Again, the cancer cells that ultimately prove fatal in prostate cancer are the *hormone-insensitive cells*. They keep right on growing, unfazed by hormonal therapy. To these cells, whether hormonal therapy comes earlier or later *does not matter*.

For an asymptomatic man, early hormonal therapy means going from feeling fine and normal to experiencing hot flashes, loss of libido and the ability to have an erection, weight gain, changes in muscle mass, skin, and hair growth, and the subtle changes in personality that accompany the loss of male hormones. The long-term effects of hormonal therapy can include osteoporosis—loss of bone density, leaving bones more brittle and easy to break—and decreases in mental acuity (discussed earlier). What's the point of going through this early, when, ultimately, you could achieve exactly the same benefit if you wait to start hormonal therapy until there is evidence of progression of disease?

The idea of early hormonal therapy appeals to many men because it's doing something rather than nothing. Many doctors, too, promote a proactive approach, telling their patients that this will "delay progression" of the disease. Actually, it takes a lot of time for a doctor to convince a man *not* to start early hormonal therapy—and unfortunately, many doctors don't have very much time to spend with their patients. If you want to attack the cancer aggressively, don't pin all your hopes on hormones. Instead, read the section below on nonhormonal approaches, and consider enrolling yourself in a clinical trial—there are many—aimed at killing the cancer cells that hormonal therapy can't touch.

Intermittent Hormonal Therapy (Intermittent Androgen Suppression)

In searching for some kind of compromise between early and late hormonal therapy, many doctors have embraced the idea of the "happy medium"—intermittent hormonal therapy.

Basically, it works like this: Men start taking hormones early—after an elevated PSA score following a radical prostatectomy, for example—before signs or symptoms of advanced cancer begin. Then, when their PSA levels drop, they stop taking them, and get a little "vacation" from treatment. The men are monitored closely, and at the first sign that the tumor is growing, they start taking the hormones again.

The major benefits of all this, advocates say, include better quality of life—recovery of sexual function, and a greater sense of well-being during the downtime between treatments. These advocates believe prostate cancer can be "cycled," like a rubber band that stretches and then—*boing!*—snaps back to a smaller state, then stretches again. And that, in this way, they can stave off the emergence of the androgen-insensitive cells that ultimately prove fatal in men with metastatic prostate cancer.

There are just a few problems here. The first, as we've discussed in this chapter, is that there's *no evidence that any form of hormonal therapy prolongs anyone's life when it's begun earlier than a man absolutely needs it.* So why would interrupted therapy work better? All the benefits of intermittent hormonal therapy—mainly, this means the better quality of life—can be had simply by *delaying* therapy until a man has signs of progression, without the serious roller-coaster effect of starting and stopping these powerful drugs.

Speaking of quality of life: Many of the men beginning the treatment are asymptomatic, with early-stage disease—men who wouldn't be considered, by many physicians, appropriate candidates for hormonal therapy in the first place. (However, these men might be excellent candidates for a trial of one of the new therapies discussed below.) For these men—many of whom have an excellent long-term outlook without any further treatment—it's hard to justify the intensive monitoring, the expense, and most of all, the life-changing repercussions of hormonal therapy without substantial proof that this on-again, off-again approach even works.

Which brings us to the second problem: *The evidence for intermittent hormonal therapy is largely theoretical.* Advocates cite experimental studies, but not solid data from randomized clinical trials in humans—mainly because there haven't been any published results yet. In one of these experimental investigations, mice were castrated when their tumor reached a certain size. When the tumor shrank to 30 percent of its original weight, scientists transplanted it into another mouse. The tumor shrank, began to grow again, and that mouse was castrated. Then, when the tumor shrank again, it was transplanted into still another mouse, and so on. The investigators inferred from this that "cycling" androgens can delay the time to tumor progression—the time before the androgen-independent cells take over and hormonal therapy no longer works.

They didn't take into consideration one very basic issue: Any time a tumor is removed and transplanted into another animal, it shrinks—because many of its cells simply don't survive the move. So the scientists were killing cells just by transplanting them—and the big benefits they cited were almost certainly from the transplantation, not from the hormone manipulation. The researchers could have avoided scientific criticism simply by giving the animals "cycles" of reversible hormone suppression. After all, this is what would be done in human patients. Investigators in another study actually did this. Their findings: Animals that were castrated or treated continuously with DES (in other words, animals given constant, *not interrupted,* therapy) survived 50 percent longer than animals on intermittent hormone suppression.

Frankly, this is not thrilling scientific evidence. In fact, it's downright weak when you consider the effects of therapy *based merely on these findings* on men's health and quality of life. So why is anyone gung ho about intermittent hormonal therapy? Why is it being enthusiastically endorsed for clinical trials? The cynical in our field might explain this rush to the intermittent therapy bandwagon by looking at other statistics. One of them is that in 1995, American men spent more than $1 billion on LHRH agonists and another $350 million on flutamide—which may explain why some drug companies seem anxious to pursue this avenue of therapy without any evidence that it prolongs life.

At this time, the only bottom line on intermittent androgen suppression (other than the financial one) is that it's an investigational form of treatment, and that it will require years—and thoughtfully designed, randomized clinical trials in actual human patients with prostate cancer—before its effectiveness can be proven.

SHOULD YOU BE IN A STUDY?

It depends on the study and the medical institution that's taking part in it. Make sure, before you enroll, that you know exactly what's being tested, how the study works—whether some patients (and perhaps yourself) will be receiving placebo treatment, for example—and whether there are any potential side effects. Generally, there are many advantages to participating in a study. Medical studies are strictly controlled, with well-defined rules (participants can stop being in the study whenever they want) and review boards that include doctors, nurses, lawyers, scientists, clergy members, and laypeople. Often, people who take part in medical studies are followed more closely, and thus receive better medical care, than the general public—and usually at little or no cost. (Sometimes, if a medication proves helpful, participants are even given a free supply as a reward for their help.)

Participating in a study often means access to new drugs that aren't yet available to others; you may get first crack at a new breakthrough. And many people who volunteer for a medical study say that they feel that they are doing something important—that their contribution will advance medical science, and that it ultimately will help other people.

"If they're motivated and feel well, patients should always explore this option," says Johns Hopkins oncologist Mario Eisenberger. "They shouldn't give up. For many patients, being in a study gives them a new outlook and new hope."

Step-Up Hormonal Therapy

This is a gradual approach to hormonal therapy—and it has great appeal to many men with micrometastases, who have no signs or symptoms of cancer progression but want to "do something" now. The idea here is to start modulating the male hormones with agents that have the fewest side effects, and then to escalate as needed, if the disease progresses. For example, as we mentioned earlier, prostate cancers don't make a lot of DHT; thus, we would not expect a drug that blocks the production of DHT—finasteride (Proscar)—to be very effective in controlling prostate cancer. And it isn't. However, it doesn't have many side effects—and so, men on "step-up" hormonal therapy start with the most benign option, finasteride. If the PSA continues to rise, or starts rising again, they move to the next level—an antiandrogen as monotherapy. If that begins to lose its effectiveness, they then add finasteride, and if that doesn't work, then add an LHRH agonist. Although there is no scientific evidence to tell us whether this "step-up" therapy—in effect, a "candy-coated" approach to hormonal therapy—is any more or less effective than any other form of treatment, it's safe to say that it's probably a lot more expensive. But it's attractive, too. Many men feel better when their PSA level falls, especially when the treatment has few side effects. It's hard to convince these men that there is no evidence that this works—nor that any form of hormonal therapy is better than delaying treatment until there are signs of cancer progression, as discussed above. And if this is what you want to do, then you should do it.

However, there are two other drawbacks, besides the expense. One is that the men who choose step-up hormonal therapy are also excellent candidates for a trial of one of the new nonhormonal therapies—and in the long run, these have a much better chance of killing the prostate cancer cells that don't give a hoot about how much, or how little, male hormone you have. Two is that it will be hard for medical science to make progress in finding ways to kill these androgen-insensitive cancer cells if the patients who could benefit most from these trials are taking hormones that make them feel better psychologically, but ultimately may not control their cancer. Remember the delayed progression that masks the silent progression of cancer, discussed above? This happens with step-up therapy, too. You may not feel it, but the cancer is still there, growing stealthily, and when it breaks out from below the medical radar screen, it can burst back into your life with a vengeance. Thus, you should ask yourself: Will the good feeling I have now, that sense of doing something positive to fight my cancer, be enough to outweigh any second-guessing I may have later—for not enrolling in a trial to fight the androgen-insensitive cancer cells when they were more vulnerable?

Hormonal Therapy: Conclusions and a Look into the Future

Hormonal therapy doesn't last forever. But this is not to say that hormonal therapy does not work. *It does work. It does prolong life, and it does ease many symptoms of advanced prostate cancer.* The message here is this: There's no evidence that giving a man early hormonal therapy—intermittent or continual—or giving more hormonal therapy than is necessary works any better than giving adequate hormonal therapy *if and when a patient needs it.* Many men are told that early hormonal therapy will "delay the progression" of the disease. Unfortunately, as we discussed above, this is not true. The only thing delayed is your *knowledge* of the progression.

Hormonal therapy does not cure prostate cancer. And if a man lives long enough, this cancer will progress. If it were simply a matter of controlling the hormone-responsive cells, we'd have it made. But it isn't; it's the tricky hormone-insensitive cells—those are the ones we must learn to kill, or at least disable. So what we need, urgently, is a better way to target this group of cells. As you will see below, many exciting new approaches to doing exactly this are being developed and tested.

WHAT ABOUT PC-SPES?

One headline screamed, "New Hope for Prostate Cancer." Another used the word "breakthrough." Many men swear by it. They're all talking about PC-SPES.

Now: What is it? Well, it's a "natural" preparation, a combination of eight herbs (most of them used in Chinese medicine), including saw palmetto (which is known to improve urinary symptoms in men with BPH). Some of these herbs are potent phytoestrogens ("phyto" means that they come from plants), and it appears that the estrogen is the key to how PC-SPES works. (Some people are surprised that this "herbal" remedy can have such a potent effect. They shouldn't be—one of the most effective herbal medicines in the world is used to treat heart disease. It's digitalis, and it comes from the leaf of a plant.)

When PC-SPES is given to men who have never received hormonal therapy, it acts like any other estrogen. It suppresses testosterone, and causes PSA to plummet in virtually all men. Like other estrogens, it can cause breast enlargement, loss of sexual function, and life-threatening blood clots in the legs, which can spread to the lungs (see the side effects of DES, above). PC-SPES is also very expensive, costing from $200 to $500 a month.

So great is the hype surrounding this drug that some men with localized disease have started taking it—in effect, hitching their wagon to this unproven star. A man with clinically localized prostate cancer (stage T1c disease) with a PSA of 8.8, who decided to delay surgery or radiation, began daily treatment with nine PC-SPES capsules a day. After three weeks, his PSA had dropped to 1.4, and after eight weeks, his PSA was less than 0.1. He has continued on a maintenance dose of six capsules, and his PSA remains undetectable. However, the man's life has changed in other ways: He has had a loss of libido, erectile dysfunction, extreme breast enlargement and tenderness, a reduction in overall body hair, edema, and a significant drop in his lipoprotein level—all of which he could have achieved with a low dose of DES, for $5 to $15 a month. Also, he may seriously compromise his odds of being cured of cancer by this effort to "delay" the disease. (As we discussed earlier in this book, hormonal therapy does not put prostate cancer on a "block of ice," because the hormone-insensitive cells keep on growing.)

Many men have been sold on PC-SPES because it can make PSA fall in about half of men who begin taking it after standard hormonal therapy has failed. However, so can DES. In a recent study from Great Britain, thirty-four men who had failed second-, third-, or fourth-line hormonal therapy received DES, 1 milligram per day, combined with 40 milligrams per day of hydrocortisone. Of the twenty-nine men who had symptoms, twenty-four experienced an improvement, and twenty-one had a decrease in PSA by greater than 50 percent, lasting an average of four to six months.

If you are considering treatment with PC-SPES, talk to your doctor first, and find a form of treatment that may be more effective and safer. (If further hormonal treatment doesn't work, then you should consider one of the new, nonhormonal treatments discussed below.)

Now, the argument from proponents of herbal medicine is, "Doctors just don't trust herbals on principle, no matter how effective they are." Not true. Doctors don't trust *anything* until it has been proven to be safe and effective. (Remember, the first rule of medicine is, "Do no harm.") In fact, says physician Michael Katz, of the March of Dimes Birth Defects Foundation, in a letter to the editor of the *New England Journal of Medicine*, "what the proponents of alternative [complementary] medicine are demanding is alternative epidemiology that would accept anecdotes as proof." Another physician, writing in the same issue of the journal, commented: "While attending a conference on alternative medicine, which was organized by one of the most respected medical schools in New York City, I realized why this conference was so popular. During the coffee breaks and lunch hour, I discovered that a large number of participants were driven to learn the new "science" in order to build an "herbalist" practice, which is outside the control of and not currently reimbursed by managed care. Many were also interested in the profitable sale of these untested products to their patients." Ouch. The message from both of these doctors—and my own advice to you—is, use the proverbial grain of salt in digesting information about any "breakthrough" product. Do your best to get past the hype.

If You're on Hormonal Therapy, How Often Should You See the Doctor?

If you're on hormonal therapy—no matter what kind, and even if you feel perfectly fine—you should be followed closely. For most men, this means that you need to see your doctor every three to six months. At every visit, you should have:

- A careful history taken, to help your doctor spot subtle symptoms— such as back pain or other bone pain, difficulty with urination, or blood in the urine—that may suggest progression of cancer;
- A physical exam—to feel for any lumps or changes in the prostate or the prostatic bed; and
- Certain laboratory tests. This is mainly blood work—a PSA test, to monitor the response to hormonal therapy, and what's called a "serum creatinine," a test to monitor kidney function. (An elevated creatinine level in the blood may signal that the cancer has silently obstructed the kidneys.)

Your PSA should fall to close to the undetectable range, and stay there for a long time. Note: Hormones play a major role in the production of PSA; thus, when the male hormones are suppressed, hardly any PSA is being made. Many men assume that having a very low PSA means the cancer is gone. Unfortunately, although the cancer has suffered a severe setback, it's still there, but the remaining cancer cells— the dreaded hormone-insensitive kind—don't make much PSA.

If your PSA stays at a very low level, you probably don't need any imaging studies, such as a bone scan or a CT scan. In fact, if a man is having a great response to hormonal therapy, a bone scan may look *worse,* because the bone, freed of cancer, is actually healing—and this new bone growth can make the bone scan light up like a Christmas tree. If, after a long period of remaining stable, your PSA starts to go up, this usually means that the tumor is beginning to grow again. It may take six months or longer after this first elevation in PSA before there are any signs or symptoms of progression, or before a CT scan or bone scan may pick up new signs of cancer.

If Your PSA Begins to Rise Now, What Should You Do?

First, let's make sure that the laboratory test is correct. Just about every doctor who treats men with prostate cancer can tell you that labs sometimes make mistakes. Have the test repeated in another laboratory. If the PSA still comes back elevated, the next step is for you and your doctor to make sure that you're receiving the maximum benefit from hormonal therapy—that it's doing the job it's supposed to do, and that it's not making things worse.

If you've been castrated, make sure that all the tissue was taken out. This is easier than it sounds; all you need is a blood test to measure your testosterone level. Similarly, if you're taking estrogen or an LHRH agonist, make sure you're getting the recommended dosage and getting your shots regularly (if you're not, the level of hormones may be fluctuating). Again, a blood test can confirm whether your testosterone level is at the crucial castrate range. In either case, if there's too much testosterone in the blood, this is probably the problem, and it can be fixed.

If your testosterone is in the castrate range and you're not on an antiandrogen, you should try taking one, to see whether this makes your PSA levels fall. Some men are helped by this. If, however, you already are taking an antiandrogen in addition to castration, estrogen, or an LHRH agonist, try stopping it (see above). In some men, going back and forth—stopping an antiandrogen, starting another one, stopping that one, restarting another one—causes repeated declines in PSA, and stretches out the time that hormonal therapy can control cancer. However, when it is clear that your PSA is no longer being controlled, it is time to act (see below).

In a few men, prostate cancer can come back without the PSA ever going up. This happens when the cancer returns as a *small-cell carcinoma*. When prostate cancer transforms itself into this kind of tumor, it behaves differently—often recurring as a large mass in the pelvis, or as metastases to unusual sites, like the liver or lung. If this is the case, a biopsy should be performed. It's important to know whether you have a small-cell carcinoma, because these cancers have a makeup similar to that of other small-cell cancers (of the lung, for example), and they respond to the same kinds of chemotherapy drugs used to treat these other small-cell tumors (see below).

What Happens if Hormonal Therapy Doesn't Seem to Be Working?

For decades, hormonal therapy has been the mainstay of systemic (treatment that affects the whole body, as opposed to "localized" treatment, which targets a particular area) therapy for prostate cancer. Hormonal therapy gave doctors a way to reach the cancer cells we knew were out there, but couldn't even see—the cells that had slipped out of the prostate and escaped to distant sites. And even though hormonal therapy doesn't work forever, it does work quite well, often for years. However, the development of a hormone-independent state—in which the cancer is no longer controlled by hormones alone—happens to most men with advanced cancer, over time. The hormones *do* keep working, on the cells they have always affected—the cells that respond to hormones. But the androgen-insensitive cells continue to grow and multiply, and develop devious new techniques, until they finally take command.

The problem is similar to what can happen with antibiotics—the development of antibiotic-resistant organisms. It happens in other diseases, too, such as AIDS; just when doctors get a handle on the slippery virus, it outwits them. On the life-and-death battlefield of serious disease, it truly is "survival of the fittest."

But we're getting better at guessing prostate cancer's next moves. As scientists have learned more about the biology of cancer, the intricate mechanisms involved in progression and metastasis—the links in the chain of advancing cancer—they have been able to develop new agents, specially designed to target these specific links. Fortunately, many new approaches are in the works, and even more are coming behind them.

Nonhormonal Approaches to Advanced Cancer

Some of these approaches are brand-new. Others have been around for a while, but never used as they're being tried now—early, when PSA first signals trouble, after radical prostatectomy or radiation therapy. Many of these nonhormonal approaches have few side effects. None causes the long-term quality of life changes of hormonal therapy. One of these drugs, someday, is going to stop prostate cancer from advancing—or maybe even cure it altogether. For the first time ever, something new has entered the picture of advanced prostate cancer. More than hope, it's optimism.

The world of advanced disease can change on a dime. Many doctors—including myself—have seen it happen just like that. As a young doctor, I served two years at the San Diego Naval Hospital, caring for young men dying of metastatic testicular cancer. The picture was grim; in those days, chemotherapy cured only 10 percent of these men. And then came a miracle. A drug called cisplatin was discovered. A scientist noticed that bacteria did not grow around the platinum electrode on a battery, and wondered whether platinum might have an effect on cancer. He developed a derivative of platinum, and tried it on a number of mice that had tumors. It didn't work. But somebody noticed something unusual about the mice in this study—they had shrunken testicles—and asked another question: Could this compound have any effect on testicular cancer? Bingo. The response was electric, as it were—all of a sudden, 70 percent of men with this terrible cancer were being cured. Young men weren't dying of testicular cancer anymore.

Men with prostate cancer should understand this story well. There is hope that through serendipity, a similar discovery will be made. It

---

WHY HASN'T STANDARD CHEMOTHERAPY WORKED WELL IN PROSTATE CANCER—AT LEAST, SO FAR?

In some cancers—leukemia is the best example—the proliferation, or growth rate, is speedy. And from a treatment standpoint, this is good—these cancers are highly susceptible to drugs that attack rapidly dividing cells. Not so with prostate cancer. Here, proliferation is sluggish—in fact, these slowpoke cells have plenty of leisure time to repair any hits sustained from chemotherapy before they divide again. It's as if the damage never occurred.

In prostate cancer, the rate of cell division, or *birth* of new cells, is very low. For example, in testicular cancer, 60 percent of the cells are proliferating; in breast cancer, the birth rate is 20 percent—but in prostate cancer, it's only 5 percent. So why is the cancer growing, if not from a cellular baby boom? The problem, instead, is that something happens to throw off the normal process of *cell death*. Many prostate cancer cells—the androgen-independent ones—have discovered the secret of immortality. So if scientists can't stop new cells from being born, maybe they can help these cells figure out how to die—or better yet, to die at a faster than normal rate. This treatment idea is being explored aggressively. Even a very slight shift in the balance can alter cancer's growth dramatically. If we could just decrease the number of cells proliferating and increase the number dying by a measly 2 percent, we could slow down the doubling time by sixty to ninety days. And this could open major new doors to controlling and even curing the disease.

could happen tomorrow. It might—if one or more of the tactics we're about to discuss proves as successful as scientists expect—be happening already.

Here, now, is a rundown of the most promising new agents. Conspicuously absent are the old chemotherapy drugs, with their "buckshot" approach—killing everything, good and bad, in range, with limited effect in prostate cancer. These new treatments work like a high-powered rifle, with only one target in its sights—prostate cancer cells. They're specifically designed to target the biological mechanisms involved in cancer progression and metastasis. They can be grouped, based on their mode of attack.

Immunotherapy

Active immunity: The idea here is to even the fight. Think of any great lopsided battle in history—like the ill-fated Charge of the Light Brigade during the Crimean War—and imagine that you could somehow change the odds. What if those valiant Englishmen, the 13th Hussars, had worn bulletproof vests—or better yet, riot gear and helmets? They would still be outnumbered, but at least they'd have a fighting chance.

In about 70 percent of men with prostate cancer, advancing disease is accompanied by a substantial drop in lymphocytes—blood cells that make antibodies, which help the body's immune system fight off disease. The result—an underpowered immune system.

To beef up the immune system, scientists turned to a substance called *granulocyte macrophage colony-stimulating factor* (GM-CSF), a growth factor that stimulates the body's normal defense system. Among other things, the GM-CSF appears to work as a growth factor for *dendritic cells*—crucial cells in the body's immune system that, in turn, stimulate *T cells*, warriors in the class of disease-fighters called *lymphocytes*, which zero in on tumor cells and eliminate them in various ways. Lymphocytes are activated by still other proteins (basically, the human body is one big string of proteins). In ingenious work, doctors at Johns Hopkins actually put GM-CSF directly into tumor cells, and have used them as a souped-up vaccine.

The early studies focused on men who underwent a radical prostatectomy, but who still were not cancer-free. These men had micrometastases, as signaled by rising PSA levels within the first year after the operation. Some scientists believe this may be the ideal time to strike—after the cancer has been dealt a devastating blow, and before it has time to recover. The early clinical trials were encouraging: In sixteen of twenty-one patients who received a low dose of vaccine, PSA levels rose more slowly, and one man experienced a seven-month partial remission—a drop in PSA. In these early trials, the vaccine proved not only safe (all drugs must first be tested to see how the body tolerates them, and whether they cause any harmful side effects), but showed promise that the body's immune system could indeed be "cranked up" to help fight cancer.

In another approach, scientists attempted to jump-start the body's immune system with a vaccine made out of something "prostate cancer-specific." There are several candidates for these vaccine-making factories; one is PMSA (prostate membrane-specific antigen), a protein that's made on the surface of prostate cells, and is highly expressed in advanced cancers. *Antigens* like PMSA are pieces of protein that must pass inspection by the body. The body says, basically, "friend or foe?" If the body decides an antigen is an enemy, it attacks by making special assassin cells to eliminate it. Although immunotherapy will probably not be able to fight "major tumor burdens"—very large, or advanced cancers—it still might do some good. In new trials, scientists will attempt to stimulate the immune system in forty men with hormone-refractory, bone-metastatic prostate cancer, in hopes of slowing down the disease, or even causing a durable remission.

As technology improves, we will certainly find better ways to boost active immunity. For example: In the field of kidney cancer, scientists have been able to achieve dramatic regression of cancer using bone marrow transplant. Here, the bone marrow from a donor produces lymphocytes that attack the tumor in the same way they would go after a foreign body. In this work, published in the *New England Journal of Medicine*, doctors did not completely eliminate the patient's own bone marrow (as they would in other bone marrow transplants). Out of nineteen patients, the doctors achieved some exciting responses, although two patients died of transplant-related causes. Inevitably, this technique will be applied in prostate cancer, and investigators will find ways to make it safer and more effective. This is just one example of the bright future ahead for immunotherapy.

Passive immunity: A second way to use immunotherapy is through what's called passive immunity, which involves antibodies. Antibodies are Y-shaped proteins, churned out by the white blood cells, or B cells. We make them at the proverbial drop of a hat. You name it—germs, viruses, parasites, any unsavory pathogen that invades the body—and these B cells get busy, creating antibodies tailor-made for each specific enemy. Here's where the antibodies' peculiar shape comes in: The antibodies use the arms of the "Y" as grappling hooks, that stick into proteins at the surface of the offending cells, and disable them.

Scientists can create antibodies to proteins such as PMSA—which is present on nearly every prostate cancer cell, in amounts that increase as the cancer becomes more aggressive—in mice. In the past, using antibodies such as this could cause a problem—an allergic reaction. The body has its own version of the old saying, "Fool me once, shame on you; fool me twice, shame on me." The first time the body is exposed to something new, it absorbs the information, and commits it to a vast memory; the body never forgets a face, or an enemy. (In fact, by the time most of us reach adulthood, we may well have antibodies that can recognize more than 100 million different foreign invaders.) The second time, if the body recognizes this intruder as an enemy, it can develop an allergic response, which may be severe. But today, scientists have overcome this roadblock, and are able to make genetically engineered, "humanized" (a hybrid of mouse and human) antibodies in mice that don't produce an allergic reaction. In exciting studies, these antibodies, called *monoclonal antibodies* (because they were all made from a single clone, in research that won the 1984 Nobel Prize), are being used to attack prostate cancer cells directly, or to attack some of the growth factor receptors on those cells. In the future, we may use these monoclonal antibodies, or MABs, to direct chemotherapy or even radiation—to lead the treatment specifically to these cancer cells. MAB therapies are being tested in many forms and stages of cancer—most spectacularly, in lymphoma patients. Antibody-tagged radioactive isotopes—tiny bursts of radiation that, directed to specific targets by the antibodies, act as "guided missiles"—have made even grapefruit-sized lymphomas shrink or disappear completely.

One of the pioneers of monoclonal antibody research is urologist Neil Bander, of the New York Hospital–Cornell University Medical

Center. Bander, who has developed a new, highly specific MAB to PMSA, has achieved remarkable success at making large tumors "melt away" in the laboratory. Now he is testing MAB treatments in several groups of patients, including men with hormone-refractory cancer. In one early trial, the MABs proved able to target all the cancer—even some tiny sites that did not show up on bone scans. Many more trials are currently under way, or in the works.

Gene Therapy

Cracking the DNA code has been, to the world of cancer research, the equivalent of discovering the Rosetta stone—the key that unlocked Egyptian hieroglyphics. With gene therapy, again, the approach is exquisitely precise: Scientists are able to program the body's DNA like a computer chip, sending it on a selective search-and-destroy mission targeted only at prostate cancer cells.

Lethal viruses: One of the most effective weapons may turn out to be a genetically engineered virus—doctored to act as a Trojan horse, slipping into the body, attaching itself to prostate cancer cells and exterminating them before they even suspect anything's amiss. On the outside, it looks like a normal virus. But on the inside, it's a revved-up, cancer-killing machine, designed to deliver its special surprise package only to prostate cancer cells.

At Johns Hopkins, scientists are testing several viruses. One is the adenovirus, an upper respiratory virus—remodeled so that it's switched on by the PSA promoter, a small stretch of DNA near the PSA gene in the body; the PSA promoter acts as a chemical switch that governs how PSA is produced. Perhaps, if prostate cancer has a saving grace, it's PSA. This enzyme, indispensable in diagnosing the disease and deciding treatment, a marker for every stage of prostate cancer, and even a predictor of its course, is an excellent target for this new chemical warfare. Scientists studying cancers elsewhere in the body—in the breast, for example, the colon, or the brain—would give their eyeteeth for a potential weapon as selective as this: Nearly every prostate cell makes PSA. The fact that it is prostate-specific means no other cells need be harmed by this virus, which enters the body "locked and loaded," in effect, and programmed to fire only at PSA's signal. It cannot be activated in other cells. With no point of entry, it just brushes past, looking for the next PSA-making cell. The virus doesn't care whether a cancer cell responds to hormones or is hormone-resistant. As long as it makes PSA, the virus will find it.

The virus—any virus—invades an unsuspecting cell, overpowers its defenses, and co-opts its machinery to do the virus's bidding. When it has consumed all the cell's resources—stripping it clean, like a locust in a wheat field—and has no more use for the cell, it destroys it and moves on. Normally, when the body realizes that a virus is on the loose, it sends its own powerful home guard—immune system warrior cells, such as those activated in immunotherapy (described above)—to fend off the intruder.

In the first adenoviral gene therapy trial, Johns Hopkins scientists Ron Rodriguez and Ted DeWeese tested the virus in men who had a local recurrence of prostate cancer after radiation treatment, detected by a rise in PSA. This was a Phase I trial, designed simply to make sure a drug is safe for patients to take—not to measure any other results, such as changes found in PSA levels or biopsies. Nonetheless, "we've certainly seen some exciting things," says DeWeese, a radiation oncologist. The virus was easily tolerated, with minimal side effects. And, "several men had significant declines in their PSA," says urologist Rodriguez. "Even in the ones who didn't—most of them have not had the increase in PSA that you would have expected."

DeWeese administered the virus using a highly accurate computer program he helped design to administer brachytherapy seeds—in fact, the technique is similar, except that instead of radioactive seeds, it's droplets of virus being placed precisely within the prostate, guided by transrectal ultrasound and a 3-D CT scan image of the prostate.

The scientists opted to inject the virus directly into the prostate (instead of into the bloodstream) because they believe it's the best means of buying extra time for the virus to work—before the body's immune system spots the invader and attempts to knock it out. "We've all been exposed thousands of times to the common cold virus," DeWeese says. "Most of us have antibodies primed and ready to strike, to mount an immune response. So while all of these patients will get an immune response at some point, at least it's delayed long enough to allow some replication of this virus, and therefore killing, to occur."

Among other things, the investigators hope to find out how much of the virus ultimately makes it out of the prostate and into the bloodstream. It may be that, if the virus demonstrates some staying power, it could help men with metastatic disease. Another exciting suggestion from this early study, and the laboratory work that preceded it, is that the virus may be effective when used even earlier—"maybe with radiation up front," says DeWeese, "to increase the amount of killing that radiation might provide."

Rodriguez has continued to improve the virus, developing "son of" viruses—second- and third-generation drugs—and exploring different means of delivering them. One of the most daring involves a powerful agent that Rodriguez admires for its ruthless, cell-killing efficiency—the diphtheria toxin (DPT). "It's a very potent cellular toxin that poisons protein synthesis," he explains. "It's among the most potent molecules known to man. As little as *one molecule* of this toxin can kill a cell." Rodriguez is working to add this deadly cocktail to the mix. Already, he has mastered the intricate feat of engineering diphtheria into the adenovirus, and now is working to make sure the virus is safe.

Unlike other agents, the diphtheria-engineered virus does not rely on cell proliferation, or division, as an ignition switch. "If you're a prostate cancer cell that's resting, and you get exposed to DPT, you're going to die." Rodriguez is also working with other prostate-specific sequences of DNA, which he has cloned. Some of these, he notes, may turn out to be more responsive to hormones; others may work best in prostate cancer that does not respond to hormonal therapy. "Advanced cancer," he explains, "is a different animal." One day, if viruses designed with these promoters prove successful, "we may be able to custom-engineer a virus to fit patients' different needs."

Activating apoptosis: Another PSA-targeted approach works like a molecular grenade that detonates only in prostate cancer cells, causing them to kill themselves. This "suicide" process is called programmed cell death, or *apoptosis*—a Greek word that refers to leaves dropping off a tree.

"We're taking advantage of two attributes of prostate cancer here," says Johns Hopkins scientist John Isaacs. "One is that it makes PSA, and the other is that PSA is an enzyme that can clip proteins, like a pair of molecular scissors." (This aspect of PSA is discussed in Chapter 5, under "Bound and Free PSA.") As part of its normal routine, PSA recognizes certain strings of amino acids, the building blocks of proteins, and cuts them up. (The specific proteins are involved in making a sperm-trapping gel, which is part of semen; PSA's main job is to break down this gel.) Isaacs and colleagues are designing a drug by genetically altering a potent toxic molecule, hooking it chemically with this protein carrier—so that it's only activated when PSA goes into its protein-clipping mode. Then the PSA, recognizing this sequence of proteins that it's supposed to cut, will, in effect, pull the pin on its own grenade: One clip and boom! Out comes the toxic molecule.

The secret weapon here is an unlikely terminator, derived from an innocuous-looking member of the parsley family. It's a compound called thapsigargin—isolated, Isaacs explains, from the *Thapsia garganica* plant, which is found in the Mediterranean. (Isaacs is working with Soren B. Christensen, the medicinal chemist from the Royal Danish School of Pharmacy who first isolated, characterized, and named thapsigargin.)

For nearly two thousand years, resin from this plant has been a staple of Arabian medicine; it's a natural irritant, easily absorbed through the skin, which can ease the pain of rheumatism. Thapsigargin works by burrowing its way into a cell and targeting a protein that acts as a calcium pump. Like someone bailing water out of a leaky rowboat, this pump keeps calcium from rising above a certain level inside a cell.

The most interesting thing here is the calcium, which also happens to be a key that turns on the engine of apoptosis. "This gives cells very specific signals to activate a process of suicide," says Isaacs. "Normally, calcium is almost ten-thousand-fold higher outside of a cell than within it. If too much of the calcium gets inside, it causes the cell to reprogram itself and activate this suicide pathway." The effect is like turning up the gauge on a pressure cooker.

Programmed cell death is certainly not a new concept. Apoptosis is fundamental to how babies develop—the way certain cells in limb buds die, for instance, so that fingers and toes can form. It's the reason a tadpole loses its tail and becomes a frog. "If you look at these developing limb buds [in an embryo], the cells that are going to live are *right next to the cells that die.*" What could control such a tightly orchestrated, developmental pattern? For a long time, it was assumed that the microenvironment around the cell basically murdered it—in other words, that a bad environment killed the cells. But it's now clear that the cells that are dying are in a very happy environment: They've got plenty of nutrients, plenty of oxygen—everything that they need to live. But they've been given a signal, and that signal says, "Don't live. Die." And they do.

Now imagine a medieval fortress under siege. The enemy is outside, but one soldier scales the walls and opens the mighty gates, and this is all it takes to change the course of battle. By interfering with the crucial pump, thapsigargin allows that calcium outside the cell to sneak inside; it reaches too high a level, disrupts the cell, and activates this pathway of death. "The DNA inside the cell's nucleus gets all chewed up, and becomes degraded to the point of not being useful for any information. The nucleus itself becomes fragmented, then the cell becomes fragmented," says Isaacs. The grand finale is an act of cannibalism: These little fragments, called apoptotic bodies, are then consumed by neighboring cells.

"The great thing about this," says Isaacs, "is that the cell has no way of preventing its own activation of this pathway." Another bonus is that this death pathway—unlike many chemotherapeutic drugs—doesn't require rapidly dividing cells. It can kill any cell, within twenty-four to seventy-two hours. At this point, all of this work has been performed in animal models, and not yet tested in humans.

Drugs That Block Tumor Invasion and Metastasis

This is the "class of drugs that make biologic sense," says Johns Hopkins oncologist Michael Carducci. They are "antimetastatic"—they put roadblocks in the way of cancer's progress, hindering it from invading other cells, or from developing new blood vessels (this is called *angiogenesis,* discussed below), or from growing at all. *Matrix metalloproteinases* (MMPs) are enzymes—produced in abundance in many cancers—that enable cancer cells to invade by clearing a path around them, and making them more mobile. They're like worker bees. Scientists believe that by blocking these enzymes, they can inhibit, or at least slow down, the spread of cancer. There is biological precedent here: When a man nicks his chin shaving, for example, white blood cells and wound-healing cells called fibroblasts charge in, deactivate these enzymes, and save the day.

A drug called marimastat, given in pill form, works in much the same way; it inhibits MMPs. It has completed early trials, led by Eisenberger and Carducci (these are to make sure the drug is safe, and to find an effective dose). Now it is being tested in patients, with the hope that it will slow down the cancer, and slow the rise of PSA indefinitely. Other drugs in this exciting category are citrus pectin (a plant fiber derived from citrus fruit), and endothelin-1.

Blocking endothelin: targeting pain, and cancer itself? University of Pittsburgh urologist Joel Nelson has learned a lot about endothelin over the last few years: As a urology fellow at Johns Hopkins, he was the first to link this chemical—made by endothelial cells, which line blood vessels—to the excruciating, debilitating pain that comes when prostate cancer invades the bone. He also tied endothelin to the unique bone damage found in some men with prostate cancer, in which the bone becomes unnaturally thick and rock-hard. And his idea that thwarting endothelin might ease terrible pain—which, for years, was simply assumed to be an inevitable part of the grim package of "bony metastases"—has led to the first clinical trials of a new endothelin-blocking agent, called an endothelin receptor antagonist.

But it may be that Nelson has only scratched the surface: Endothelin may turn out to be an even bigger behind-the-scenes player in prostate cancer than anybody realized. And it just might be that blocking endothelin can alter the course of prostate cancer itself.

Endothelin is a vasoconstrictor, the most powerful one ever discovered. It is found in the bloodstream: In a heart attack, endothelin is one of several chemicals that cause an artery to spasm, or slam shut—cutting off the supply of blood and oxygen to tissue, resulting in terrible, sometimes crushing pain. But endothelin's concentrations are highest—about five hundred times greater—in semen; part of this fluid is contributed by the prostate.

Chemically, endothelin bears a striking resemblance to snake venom, and to apamin—"the compound that hurts so much when you get stung by a bee. Endothelin is painful when it's given in the right doses to humans," says Nelson. "Is it possible that some of the bone pain that men experience in advanced prostate cancer is because the cancerous cells are secreting something which is very similar to snake venom?" And is it possible to spare patients this terrible ordeal by cutting off the supply of endothelin?

So far, the early clinical trials of the endothelin-blocking agent

Nelson helped design—any trials of a new drug must first prove that it does no harm, and find a dosage that's safe for patients to take—have found that "the drug is very safe, very well tolerated," Nelson says. The drug, given to men and women with advanced cancer that had metastasized to the bone, did indeed seem to relieve pain, as measured by a significant decrease in patients' need for morphine or similar painkillers. (However, because there was no control group of patients taking placebos in these early studies, Nelson cautions that further studies are needed to determine just how effective the endothelin-blocker is in easing pain.) "If we can improve this terrible pain and make people feel better, we can make a major improvement in quality of life for these patients," Nelson says.

But he hopes for even more. The healthy prostate makes endothelin; the cancerous prostate does, too, even during hormonal therapy—and this is of great interest to Nelson. Because endothelin is impervious to hormones—just like the hormone-insensitive cells in advanced prostate cancer—is it possible that blocking endothelin can also somehow slow the growth of cancer, and prevent its damage? In laboratory studies, he and colleagues found that cancerous mice with higher levels of endothelin developed significantly more new bone growth (similar to the bone changes found in men with advanced prostate cancer) than other mice—and mice given an endothelin-blocker seemed to be protected against this growth.

The early clinical trials of the endothelin-blocker produced another exciting finding: a drop in PSA levels in 68 percent of men with prostate cancer. In some men, this decline was small—a decrease, for example, from 800 to 780. But in other men, PSA levels plummeted: One man's PSA shot down from 880 to 440 within a week; in two men, the PSA drop was nearly 90 percent. (It may be that some prostate cancers—which are notoriously variable in their makeup of cells, and their susceptibility to various forms of treatments—contain more endothelin, or are more affected by an endothelin-blocker, than others. If this proves true, perhaps scientists can one day predict who will be most greatly helped by this kind of drug.)

The next step is to find out whether the endothelin-blocker can go the distance in fighting the cancer itself. Already, Nelson's laboratory work has shown that endothelin inhibits cell death—that cells given endothelin are less vulnerable to chemotherapy, that they don't die as readily as other cells. "Obviously, we'd like cancer cells to die," he says. "If we can block endothelin's ability to let cancer cells survive, it may increase the effects of chemotherapy or hormonal therapy."

Angiogenesis Inhibitors

One way to stop cancer—cut off the supply line: The idea here is to put cancer on a leash. It may not die, but it won't get any bigger, either. There is great excitement in the scientific community about drugs that can accomplish this. They are called *angiogenesis inhibitors.*

Like Roman soldiers, advancing cancers pave the way before them, laying down a track of new blood vessels. This guarantees a ready-made supply of nutrients—nourishing meals for the road—which, it seems, the cancers absolutely cannot do without. Destroy this infrastructure, cut off the supply line, block these new blood vessels—and the cancer cells starve.

Cancer cells make new blood vessels grow by subverting a normal process involved in wound healing. "Usually, once you become an adult, your blood supply is pretty stable, and—except when your body's trying to repair an injury—you don't really need new blood vessels," explains Johns Hopkins oncologist John Isaacs. "But in order for a cancer to grow, it has to stimulate its host to do a lot of things for it. A cancer isn't an autonomous machine that can grow anywhere; it's not like an air fern that just needs sunlight and water. It's very dependent on its host, and one of the major reasons why is because it needs vigorous growth of new blood vessels."

This process is called angiogenesis—and drugs to block it, angiogenesis inhibitors, already exist. The good thing about these drugs, Isaacs says, is that "your other blood vessels—supplying your heart, lungs, brain, and normal tissue—are already fully developed. Inhibitors of angiogenesis don't really produce any damage to them. They target the blood vessels *only in cancerous areas.*"

Isaacs, Eisenberger, and Carducci have been working with an angiogenesis inhibitor called linomide, which has many qualities of a "dream" drug. It's inexpensive and already available, it can be given in pill form, it has low toxicity and hardly any side effects—and it does a beautiful job of stalling tumor growth. Best of all, "there's really no way the cancer cell can become resistant to its requirement for blood vessels." That would be like a lung cell becoming resistant to oxygen.

"The disadvantage is that it's not something you could take only once and then never take again," Isaacs continues. "The blood vessels are constantly being stimulated to grow by the tumor, so you'd have to take this chronically—like someone with high blood pressure who takes medication every day." But many men might find this a tiny price to pay for the potential benefits—putting a cancer's growth in slow motion for years, perhaps even decades. "Say a man has very limited, micro-metastatic disease," says Isaacs. "We know that, untreated, it might take five or six years (or longer) for this cancer to produce symptoms. But an antiangiogenic medication might be able to prevent that from happening for twenty years. If the man is sixty years old, that may allow him to not die from prostate cancer. He may still have prostate cancer cells in his body—this doesn't eliminate all of them—but it will allow him to survive his cancer." The advantage of these drugs is that they only block the formation of new vessels—they don't affect established vessels. And new vessels are the lifeblood, literally, of tumors. Unfortunately, however, they are also forming in the heart, all the time, as a natural way to bypass blocked vessels. There is concern that this may be a major problem in the widespread use of these drugs against cancer, and doctors are approaching studies of them in humans with great caution.

Angiogenesis inhibitors are being tested in many forms of cancer. Scientists believe they will work best on men with micrometastases, and that starting these drugs once cancer has become entrenched—when it starts producing such symptoms as bone pain—would be like closing the proverbial barn door after the horse has already galloped away: too little, too late. "If a man has very extensive disease, these drugs won't cause the tumor to melt away," explains Isaacs. (Another approach, such as gene therapy, may prove more effective for these men.) It may be that angiogenesis inhibitors will prove most effective when combined with other forms of treatment.

Some angiogenesis inhitors being tested in prostate cancer, at several centers around the country, include TNP-470, CM-101, thalidomide, tecogalan, angiostatin, and endostatin. Also, drugs in other categories seem to thwart angiogenesis as well.

Differentiating Agents

Here again, the idea is to slow down the cancer, to tame it—ideally, to make it revert to its former, slow-growing self. "Every cancer has cells that are dividing, and cells that are dying," says Eisenberger. "If the cells are proliferating very actively—much more than the rate of dying—then the cancer is growing." Differentiating agents keep cancer in check by slowing down the booming birth rate, giving the death rate a chance to catch up. "This is not conventional chemotherapy," adds Eisenberger. "It's not one of those drugs that you give and destroy everything, and then hope that the healthy things come back very quickly and the cancer cells will not recover. It's much more selective."

Differentiating agents that show promise: Differentiating agents that have worked well in early experiments include retinoids (vitamin A derivatives), vitamin D derivatives, and butyrates. In Chapter 3, we talked about vitamin D's role in discouraging cancer; in laboratory studies, it causes cells in culture to revert to a more differentiated state. Potent analogs of vitamin D are being tested to see whether they may work in men with more advanced disease. However—just as we discussed in Chapter 3, when it comes to preventing cancer—calcium may limit the effectiveness of these drugs. Another receptor on cells that blocks growth and promotes differentiation is known as PPAR-gamma (peroxisome proliferator-activated receptor gamma). The drug troglitazone (which was used to treat diabetes) activates this receptor, and clinical trials with this compound are in progress. There is some evidence that this receptor is activated by fatty acids; more on this in the diet section, below.

There are several studies involving the drug phenylbutyrate, for men with hormone-refractory prostate cancer. Phenylbutyrate is a "differentiating agent," which works by putting cancer's growth, or proliferation, in slow motion. Carducci and colleagues have shown that together with vitamin A (which slows down cancer's growth; low levels of vitamin A are believed to increase a man's susceptibility to prostate cancer), phenylbutyrate can hamper the growth of new blood vessels, and can shrink tumors and prevent them from progressing. In another study, phenylbutyrate will be combined with azacytidine, a drug that can reverse some of cancer's expedient genetic changes. "Cancers turn off certain genes that can inhibit cancer growth," says Carducci. "Azacytidine can turn those genes back on, and when you combine that with phenylbutyrate, you increase the likelihood that these genes will stay on, and give men a better chance to fight the cancer."

Drugs That Inhibit Signal Transduction and Cell-to-Cell Interaction Mechanisms

Cells talk to each other, through a bunch of signaling mechanisms involving highly specific receptors. There are several ways to interfere with these signals—to block the transmissions, or throw "static" in the mix, or change the message. Scientists have decoded some of these transmissions; in breast cancer, for example, we know that one of these receptors is HER-2. A "humanized" monoclonal antibody (like the MABs discussed above) has been approved by the Food and Drug Administration as a treatment of breast cancer. This same compound, in combination with several others, is also being tested in prostate cancer. Similar approaches for substances called growth factors, chemical switches that help promote cell division (some of which are believed to spur prostate cancer's progress) such as epidermal growth factor, are also under way.

Chemotherapy

The accepted thinking, until recently, has been that chemotherapy doesn't work in prostate cancer—and in many respects (such as the slow nature of prostate cancer cell proliferation, discussed above), this is largely true. However, in the past, doctors didn't give it much of a chance to work, either. The men who were felt to be candidates for chemotherapy often had what's called "poor performance status." Even the name of this category registers defeat. Here, chemotherapy was the last resort, the "Hail Mary pass." These men were in pain, often debilitated; they had lost weight, and were too weak to tolerate strong doses of chemotherapy. Thus, we have to admit that chemotherapy really wasn't given a fair shot—and we do not know for sure that in other, less beaten-down patients, it might not have worked better.

Today, as we've mentioned above, chemotherapy is being viewed in a new light. It's now being considered for men who are not in pain, who have a much smaller, more manageable tumor burden—in other words, for men with a "good performance status." We also have a better marker to help us here—once again, our invaluable friend PSA. In years past, it was hard to know whether the cancer was responding because the markers we did have—bone scans, for instance—were crude in comparison, with much room for ambiguity. PSA lets us be much more objective—and basically, we're rewriting the textbooks in this field. Doctors now are getting smarter about how to use these drugs.

For example: Johns Hopkins oncologists Mario Eisenberger and Michael Carducci are studying drugs in the taxane family (which includes the drug Taxol, shown to help women with ovarian cancer). One of them, Taxotere, is being studied in combination with Emcyt— an estrogen-related drug known to diminish testosterone and kill cancer cells, but which has caused undesirable side effects including nausea, heart problems, and a higher risk of blood clots. "Virtually all studies using the combination of Taxotere and Emcyt have shown a consistent response in patients with widespread disease, ranging between 30 and 70 percent," says Eisenberger. "But the side effects of Emcyt are very prominent, because men have to take it daily." Eisenberger developed a new protocol, in which Emcyt is given for one day only in five divided doses, along with Taxotere. "This abbreviated exposure to Emcyt has substantially improved the tolerance of this combination," Eisenberger says. Emcyt and Taxotere are repeated every three weeks, for a total of six times. "We're observing a high response rate, about 50 percent, and our next objective is build on that." In some patients, results have been dramatic: PSA levels have dropped by at least 50 percent, pain has decreased significantly, and metastases—even in the lymph nodes and liver—have shrunk.

New drug combinations such as these are being developed almost every day. However, until now, the major benefits have been in improving the quality of life—particularly with combinations of mitoxandrone and prednisone, which has been shown to reduce pain. So far, none of these agents has shown a significant improvement in survival, and no regimen today could be considered standard therapy for the disease. However, the recent success of some of these combinations gives us great hope that—as we develop better drugs and get smarter in using them, and as more men enroll in clinical trials before cancer has progressed—we should be able to see a significant impact on length, as well as quality, of life.

The Exception to Standard Chemotherapy: Small-Cell Carcinoma

Small-cell carcinoma is different from "regular" prostate cancer in many ways, although at first it looks just the same. Typically, a man who has small-cell carcinoma of the prostate appears to have the usual prostate cancer, and may undergo surgery or radiation to cure it. Sometimes, however, the disease returns—with a vengeance. Instead of a few stray cells causing a detectable PSA, small-cell carcinoma bursts back on the scene as a rapidly growing, soft-tissue mass, often in the prostate bed. Worse, this is often quickly followed by spots of cancer in the lungs, liver, bone, and brain—and throughout all of this, a man may have only a low PSA. The diagnosis of small-cell can be confirmed with a biopsy of one of these areas. It is crucial to know whether you have this form of prostate cancer, because the same drugs that work on small-cell carcinoma elsewhere in the body work here as well. Many doctors prescribe combinations of cisplatin or carboplatin and Etoposide, Taxol, Taxotere, and topotecan. Radiation can be very effective in targeting isolated metastases as well.

Help if You're in Pain

Another issue in advanced cancer is the day-to-day business of palliative treatment—easing symptoms and pain, and keeping up nutrition in men who don't feel like eating. In this area of treatment, thankfully, there *is* much that can be done, and *you have a right to demand everything possible*—medication or a procedure to ease pain or symptoms of urinary obstruction—to make your life better. Many men are amazed at how much better they feel when the *individual* symptoms of advanced prostate cancer are addressed and eased. And the intangible benefits of simply feeling more like your old self again—being able to go back to work, play a round of golf, or attend a family gathering—are beyond price.

"Pain is very closely associated with quality of life," says Johns Hopkins oncologist Mario Eisenberger. "People in pain have a reduced appetite; they lose weight. They're often depressed. Sometimes they're bedridden, the pain is so bad. If we control the pain aggressively, we often see patients getting stronger and eating better. Aggressive pain management is clearly to the patient's benefit."

It's not only beneficial, it's your *right* as a patient not to suffer. Far too many men with advanced prostate cancer endure excruciating pain in the course of their disease. Several studies have shown that an average of 72 percent of men with advanced prostate cancer are in pain. In one study of 201 men with prostate cancer, 47 percent reported feeling pain that ranged from "moderate to very bad"— *despite the use of painkillers.* This tells us several things. One is that, as diseases go, prostate cancer is more painful than most. Its particular patterns of spreading—metastases to bone, and particularly to the spine—make it second only to cervical cancer in terms of severe pain. But this study also shows us something else: These 201 men were on analgesics—painkillers—yet they still hurt. Some of them even felt miserable pain. *Does this mean that painkillers don't work? No. It means the doctors treating these men weren't giving them enough medication to make them comfortable.*

There is no excuse for that. And often, both sides—doctors as well as patients—are at fault. An article by University of Colorado scientists cited some reasons why prostate cancer patients often are undermedicated.

Here are some of the reasons why doctors may not give enough pain medication: One is that many doctors just don't learn enough about pain medication in medical school and in their subsequent professional training; they learn how to save or prolong lives, but not always how to make their patients comfortable. (This situation is getting better, as medical schools and continuing education courses are doing a better job teaching doctors how to manage patients' pain.)

But perhaps a bigger problem—and this also has to do with the way health care professionals are educated—is the very real fear that patients will get addicted. *This is hogwash.* The sole purpose of these drugs is to alleviate pain, and frankly, few patients need these medications more desperately than people with cancer—especially men with metastatic prostate cancer whose pain is extreme.

And yet every day all over this country, this study showed, some doctors prescribe painkillers at inadequate dosages; some nurses withhold doses of painkillers; and some pharmacists refuse to provide drugs.

In addition, some doctors worry about controlling the side effects of analgesics (see below). They worry about inadvertently precipitating a patient's death—or worse, being an unwitting part in a patient's suicide attempt—if he overdoses.

Other problems listed in this study come under the category of communication failure. Some guidelines for drug dosages (printed in medical reference books and other sources) are not appropriate for the particular intensity of cancer pain. And sometimes—this is increasingly common—if a patient is being looked after by a group of physicians, there may not be a clear understanding of who's responsible for pain management. The pain may "fall through the cracks."

You're a patient; what can you do? If you're suffering terrible pain, talk to your physician. If you're being treated by a group practice, demand that one doctor oversee your pain and other symptoms. If you're still not satisfied with the care you're getting, look for another doctor—preferably, someone who treats many cancer patients and is attuned to their particular, intense pain.

Another option is to contact the National Hospice Organization, a group whose goal is to "enable patients to carry on an alert, pain-free life and to manage other symptoms," so their days "may be spent with dignity and quality at home or in a home-like setting." (For more on this, see "Where to Get Help," at the end of this book.)

Most hospice programs—and there are hundreds throughout the country—are directed by physicians, and care is administered by a spectrum of health care professionals, including nurses, psychologists, members of the clergy, and social workers. Care is available twenty-four hours a day, every day, and it is centered around patients and their families.

There are also some regulatory issues, the University of Colorado study showed. When potentially addictive narcotics (strong painkillers like morphine) are involved, so is the government. That's why most of these drugs are called "controlled substances." Some governmental red tape can include limits on refills; however, this is not an insurmountable difficulty—it just means patients need to get their doctors to write new prescriptions when their medication runs out.

But finally, the study showed a variety of reasons why the *patients themselves* didn't ask for adequate pain medication. Some men aren't very good at expressing their symptoms, or conveying the depth of their pain, the researchers found. Some men feel it isn't "macho" to admit that their pain is intolerable. (If you have a problem with this, it may help to take along a family member who feels no such hesitation when you go to see the doctor.) Other men are afraid of becoming addicted—and some of these men aren't helped any when zealous family members urge them to "just say no" to drugs!

Some men believe that the pain is just an inevitable part of having the cancer and that nothing can be done to help them. Others worry about the pain yet to come, and want to save the "big guns," the strongest medications, until the pain becomes intolerable. (Actually, with heavy-duty painkillers like morphine, relief *always* comes when doctors boost the dosage, so there is nothing to be gained by seeing how much pain you can stand.) Some men don't want to be labeled as "bad" patients by complaining about their pain. And finally, the study said, some men—ever the providers—worry that costly pain medication will use up all their families' resources. For these men, methadone may be a good option—at around $30 a month, it's the cheapest narcotic.

The bottom line is that you—or a loved one with prostate cancer— do not need to suffer terrible pain. There is help available. Take it.

Drugs for pain: It makes sense to treat each level and kind of pain differently. At the lowest level is mild pain that responds to aspirin, acetaminophen (Tylenol), or ibuprofen (Advil or Motrin). Next come opiates, drugs such as codeine. As opiates go, these drugs are considered weak. In terms of pain relief, they can't hold a candle to high-powered opiates such as morphine—the highest rung on the pain relief ladder. (However, these milder opiates generally are sufficient to ease moderate pain.) The biggest advantage to strong opiates is "their lack of ceiling effect," as one study puts it. "Increasing the dose always increases the pain relief," although it also can increase the side effects.

In addition, other drugs not generally classified as painkillers— particularly corticosteroids—have proved helpful in reducing inflammation and bringing relief from some spinal pain. Ask your doctor if one of these drugs might be right for you.

If you are elderly, have other health problems, or are taking other medications, certain painkillers may have a stronger effect on you than on other men. Be sure to discuss these factors, the side effects of various drugs, and the form in which you should take these drugs—a pill, or liquid, rectal suppository, skin patch, or shot—with your doctor. If you need additional information, your pharmacist also may be able to provide you with the package insert sheets for various drugs. These generally are impenetrable, are written in tiny print, and confusing—they contain more information than most people want to know. They also tend to list every possible side effect, even the unlikely ones. However, some people find this information helpful.

(For more sources of information, see "Where to Get Help," at the end of this book.)

Complementary approaches to pain management: Talk to your doctor before you try any treatment, even if seems "natural." Having said that, many people benefit from other, nontraditional forms of pain management, including prayer and meditation (discussed below), acupuncture, deep breathing, aromatherapy, relaxation techniques, massage therapy, biofeedback, hypnosis, yoga, and even laughter (also called humor therapy). Advocates of these therapies cite many good effects. They can lower blood pressure; reduce stress hormones, which cause the arteries to tighten; slow the heart rate; block or interfere with pain signals; stimulate the immune system; cause the body to release endorphins—its own natural painkillers—improve blood circulation. Most importantly, the above therapies are not harmful. And all of these benefits—particularly those to the cardiovascular system—can improve your quality of life.

Drugs for milder pain: Listed here are some nonsteroidal anti-inflammatory drugs (NSAIDS) and some of their brand names. (Just because we don't mention the brand name here doesn't mean it isn't a good drug.) Over-the-counter drugs include aspirin; acetaminophen (brand names include Tylenol and Datril); and ibuprofen (brand names include Motrin, Advil, and Nuprin). Prescription drugs include diflunisal (Dolobid); choline magnesium trisalicylate (Trisilate); salsalate (Disalcid); naproxen (Naprosyn); naproxen sodium (Anaprox); indomethacin (Indocin); sulindac (Clinoril); and ketorolac (Toradol).

Drugs for moderate to severe pain: Here are prescription drugs, and some of their brand names. (Again, not all brand names are mentioned here.) They include fentanyl (Duragesic); propoxyphene (Darvon, Darvocet); codeine (Tylenol with codeine); oxycodone (Tylox, Percocet, Percodan); meperidine (Demerol); methadone (Dolophine); hydromorphone (Dilaudid); and morphine (Roxanol).

Treating Specific Pain

Until recently, a widespread treatment called "hemi-body" irradiation commonly was used to ease pain in prostate cancer patients with metastases to bone in several places. Hemi-body irradiation involved what radiologists call "wide fields" of radiation—large expanses of the body, and comparatively high doses of radiation. The problem was that this often wiped out key blood-forming cells in the bone marrow and compromised the body's immune system, resulting in such complications as infections and the need for transfusions.

Now, for pain that is concentrated in one area—a portion of the spine, for instance—more specific pain treatment is a far better approach. Some of these are discussed below.

Spot radiation: This is localized external-beam radiation treatment, targeted at one or several painful bone metastases. It won't prevent new metastases from cropping up in bone, but it generally helps ease pain in the sites it does treat. Spot radiation often results in several months of dramatic relief from pain, and it helps prevent spinal cord compression (see below). In recent studies, 55 percent of patients received complete relief from pain, 33 percent had partial relief, and only 12 percent had little or no response.

Radioactive strontium: Strontium-89, a radioactive isotope injected into the body as an outpatient procedure, is specially tailored for bone pain. Like calcium, it is taken up immediately by bone, as water is absorbed by a sponge—except this compound tends to zoom right past healthy bone and zero in on metastatic cancer. (Strontium-89 is soaked up by tumor in bone, instead of bone marrow, at a ratio of ten to one.) Relief from pain has been reported in from half to 80 percent of patients

Strontium-89 has a long half-life—fifty-one days—in the body; a single shot of the compound has proved effective at relieving pain for an average of six months. One advantage of this, as compared to spot radiation, is that it acts on *new sites of metastasis* that crop up while it stays in the body, as well as the older sites of cancer it originally was intended to treat. A European study suggests that strontium-89 may be even more effective if it's given earlier, before bone pain develops; this may help prevent progression of bony metastases, and avoid the need for spot radiation.

Also, strontium-89 can be used in combination with spot radiation. In one study, doctors found that this combined approach—strontium-89 plus spot radiation—delayed progression of pain seven months longer than radiation alone.

Side effects: The few side effects associated with strontium-89

include the potential for bone marrow damage; this is characterized by a drop in platelets. Also, some men report a mild increase in pain for the first couple of days after receiving the injection; this can be controlled with other pain medication. And a safety note: Because this radioactive substance is excreted in the urine, for the first forty-eight hours after receiving the injection urine must be taken care of in a certain way; this means you must urinate into a special container—not into the toilet—and dispose of this as directed by your doctor.

Bisphosphonates: In early studies, drugs in this group, particularly pamidronate, also have shown promise in easing the pain of bone metastases in other forms of cancer.

When Additional Treatment May Be Needed

In addition to causing extreme pain, metastases of cancer to bone can cause two other catastrophic complications—spinal cord compression and pathologic fracture.

Spinal cord compression: About a third of men with metastatic prostate cancer may be at risk for spinal cord compression—when cancer eats away at the spine, causing part of the spinal column to collapse, trapping and sometimes crushing nearby nerves. If you have severe pain in your back that accompanies leg weakness, loss of sensation (often beginning with numbness or tingling in the toes), trouble walking, constipation, or urinary retention, you may be at risk, and you need an MRI scan right away. *An MRI scan is essential—it gives details of the spinal cord and can show early signs of compression.* If spinal cord compression is an immediate danger, the MRI will show the cancer invading the dura, the membrane surrounding the spinal cord; this is called extradural compression. If your hospital doesn't have an MRI machine, it's worth it to make arrangements to travel to another hospital. *This is a very serious problem—a true emergency—and it requires aggressive, immediate treatment!* It is far better to treat potential spinal cord compression early than to try and repair the damage after it happens.

Patients in imminent danger of spinal cord compression should be treated with large doses of corticosteroids (usually a drug called Decadron) for forty-eight hours. Then, depending on how your body responds to this, your doctor will make a decision on what to do next—this could mean spot radiation treatment to the spine, or something called surgical decompression, an operation to ease the cancer's pressure on the spinal cord.

If you have not yet begun hormonal therapy, now is an excellent time to begin—and fast—with immediate castration or treatment with an antiandrogen (see above). Giving an LHRH agonist alone in this situation is not a good idea, because it can cause a surge in testosterone that could aggravate the cancer sitting so precariously in the spine. This may be a unique job for drugs called LHRH antagonists, when they are approved for use.

Spinal cord compression is yet another blow in a series of unpleasant complications of prostate cancer, and it has the greatest potential to ruin quality of life—it can lead to paralysis, with an accompanying loss of bowel and bladder function. Most significantly, it can result in the loss of a patient's independence and feeling of dignity.

If you begin to feel any of the warning signs mentioned above, *call your doctor immediately; don't wait until your next scheduled appointment!* This may mean the difference between remaining able to walk and being bedridden.

Pathologic fracture: When cancer invades bones, they become brittle. Brittle bones break. Therefore, men with metastatic prostate cancer are prone to broken bones (called pathologic fractures). Most susceptible are bones that bear much of the body's weight, in the hip and thigh. Sometimes, doctors can take steps to protect bones at risk—putting pins in the hipbone to strengthen it, for example. Such steps are a good idea when a bone has a large area of cancer (greater than 3 centimeters in diameter) that takes up at least half of the bone's outer shell.

Other Complications

Fatigue: Develop a healthy respect for fatigue. For many people with cancer—any kind of cancer—it's a ubiquitous shadow. Hard to measure, and sometimes hard to see (particularly in men who make the extra effort not to show discomfort or admit any perceived weakness), fatigue can have profound effects. Wendy S. Harpham, a physician who has experienced this "on both sides of the stethoscope," in caring for patients and in her own battle as a long-term survivor of non-Hodgkin's lymphoma, coined the term "post-cancer fatigue." As she recently observed in the journal *CA—A Cancer Journal for Clinicians,* this fatigue can manifest itself in unexpected ways—difficulty concentrating or learning new information, forgetfulness, irritability or emotional swings, clumsiness, malaise, loss of interest in the world in general, miscommunication, mistakes, or decreased sexual desire. "Unlike the tiredness that healthy people feel, this fatigue is more difficult for patients to ignore, often impairs patients' ability to function well, and is not relieved with one night's rest. . . . The underlying physical problem . . . is that extra effort is required for even normal activities and social interactions." Because your energy levels may fluctuate from one day to the next, or even from hour to hour, this may affect your ability to "pull your weight" at home or work—and this, in turn, may heap guilt or feelings of inadequacy on top of your other burdens. It may inevitably affect your family and colleagues as well. "The situation may be compounded," Harpham adds, "if well partners, caregivers, or coworkers run out of steam. No matter how tired healthy people may be, they feel they can't complain or take a rest because [cancer] survivors are always more tired."

If any of this description strikes a familiar chord, talk about it with the people in your life, Harpham advises—so they can understand what's going on. A "tense facial expression or body language may cause bosses, friends, co-workers, and family members to believe that [you're] angry, sad, or upset when, in fact, simple tiredness is the culprit. Children may worry, mistakenly, that their parents are angry with them." Fatigue can fuel anxiety as well, and magnify everything. But learning to recognize fatigue for what it is—and taking a few necessary steps to accommodate it, instead of becoming frustrated with what you can't do—can help many patients and their families deal with this problem. For more help, talk to your doctor.

Urinary tract obstruction: If you're having any of these symptoms—weak urine flow; hesitancy in starting urination; a need to push or strain to get urine to flow; intermittent urine stream (starts and stops several times); difficulty in stopping urination; dribbling after urination; a sense of not being able to empty the bladder completely; or not being able to urinate at all—it's probable that the cancer has become extensive enough to block your urinary tract. Several procedures are available to ease these symptoms, including a TURP procedure or the placement of stents.

Weight loss: What's wrong with losing weight, particularly if you've spent the better part of your life trying to do just that? The problem here is that people who have cancer need to eat. Losing weight means losing strength and the body's reserve for fighting off illness.

No appetite? Able to eat just a little at a time? The thought of vitamins makes you gag? Then eat less, more often—have small, nutritious snacks throughout the day. Make every calorie count. Empty calories in sugared iced tea or soda won't do your body as much good as the calories in juice, for instance; the same goes for the empty calories in a doughnut versus the calories in a muffin or slice of banana bread. Finally, if you just can't force yourself to eat as much food as your body needs, you may want to try a calorie-packed liquid nutrition supplement like Ensure or Sustacal. Most hospitals have nutritionists available to help you solve dietary problems like these. That's what these people are there for—let them help!

In severe cases of weight loss, doctors can insert a gastrostomy tube, which bypasses the upper digestive tract and allows patients to get much needed nutrition in liquid form. This tube provides a painless route for food to get to your stomach. It's comfortable and discreet—hidden by clothes—and it can be removed when your appetite comes back and you don't need it anymore.

Constipation: This is another big problem for many men taking strong painkillers like morphine, which sedate the digestive tract as they relieve pain. Many doctors prescribe mild laxatives or stool softeners at the same time they prescribe opiate analgesics. Another option is adding fiber supplements to your diet; these are available in a variety of forms, including mixtures you can add to fruit juice. You don't have to have a bowel movement every day, but you should be having one every two to three days—and when it does happen, it should not be uncomfortable.

PROSTATE CANCER AND DEPRESSION

Here are some of the things you already have to cope with—stress, fear, anger, anxiety, sweating out one PSA test after another, pain, fatigue, uncertainty. And the cancer itself. But at some point, an estimated one in four cancer patients battle depression as well. Although it's common, this is not a normal part of cancer, and it can be treated. Not treating depression—in a stoic attempt to "ride it out," or "snap out of it"—can even shorten your life. This is something beyond the normal sadness that accompanies having cancer.

If you have any of these symptoms, see your doctor: sadness that won't go away; sleeping much more, or much less, than normal; waking early in the morning, worried, and being unable to go back to sleep; inability to be happy; eating much more, or much less, than normal; feeling tired all the time; inability to concentrate or make decisions; restlessness; listlessness; not wanting to participate in normal activities; feelings of worthlessness, helplessness, and guilt; thinking often about death or suicide.

The vast majority of people suffering from depression can be treated successfully. Because the problem—believed to stem from a biochemical imbalance, or faulty communication in brain cells—differs in everyone, it may take a bit of trial and error for you and your doctor to find the treatment that works best. Be patient, and don't give up. It may also help for you to talk to other men who are going through this. Ask your doctor about support groups in your area. (For more, see "Where to Get Help," at the end of this book.)

Complementary Medicine

In Chapter 4, we discussed many dietary approaches to preventing prostate cancer. Although the situation is different, the caveat of treating yourself still applies. Just because something is "complementary," or "alternative," and you can buy it in a "health" food store, doesn't mean it can't hurt you. Remember, you can overdose on anything, if you get too much of it. Anything can be toxic, if taken improperly. Complementary medicine can include "lifestyle therapy" (some approaches are mentioned above in the section on pain) and dietary changes. At a minimum, these lifestyle approaches (including spirituality and prayer, discussed below) can change the way you perceive your illness. They can help you cope better, and there is a cascade of good events that can come from this—eating better, for one thing, becoming more rested, feeling stronger, and having a greater sense of well-being.

Changing your diet may help slow the course of prostate cancer, but nobody knows for sure yet. There is evidence to support this, which we'll discuss below. On the other hand, as we discussed above, it is dangerous to lose too much weight; this could backfire, and seriously impede your body's ability to fight cancer. Also, studies suggest that as many as two thirds of patients who use alternative therapies don't tell their doctors. This is bad; alternative therapies (even the "natural" remedies such as plant extracts or botanicals) can change the effectiveness of other medications, and cause side effects. If you choose to augment your diet with any supplements, be sure to tell your doctor.

The Mind-Body Connection

The mind has a tremendous—and largely untapped—ability to influence the body, for bad as well as good. With this in mind, let's take a moment to dispel some guilt. There are a lot of books out there—and countless seminars, articles, and self-help pamphlets— selling the idea that with the right attitude, mental state, spiritual serenity, or even diet, you can heal yourself or control your illness. Okay—in fact, we'll explore this briefly in a minute. But the flip side of this argument is that if your illness progresses, somehow you've messed up, that you're to blame—not eaten enough vegetables, taken the right multivitamins or supplements, gotten enough rest or exercise, or just generally allowed negativity to compromise your health. This definitely is not true.

"The average patient generally does not have a clear grasp of the molecular biology of carcinogenesis," writes physician and cancer survivor Wendy Harpham, in *CA—A Cancer Journal for Clinicians.* "Even to those patients who understand that recurrence is due to mutated cells that escaped the earlier round(s) of cancer therapy, the possibility of having accelerated the recurrence can be disturbing. Just as believers in mind-over-matter worry that negative thoughts can cause cancer cells to multiply, those who want to believe that proper actions can control outcome worry . . . that they've set themselves up for progression of disease." Too often with cancer, Harpham adds, a vicious cycle of fatigue and anxiety can set in, each feeding off the other.

British evangelist David Watson, who wrote about his own battle with cancer in the book *Fear No Evil,* points out how unproductive such thinking is: "Many times I have talked with those who are seriously ill, and I have found them anxiously wondering what they had done to bring about their condition. They blame themselves; or if they cannot live with that, they project their guilt on to others or God. It's someone's fault! The trouble is that either feelings of guilt, which are often imaginary, or direct accusations, which are often unfair, only encourage the sickness. Both hinder healing."

Above, we mentioned some therapeutic options that generally come under the heading of "alternative," or "complementary" medicine (although these practices, many of them traditionally Eastern, are becoming increasingly respected by Western physicians). All of these have been helpful to somebody; and the way they help one person may not be the way they prove beneficial to you. But we know that using your *mind* to lower your blood pressure, to facilitate deep breathing and relaxation, can help your *body* in its battle with cancer. We also know that the "lone wolf" does not do as well as the man who has many connections—who is married, who has good relationships with family and friends, who goes to church or synagogue. Many studies have confirmed the importance of emotional connection— loving support—in good health. As Tedd Mitchell, M.D., director of the Cooper Clinic's Wellness Program, recently observed in a national magazine, "We are made not to live alone, but to interact regularly with others. . . . In my medical practice, it seems that patients with strong family ties cope better with illness."

Now, what about faith, prayer, and spirituality? If you are religious—whatever your religion—you probably feel great comfort in knowing that you're not alone, that God is always with you. You can draw strength from prayer and from the prayers of others, and from seeking peace. You can surrender the burdens of illness, anxiety, fear, fatigue, and uncertainty—trade them all in for a greater serenity about the future.

Note: If you are not religious, but thinking about it, now is the perfect time to explore your spirituality. There are excellent reasons to support this decision—numerous studies have shown that, among other benefits, religious people—who put their faith in something larger than themselves—live longer, have lower blood pressure, need fewer pain medications. But if you are not interested, then you should not feel pressured; extra pressure is the last thing you need in your life right now. You should be allowed that freedom, and family members and friends should respect your wishes. (However, you still may want to explore one or more of the complementary forms of therapy mentioned above, for stress reduction, relief of pain, and an improved sense of well-being.)

So: If you pray for God to take away your cancer, will you be healed? Maybe. But many religious leaders say that the better, far more effective, prayer is the "Thy will be done" kind—because you don't know the big plan for your life (if you believe there is one, that is). Nobody does. It may help for you to talk about this with your doctor as well, if you feel comfortable doing so. Ask your doctor if he or she believes in God, and in prayer. You can also direct your prayers for greater good—to help the doctors taking care of you, the scientists working to find the cure, and all the men with prostate cancer, and their families.

Can Changing Your Diet Affect Your Cancer?

In Chapters 3 and 4, we discussed the strong circumstantial evidence linking the development of prostate cancer to dietary factors. It also appears that diet can influence the development of prostate cancer throughout an adult's lifetime. To boil down the facts:

- At autopsy, between 30 and 50 percent of men around the world— even in Asia, where prostate cancer is very rare—are found to have small amounts of prostate cancer.
- The lifetime risk of developing prostate cancer for men living in Asia is 2 percent. In the United States, it's much higher—16 percent.
- When an Asian man moves to a Western country, within twenty-five years, his risk of developing prostate cancer nears that of a Caucasian man in North America.

This suggests that the factors that cause prostate cancer to begin are common in all cultures. Something about our Western diet promotes these small areas of cancer to grow large enough to need treatment— but something about the Asian diet seems to prevent this progression of cancer.

Based on these facts, many men believe that once they have prostate cancer, they can slow it down or cause it to reverse itself by changing their diet. One of the most intelligent and vocal advocates of this is Michael Milken, who at the age of forty-seven was diagnosed with advanced prostate cancer. His story is well known, because he has devoted his life and considerable resources to fighting this disease, and finding a cure. He has also changed his diet; he drastically reduced the amount of fat he eats (to 9 grams a day), and stopped eating desserts and most dairy products. Furthermore, because the Asian diet is rich in soy protein, he made this a staple of his diet, substituting tofu or tempeh for meat, and mixing soy protein isolate powder with water or fruit juice. To make his spartan diet more palatable, he worked closely with Chef Beth Ginsberg to create tasty meals. (These are in *The Taste for Living Cookbooks*, by Ginsberg and Milken.) The idea of finding a "cancer-fighting" diet strongly appeals to many men.

In fact, many men with prostate cancer spend a lot of time at the health food store, loading up on dietary supplements such as saw palmetto and zinc. Although it's probably not a bad idea to take vitamin E and selenium (see Chapter 4), there is no good evidence that other supplements or herbals will help slow down the progression of established cancer.

Thus, the verdict on diet and advanced prostate cancer is: We don't know yet. There has been no scientific, objective study to examine this approach. We do know that in breast cancer—a disease that seems to parallel prostate cancer, with its low rates in Asian women, and increase in risk when Asian women migrate to Western countries—the consumption of fat, red meat, or fiber after diagnosis has not been found to lengthen or shorten life. As we discussed in Chapter 3, prostate cancer is believed to happen because of oxidative damage to DNA. Hit after hit—mainly from eating too many "bad" things, or not enough "good" things—causes a series of irreversible mutations in DNA, which in turn lead to cancer.

It is not reasonable to assume that diet can reverse cancer after the fact—that it can "unring the bell." The best example of this is smoking—we know it causes lung cancer, but it's impossible to make lung cancer go away by stopping smoking. There are a number of studies that suggest that soy and rye bran can inhibit the development of tumors. However, in most of these studies, treatment with soy must begin at the time the tumors are implanted into the animals. Soy and bran contain significant amounts of phytoestrogens, and these plant-derived estrogens can act like other estrogens and suppress testosterone. Also, some of these cancer cell lines can respond to estrogen itself. Thus, it's unclear whether these experimental studies can accurately predict what would happen to a man who has an established cancer.

Having said all that: There are some reasons to believe that changing your diet may help. In the nonhormonal treatment section above, we mentioned a receptor on cancer cells called PPAR-γ (pronounced "gamma"). When it's activated, this receptor causes prostate cancer cells to become more differentiated. There is some evidence that fatty acids in the blood may interact with this receptor.

Also, several studies have suggested that when animals are fed a fat-free diet, experimental prostate cancers grow more slowly. And arachidonic acid, an omega-6 polyunsaturated fatty acid, is known to stimulate the growth of prostate cancer cells in tissue culture.

So what's the bottom line? If you want to change your diet to reduce the intake of fat, and increase your intake of soy, you should do it. But be careful not to lose too much weight too quickly. A rapid, 10 percent drop in your weight can compromise your immune system—which may be the major self-defense mechanism that is holding your cancer in check.

NOTE FOR WIVES, PARTNERS, AND CAREGIVERS: TAKE CARE OF YOUR OWN HEALTH, TOO

Alice B. Baldwin, whose husband had a successful radical prostatectomy (but who died a few years later of colon cancer), became a reluctant expert on coping with a husband's illness. She has some excellent advice to offer wives on this subject. "You may be tempted to skip meals, to lose sleep, to forgo exercise, to drive in bad weather, and generally to ignore your own health," particularly if your husband is hospitalized.

But neglecting your own health now may mean you won't have enough strength and stamina left over for the longer haul. "Recognizing your needs and fulfilling them as adequately as circumstances permit is your obligation not only to yourself, but also to your spouse and to all who love you."

• *Eat right, and take a multivitamin.* Baldwin learned this the hard way during her husband's recovery from liver surgery. "Because of my concern for his welfare, I skipped meals off and on for a few days. Suddenly, the corridor blurred, and I found myself gripping a water cooler to keep from falling. For a few awful moments, I was afraid I would faint. In a few minutes I felt better, and after eating a light lunch, I was perfectly all right. I realized what a serious mistake I'd made by skipping those meals." If you can't take time for a regular lunch, be prepared, with energy-boosting snacks such as boxes of juice, cheese and crackers, raisins, peanuts, and granola bars. Just don't let yourself become run-down.

• *Keep track of your weight.* "We all react differently to stress, but you should note and quickly correct gains or losses of more than a few pounds."

• *Get some exercise.* Take a walk once or twice a day. You'll need your own strength and resilience now more than ever.

• *Get some sleep.* Your odds of sleeping better will improve if you keep up an adequate diet and get some exercise. Recognize that stress interferes with your body's normal patterns, and snooze when you can—even if it's not when you're used to resting. Relaxation techniques—listening to peaceful music, visualizing pleasant scenes, breathing deeply—may help you unwind. If it helps, "remind yourself that you've done the best you could; your spouse and the medical staff have done the best they could; and now the day has ended," says Baldwin, although she admits that some nights she was simply too upset to sleep. "My husband's condition, his doctors' anxieties, my fears of the future all outweighed my physical and emotional exhaustion. Even as I write this sentence, my stomach muscles tighten, my throat constricts, my palms begin to sweat, and I remember exactly how scared I felt."

• *Ask family and friends for help—particularly if you're commuting to the hospital or doctor's office on unfamiliar roads or in heavy traffic.* "At the hospital, you will benefit from their handholding and emotional support; on the road, they can handle the tricky turns."

• *Check your own daily vital signs.* Baldwin recommends asking yourself some basic questions every day, including: How do I feel today? Why do I feel that way? Tomorrow, I will take care of my need for (fill in the blank). What concern interfered with my sleep?

Finally, when the treatment is over, and life is getting back to normal, *realize that your relationship has altered in subtle but significant ways*, Baldwin says. "If we did not actually love one another more than we did before the illness, we now cherished one another more fully. Our children and our relationships with them were similarly changed. Perhaps the experiences we shared accelerated our normal maturation and led us all to appreciate one another more deeply.

"I recognize that I was physically and emotionally drained, and that I lost much of my resilience. Evidently this was obvious to our children, because I detected them going to new lengths to protect and to help me. My gratitude to them was tempered by my concern for them. Discussing this with the youngest, a recent college graduate, I said: 'We do not want our lives to interfere with your life,' and she replied, 'Your lives are part of my life.' "

Glossary: A Guide to Medical Language of the Prostate, from A to Z

Note: Most of the words here are nouns; where we thought it necessary, we indicated otherwise.

A

Ablation: to "get rid of." Cryoablation, for example, means using freezing temperatures to get rid of prostate cancer. Hormonal ablation means getting rid of the hormones that nourish a prostate tumor.

Acid phosphatase: an enzyme that, like PSA, is secreted by the prostate. Elevated acid phosphatase levels can signal that something is wrong with the prostate.

Acute bacterial prostatitis: a form of prostatitis associated with urinary tract infections, positive cultures that identify bacteria in the prostate, and an abundance of white blood cells in prostatic secretions. Acute bacterial prostatitis comes on suddenly, accompanied by fever and symptoms that demand prompt treatment.

Adrenal androgens: weak male hormones made by the adrenal glands. These include androstenedione, dehydroepiandrosterone (DHEA), and dehydroepiandrosterone sulfate (DHEAS), plus small amounts of testosterone. They are minor players, believed to make up only 5 percent or less of the total androgen stimulation to the prostate. Their total effect on the prostate is a controversial issue.

Age-specific PSA levels: a new way to evaluate PSA tests, using a man's age to determine the significance of his PSA reading.

Alpha blockers: drugs, originally designed to treat hypertension, that act on the prostate by relaxing smooth muscle tissue.

Alpha-linolenic acid: among the omega-3 class of polyunsaturated fats, but it's a "bad" one, found in red meats, margarine, cooking oils, and mayonnaise.

Analgesics: painkillers.

Analog: a synthetic lookalike of a drug or body chemical.

Anal stricture: tight scar tissue that can interfere with a bowel movement.

Anastomosis: the site where two structures are surgically reconnected after an organ has been removed. After radical prostatectomy, this refers to the connection between the reconstructed bladder neck and urethra.

Androgen-dependent, or -sensitive cells: cells in prostate cancer that are nourished by hormones, which can shrink dramatically when the hormones that nourish the prostate are shut off.

Androgen-independent, or -insensitive cells: cells in prostate cancer that are *not* nourished by hormones, and therefore don't respond to hormone therapy.

Androgens: male hormones such as testosterone.

Angiogenesis: the process of forming new blood vessels. Advancing cancer paves the way ahead with new blood vessels. The idea behind drugs to block this process, called angiogenesis inhibitors, is to starve cancer by cutting off its supply line. Cancer may not die, but it won't get any bigger, either.

Anti-androgens: drugs such as bicalutamide and flutamide, used in hormone therapy to treat prostate cancer. These drugs block the effects of testosterone and DHT on the prostate cell by neutralizing their effect (they prevent testosterone and DHT from binding to the androgen receptor).

Antibiotics: drugs that kill bacteria.

Anticholinergic drugs: a group of drugs whose side effects include hindering urination. These may help some men with incontinence.

Anticoagulants: medications that help prevent the blood from clotting.

Anti-metastatic drugs: drugs that put roadblocks in the way of cancer's progress, discouraging it from invading other cells or from developing new blood vessels (this process is called angiogenesis).

Antimicrobial drugs: bacteria-killing drugs, such as antibiotics.

Apoptosis: also called "programmed cell death," the process by which cells kill themselves.

Arachidonic acid: an unsaturated fatty acid found in red meats, whole milk and cheese, and egg yolks.

Arterial *(adj.):* relating to the arteries.

Artificial sphincter: an implanted device used to treat incontinence that has persisted for a year or longer and shows no signs of improving on its own.

Asymptomatic *(adj.):* experiencing no symptoms. A man with asymptomatic prostate cancer doesn't notice anything out of the ordinary; he feels fine.

Atypical *(adj.):* a finding on biopsy; this means the cells do not look normal but are not necessarily cancerous.

B

Benign: harmless; not cancerous, not fatal.

Benign prostatic hyperplasia: see **BPH**.

Biopsy of the prostate: a means of sampling prostate tissue so it can be checked for the presence of cancer; this is done with the help of transrectal ultrasound.

Bladder: a hollow, muscular reservoir that functions as a holding tank for urine.

Bladder neck contracture: constriction of the bladder neck, caused by scar tissue. This can impede urine flow.

Bladder spasms: painful, uncontrollable contractions of the bladder.

Bladder stones: tiny formations made when crystals of uric acid or calcium precipitate into the urine.

"Bloodless field": a surgical term that means controlling bleeding within a patient, to give surgeons a better field of vision as they perform an operation.

Blood-prostate barrier: a membrane that prevents many substances—including antibiotics—from entering the prostate. This barrier breaks down during bacterial prostatitis, permitting most antibiotics to enter.

Bone scan: also called radionuclide scintigraphy. In a bone scan, doctors inject into the bloodstream a radioactive tracer, a chemical that's attracted, like a magnet, specifically to bone. The bone scan is an excellent means of finding out whether prostate cancer has spread to bone.

"Bound" PSA: PSA molecules in the bloodstream that are chemically tied to proteins. Other PSA molecules are without these chemical ties; these are called "free." If a man has a PSA test and most of the PSA is bound, the PSA elevation is probably coming from cancer.

BPH: benign prostatic hyperplasia, or enlargement of the prostate. A benign condition that occurs in most older men when prostate tissue begins to grow around the urethra, gradually compressing it and hindering urine flow.

BPSA: This is a particular form of free PSA produced by the prostate's transition zone, a thin ring of tissue that surrounds the urethra, in BPH. BPSA is more of a marker for BPH than for cancer.

BUN test: the blood-urea-nitrogen test, a blood test to check kidney function.

C

Calculi: see **prostatic calculi.**

Capsule of the prostate: the outer wall of the prostate gland.

Castrate range: the level to which testosterone drops after orchiectomy. This is an important point of comparison in monitoring hormone therapy, as certain drugs are judged by their ability to reduce testosterone to this range.

Castration: see **orchiectomy.**

Catheter: a tube used for drainage or irrigation, most commonly to drain urine out of the bladder.

Cell division: how the body's cells multiply. A single cell divides in two. Then those two cells divide in two, and so on.

Chemical castration: the use of drugs to accomplish the same effect as orchiectomy—that is, to lower testosterone to the critical "castrate range."

Chemotherapeutic drugs: a host of cell-killing drugs used to treat many forms of cancer.

Chronic bacterial prostatitis: a form of prostatitis associated with urinary tract infections, positive cultures that identify bacteria in the prostate, and an abundance of white blood cells in prostatic secretions. This can be a recurring illness, coming back periodically for years after an initial episode of acute bacterial prostatitis.

Chronic prostatitis/chronic pelvic pain syndrome: the most mysterious category of prostatitis. Nobody knows what causes the symptoms in this group (which used to be named by what it was not, "nonbacterial" prostatitis), and antibiotics don't help at all. In some men, the prostate may not even be the problem—the pain and other symptoms may be a result of spasms elsewhere in the pelvis, rectum, or lower back. This category has two subgroups—inflammatory and noninflammatory, based on whether any white blood cells (also called inflammatory cells) can be found in the prostatic fluid.

Clinical stage of prostate cancer: an estimation of the extent of a man's cancer, based on factors such as the digital rectal exam, the PSA test, and bone scan. Pathologic stage is much more certain, but this can only be determined when a pathologist examines actual prostate tissue after surgery.

Clonal selection: the process whereby the most poorly differentiated, rapidly growing, aggressive cells overtake the slower, well-differentiated cells as a tumor progresses.

"Complexed" PSA: another way of looking at the separation of bound from free PSA. A new assay measures the amount of PSA bound to the particular protein that binds it—a protein called alpha-1-antichymotrypsin (ACT).

Conformal radiation therapy: a technique for delivering external-beam radiation, which maximizes the dose of radiation to the prostate tumor, while keeping the risk of damaging nearby tissue to a minimum.

Corpora cavernosa and corpus spongiosum: spongy chambers in the penis that become engorged with blood during an erection.

Creatinine test: a blood test (also called a serum creatinine test) that checks for impairment of kidney function.

Cryoablation, cryotherapy: using extremely cold liquid nitrogen to freeze the entire prostate, causing cancer cells within the gland to rupture as they begin to thaw.

CT (computed tomography) scan: a circular series of X-ray pictures taken by a machine that goes around the body. A computer puts the pictures together, generating images that, as in an MRI, are like slices of anatomy.

Cystometry: a test to measure bladder pressure and function, done by passing a small catheter through the urethra into the bladder. Changes in pressure are monitored as the bladder fills with water.

Cystoscope: a tiny, lighted tube that works like a periscope on a submarine. In cystoscopy, it is inserted in the tip of the anesthetized penis and threaded through the urethra into the bladder; this allows the doctor to inspect the bladder, prostate, and urethra for abnormalities.

D

Deep venous thrombosis: blood clots that form in the deep veins of the legs, a potential complication of major surgery such as radical prostatectomy. At best, these clots can be painful. At worst they can be fatal, if a chunk of a blood clot in the leg breaks free and shoots up to the lungs. These should be treated immediately.

DES: see **estrogens.**

DHT (dihydrotestosterone): the active form of male hormone in the prostate. It is made when testosterone is transformed by an enzyme called 5-alpha reductase.

DIC: disseminated intravascular coagulation, a blood-clotting disorder that develops in some men with advanced prostate cancer.

Differentiating agents: drugs that work by slowing down cancer's rate of growth.

Differentiation of prostate cancer cells: how cancer cells look under the microscope. Well-differentiated cells have distinct, clearly defined borders and clear centers, and their growth is relatively slow and orderly. Everything about poorly differentiated cells is murkier, not so well defined. As cancer progresses, these poorly differentiated cells seem to melt together and form solid, nasty blobs of malignancy. These are the most aggressive cells in a tumor, and they are given a high grade (8, 9, 10) in the Gleason scoring system. Well-differentiated cells are called low-grade (2, 3, 4). Moderately well-differentiated cells fall right in between (5, 6, 7), and it's hard to predict what these cells will do.

Digital rectal exam (DRE): a very important part of the physical examination, in which a doctor's gloved, lubricated finger is inserted into the rectum to feel for lumps, enlargement, or areas of hardness that might indicate the presence of cancer. It is uncomfortable but not painful, and it's generally brief, lasting less than a minute.

Diuretics: drugs that work by altering the way the body metabolizes sodium; this causes the kidneys to absorb less water, so more of it leaves the body in the form of urine. For most people, diuretics mean more frequent urination and a more forceful stream. They can be disastrous for a man with BPH.

Diverticula: pockets of the bladder lining that poke out like balloons through the bladder wall. (A single one of these is called a diverticulum.)

DNA: the "genetic blueprint," vital information contained in the nucleus of every cell.

Dorsiflexion exercises: pumping the feet up and down to exercise the calf muscles, a good exercise immediately after surgery.

Double-blind study: a study in which neither the doctor nor the patient knows who's receiving placebo or the standard medication, or who's receiving the new medication being tested.

"Dry" ejaculation: also known as retrograde ejaculation. This is a complication of some prostate procedures, including TURP. For most men, this has no effect on the pleasant sensation of orgasm. Dry ejaculation is pretty much what it sounds like: semen is not expelled out the urethra when a man reaches sexual climax. Instead, it goes the other way—back into the bladder. This happens because part of the bladder neck—a muscular valve, whose job is to slam shut at the time of ejaculation, forcing semen out the urethra—is often resected along with the prostate tissue. When this area is damaged or missing, there's nothing to prevent semen from heading the wrong way. This also occurs after a radical prostatectomy or radiation therapy, because the prostate and seminal vesicles, which make the fluid, are either removed or "dried up."

E

Edema: swelling caused by fluid retention.

Ejaculate *(noun):* semen, the fluid that exits the body during ejaculation, or sexual climax. "Ejaculate" also is a verb.

Ejaculation: emission of semen at the climax of sexual intercourse.

Endothelin: a chemical that's believed to be the culprit in the excruciating, debilitating pain that comes when prostate cancer invades the bone. Endothelin-blocking drugs are now being tested.

Epididymis: the "greenhouse" where sperm mature and are stored until orgasm.

Epididymitis: an infection of the epididymis. This may occur after a surgical procedure that damages the ejaculatory ducts, allowing infected urine to "back up" into the vas deferens.

Epidural anesthesia: a local anesthetic administered through a tiny plastic tube, inserted between the vertebrae of the spine, near the small of the back. The epidural anesthetic bathes the area outside the membrane lining the spinal cord, temporarily numbing the nerves in the lower body. Unlike spinal anesthesia, which comes in one dose, epidural anesthesia can be given continuously. The area of numbness can be adjusted; so can the degree of pain relief.

Epithelial cells: cells in the glandular tissue of the prostate, which secrete fluid that becomes part of semen.

Erectile dysfunction (ED): the inability to have an erection sufficient for sexual intercourse.

Estrogens: female hormones. Estrogens block the release of a signal transmitted by the pituitary gland called luteinizing hormone (LH), which stimulates testosterone. Oral estrogens, taken as hormone therapy by men with prostate cancer, reduce testosterone to the crucial castrate range. The main oral estrogens is DES (diethylstilbestrol).

Excise *(verb):* to cut out, to remove surgically.

External-beam radiation therapy: a curative treatment for prostate cancer. It involves beaming X-ray energy into a prostate tumor from the outside, a few minutes at a time, over the course of several weeks.

F

Fascia: a thin blanket of connective tissue.

5-alpha reductase: enzymes in the prostate that convert testosterone to DHT.

5-alpha reductase inhibitors: drugs that block the formation of DHT. This causes the prostate to shrink and improves the obstructive symptoms of BPH. These drugs do not affect levels of testosterone, the hormone responsible for a man's libido and sexual function.

Fluoroscopy: an X-ray image that appears live on a TV screen instead of as a still photograph.

Foley catheter: a catheter inserted in the penis and threaded through the urethra to the bladder, where it's anchored in place with a tiny, inflated balloon. It removes urine from the body; it also can be used for irrigation, to prevent blood clots.

Following expectantly: see **watchful waiting.**

"Free" PSA: PSA (this is also called "percent free" PSA) that is not chemically bound to proteins in the bloodstream. If a man has an elevated PSA and most of the PSA is "free," then the elevation is probably due to BPH.

Frozen sections: In a staging pelvic lymphadenectomy, lymph nodes are removed, then rushed to a pathologist for frozen-section analysis to check for cancer. This is pretty much what it sounds like: The tissue is frozen, then sliced into very thin sections to be examined under the microscope.

FSH: follicle-stimulating hormone, made along with LH by the pituitary gland. FSH has its major effect on sperm production.

G

Gene therapy: one of the most exciting "nonhormonal" areas of treatment of advanced prostate cancer. Scientists are now able to program the body's DNA like a computer chip, sending it on a selective search-and-destroy mission targeted only at prostate cancer cells.

Genetic drift: As a cancer progresses, as its cells double over and over again, the DNA becomes less stable. The cancer develops new mutations; it becomes more aggressive. As the tumor progresses, well-differentiated cells deteriorate into poorly differentiated cells. This downslide is called genetic drift.

Genetic susceptibility: a complex of genetic factors that creates a more hospitable atmosphere for cancer.

Gleason score: a way to classify the grade of cancer, based on how it looks under the microscope. Cells that are well-differentiated are given a low grade (2, 3, 4); poorly differentiated cells are given a high grade (8, 9, 10). Moderately well-differentiated cells fall right in the middle. See also **differentiation of prostate cancer cells.**

Glutathione-S transferase-π (pronounced "pie," called GST-π for short): an important enzyme that helps prevent oxidative damage, which can lead to prostate cancer.

Grade of prostate cancer: see **Gleason score.**

Growth factors: substances that activate processes that promote cell division.

Gynecomastia: tenderness, pain, or swelling of the breasts in men. This is a common, easily treatable side effect of some forms of hormone therapy for prostate cancer.

H

Hemi-body irradiation: a once-common form of radiation treatment to ease pain in prostate cancer patients with metastases to bone in several places. It involves irradiating large expanses of the body.

Hereditary prostate cancer (HPC): HPC is present in families if there are three first-degree relatives (a father or brothers) who develop prostate cancer—or two first-degree relatives, if both developed it before age fifty-five—or if prostate cancer has occurred in three generations in the family (grandfather, father, son). HPC can be inherited from either side of the family.

Heterogeneity: the state of being diverse, varied. Not uniform. In prostate cancer and BPH, heterogeneity refers to a "melting pot" of cells, all jockeying for position in one area.

High-dose rate (HDR)brachytherapy: Also called "temporary" brachytherapy, this is usually given along with external-beam radiation. As its name suggests, the seeds don't stay in; they're removed at the end of each treatment session.

hK2 (human kallikrein-2): an enzyme made by the prostate that's a "cousin" of PSA.

Hormone-dependent, -sensitive: see **androgen-dependent, -sensitive.**

Hormone-independent, -insensitive: see **androgen-independent, -insensitive.**

Hormone-refractory prostate cancer: metastatic prostate cancer that has returned after months or years of being controlled by hormonal therapy.

Hormonal therapy: the use of hormones to treat advanced prostate cancer. Hormone therapy is aimed at shutting down the hormones that nourish the prostate. Some cells in a prostate tumor are responsive to this, and some aren't.

Hot flash: a sudden rush of warmth in the face, neck, upper chest, and back, lasting from a few seconds to an hour; a side effect of some hormonal treatments for prostate cancer. Although hot flashes aren't harmful to a man's health, they can be bothersome.

Hydrogenation: a means of preserving food. Hydrogenation helps keep Crisco solid at room temperature. Hydrogenated foods raise your cholesterol level and may contribute to oxidative damage.

Hyperplasia: an increase in the number of cells in the prostate.

Hyper-reflexive *(adj):* overly reactive; spastic.

I

Imaging *(verb):* seeing and taking pictures inside the body, using various forms of energy including ultrasound, magnetic resonance (MRI), and X-rays.

Immunotherapy: treatments designed to maximize the immune system's ability to fight cancer.

Impotence: the inability to have an erection. Also called erectile dysfunction, in most cases this is very treatable.

Incidental prostate cancer: small clusters of cancer cells, an apparently dormant form of cancer that resides in millions of men. In some men, this cancer never poses a danger. In others, however, it eventually does.

Incontinence: unintentional leakage of urine; this also is called urinary incontinence. (Another kind of incontinence, bowel or fecal incontinence, means having an unintentional bowel movement.)

"Infectious" prostatitis: a term some doctors use in describing bacterial prostatitis. Bacterial prostatitis is not infectious; men can continue a normal sex life without worrying about giving the disease to someone else.

Insulin-like growth factors: a class of hormones that may influence the development of prostate cancer.

Intensity-modulated radiation therapy: An approach to external-beam radiation, in which X-ray beams converge on a selected target. The intensity can be turned up, to blast the cancer, or down, to spare normal tissue.

Intermittent hormonal therapy (also called intermittent androgen suppression): In this plan, men start taking hormones early, before signs or symptoms of advanced cancer begin. Then, when their PSA levels drop, they stop taking them and get a little "vacation" from treatment. The men are monitored closely, and at the first sign that the tumor is growing, they start taking the hormones again.

Interstitial brachytherapy: implanting radioactive "seeds," or minute radioactive chunks of material, in the prostate to kill cancer.

Intra-abdominal *(adj.):* in the abdomen.

Intraurethral *(adj.):* in the urethra.

Intraurethral therapy: a form of pharmacological treatment for men with ED, using agents that can be placed directly into the urethra. One of these is called MUSE, a tiny suppository.

Invasive *(adj.):* Invasive surgery means an incision is involved; the body is physically entered. In minimally invasive surgery, this incision may be a hole as small as a dime, or there may be no incision at all if the body's own passageways—such as the urethra in the TURP procedure—are used. A *noninvasive procedure* does not invade the body at all; many forms of imaging are noninvasive.

Irritative symptoms in BPH: These include frequent urination, especially at night, a strong sense of urgency in urination, inability to postpone urination, and sleep disrupted by the need to urinate.

Isoflavones: phytochemicals in soy; one of these is *genistein,* which may help fight cancer.

IV: an abbreviation for *intravenous,* which means, literally, "through the veins." Medication, fluids, or nutrition supplements can be administered this way.

IVP (intravenous pyelogram): an X-ray of the urinary tract, which works like a glow-in-the-dark picture: A special dye is injected, making urine visible, and its path from the kidneys and out of the body easily traceable—and any blockage easy to see. Some men have severe allergic reactions to this dye.

K

Kidneys: the body's main filters. They cleanse the body of impurities and, at the same time, salvage and recycle useful materials.

L

Laparoscopic pelvic lymphadenectomy: dissection of the lymph nodes as a means of staging prostate cancer. Laparoscopic surgery is minimally invasive; there's a tiny incision, and much of the surgery is conducted through "telescopes."

Latent *(adj.):* dormant; passive.

Lateral lobe enlargement: a form of BPH that results when prostate tissue compresses the urethra from the sides.

Libido: sex drive.

LH: luteinizing hormone, a chemical signal transmitted by the pituitary. LH motivates the testes to make testosterone.

LHRH: luteinizing hormone-releasing hormone (also called GnRH, for gonadotropin-releasing hormone), a chemical signal made in the brain by the hypothalamus. LHRH tells the pituitary gland to make LH and FSH.

LHRH agonists: synthetic lookalikes of the body's chemical LHRH. These drugs shut down the pituitary's production of the hormone called LH.

Linoleic acid: found in corn oils, baked goods, and many snack foods.

Localized prostate cancer: cancer that is confined within the prostate, and therefore considered curable.

Local recurrence of cancer: when cancer returns to the prostate or nearby tissue after treatment.

Lycopoene: an antioxidant—found in tomatoes, red grapefruits, watermelons, and berries—that fights oxidative damage, which may lead to prostate cancer.

M

Metastasis, metastases, metastatic: A metastasis is a chunk of cancer that has broken off from the main tumor and established itself elsewhere. A distant metastasis means this new site of cancer is far from its point of origin. The word *metastases* is plural, and *metastatic* is an adjective that refers to a metastasis.

Micrometastases: tiny, invisible (and undetectable) offshoots of prostate cancer.

Middle lobe enlargement: a type of BPH in which a lobe of prostate tissue grows up inside the bladder. When it reaches a critical size, it can block the opening of the bladder neck like a cork in a bottle. This explains how some men with a "small prostate on rectal exam" can develop major symptoms of urinary obstruction.

Minilap: mini-laparotomy staging pelvic lymphadenectomy. The minilap begins with an incision slightly larger than in the laparoscopic pelvic lymphadenectomy. If there's cancer in the lymph nodes, the incision is closed. But if the lymph nodes are cancer-free, this incision is lengthened and the radical retropubic prostatectomy is performed under the same anesthetic.

Monounsaturated fats: some "good" fats, not linked to prostate cancer. Olive oil is a monounsaturated fat.

MRI (magnetic resonance imaging): a means of imaging that's painless, noninvasive, and does not use X-rays. It is time-consuming, however, often lasting about forty-five minutes. MRI gives a three-dimensional scan of the body, producing images that are like slices of anatomy.

N

"Nerve-sparing" radical prostatectomy: what some doctors call the anatomical approach to radical retropubic prostatectomy; they're referring to important modifications that reduce blood loss and allow men to remain potent and continent after radical prostatectomy.

Neurogenic bladder: trouble in the bladder caused by a neurological problem such as Parkinson's disease.

Neurotransmitters: chemical messengers, signals sent from a transmitter in one nerve cell to a receptor in another.

Neurovascular bundles: cordlike structures that run down the side of the prostate near the rectum. The bundles contain microscopic nerves that are essential for erection; they also contain arteries and veins that help surgeons identify the location of these nerves.

Nitric oxide: a substance released by nerve endings during erection, causing the smooth muscle tissue in the penis to relax.

Nutraceuticals: drugs extracted from specific nutrients.

Nocturia: frequent urination during the night. A man has nocturia if he has to get up several times a night to go to the bathroom; this is often a symptom of BPH.

Nocturnal penile tumescence test: an evaluation to determine whether a man has erections at night while he sleeps.

"Nonhormonal" therapy: exciting new treatments for advanced prostate cancer. Unlike the "buckshot" approach of traditional chemotherapy, they work like a high-powered rifle, with only one target—prostate cancer cells. They're specifically designed to target the biological mechanisms involved in cancer progression and metastasis.

Noninvasive *(adj.):* not invasive; in other words, there's no incision.

O

Obstructive symptoms in BPH: These include weak urine flow, hesitancy in starting urination, a need to push or strain to get urine to flow, intermittent urine stream (starts and stops several times), difficulty in stopping urination, "dribbling" after urination, a sense of not being able to empty the bladder completely, and not being able to urinate at all.

Omega-3 fats: the kind found in fish oils, which may be helpful in preventing coronary artery disease and are not linked to prostate cancer.

Orchiectomy: surgical castration. A form of hormone therapy, involving removal of all or part of the testicles. This causes testosterone to fall to the "castrate range."

Orgasm: the climax of sexual intercourse.

Overflow incontinence: when urine leaks out because the bladder is too full to hold any more.

Oxidative damage: incremental damage caused over many years, as free radicals (a toxic byproduct of everyday metabolism) attack the DNA in cells, causing mutations that lead to cancer.

P

Palliate *(verb):* to ease or relieve. Palliative treatment makes symptoms, and therefore quality of life, better—even though it may do nothing to cure the underlying cause of these symptoms.

Palpable *(adj.):* tangible. Palpable cancer in the prostate means there's a lump, lesion, or nodule that a doctor's gloved finger can feel during a digital rectal exam.

Pathologic fracture: When cancer invades bones, they become brittle. Brittle bones break. Therefore, men with metastatic prostate cancer are prone to broken bones, called pathologic fractures. Most susceptible are the bones that bear much of the body's weight, in the hip and thigh.

Pathologic stage of cancer: the definitive extent of a man's prostate cancer. (The possibilities include organ-confined cancer, capsular penetration, positive surgical margins, invasion of the seminal vesicles, and/or involvement of the pelvic lymph nodes.) This is determined after prostate surgery when a pathologist examines the actual prostate specimen and dissected tissue from the nearby lymph nodes—instead of merely making guesses about how far the cancer has spread based on test results and a few cells from biopsies.

Pathologist: a doctor who studies cells, tissue, and organs, and makes determinations about them—answering such questions as "Is there cancer here?" and "Was all the cancer removed?"

PC-SPES: a "natural" preparation, a combination of eight herbs, most of them used in Chinese medicine. Some of these herbs are potent phyto-estrogens (the word *phyto* means that they come from plants), and it appears that the estrogen is the key to how PC-SPES works.

Penile *(adj.):* relating to the penis.

Penile implants: bendable, inflatable, or mechanical prostheses that enable an impotent man to have erections and a normal sex life.

Perforation: puncture.

Perineum: the area between the scrotum and rectum.

Perineural invasion: a biopsy term, meaning that prostate cancer has been found in the spaces around the nerves near the edge of the prostate. Because cancer that has penetrated the capsule can still be cured, perineural invasion has no long-term impact on a man's long-term outlook.

Peripheral zone: the largest part of the prostate and the area where most prostate cancer occurs.

Periprostatic tissue: tissue just outside the prostate.

Peyronie's disease: a disorder of the connective tissue within the penis that can cause curvature during erection.

Phosphodiesterase inhibitors: drugs such as Viagra that can help facilitate an erection.

Phytochemicals: chemicals derived from plants.

Phyto-estrogens: estrogens derived from plants. The prefix *phyto* means "coming from plants."

PIN (prostatic intraepithelial neoplasia): abnormal cells, found in a needle biopsy, that are strongly linked to prostate cancer.

Placebo: a "sugar pill," often taken by participants in a medical study. Patients taking a placebo are compared to patients taking actual medications.

Placebo effect: a phenomenon that happens often in medical studies, in which patients taking a placebo have an inexplicable improvement in symptoms.

PMSA: prostate-membrane specific antigen, a protein that is made on the surface of prostate cells.

Polyphenols: chemicals found in black and green teas, known to have cancer-fighting properties.

Polyunsaturated fats: These are found in vegetable oils (corn oil, safflower oil, and other cooking oils), nuts and seeds, fish oils, and margarine. There are a lot of these polyunsaturated fats, and some are worse than others.

Pressure-flow studies: tests to monitor bladder pressure changes as a man urinates.

Proliferation: spread, or growth, as in "proliferation of cancer."

Prostate: a muscular, walnut-shaped gland about an inch and a half long that sits directly under the bladder. Its main function is to make part of the fluid for semen. (*Note:* "Prostate" is often confused with the adjective "prostrate," which means lying facedown, or being exhausted.)

Prostatectomy: an operation to remove all or part of the prostate.

Prostate massage: an important test for prostatitis, done during a digital rectal exam. A doctor vigorously massages or presses on the prostate to express, or force, fluid out of the prostate and into the urethra. It then is collected on a glass slide and examined under a microscope.

Prostate-specific antigen: see **PSA.**

Prostatic *(adj.):* relating to the prostate.

Prostatic abscess: localized accumulation of pus, like a pimple, under pressure in the prostate.

Prostatic calculi: the prostate's version of gallstones or kidney stones. They're usually tiny and harmless. But when they get infected, as they often do in men with chronic bacterial prostatitis, they can cause an infection to persist, and symptoms of urinary tract infections and prostatitis to return again and again.

Prostatic urethra: the part of the urethra that runs through the prostate.

Prostatitis: inflammation of the prostate.

Prostatosis: a vague, unhelpful term that means simply "a condition of the prostate."

Prosthesis: an artificial replacement for part of the body that is either missing or not functioning properly.

Proton-beam radiation: This approach to external-beam radiation therapy uses charged particles instead of electromagnetic waves. The proton beam shoots in a straight line, but it can be stopped abruptly—for example, at the delicate rectal wall, just on the other side of the prostate, so the fragile tissue in the rectum can be spared.

PSA: prostate-specific antigen, an enzyme made by the prostate. Levels of PSA can be checked in a simple blood test; elevated amounts of PSA in the blood can signal prostate cancer.

PSA density: the blood PSA score divided by the volume of the prostate, as determined by transrectal ultrasound.

PSA velocity: PSA's rate of change from year to year.

Psychogenic erectile dysfunction: erection problems that are psychological, not physiological, in nature. Doctors making this ruling if a man can't produce an erection during sexual activity but has several a night while he sleeps.

Pulmonary embolus: a blood clot in the lungs, a potential complication of radical prostatectomy. This is extremely serious and can be fatal.

Pulsed Doppler evaluation: a test that uses high-resolution ultrasound to evaluate the arteries' blood supply to the penis.

Q

Quality of life: Basically, this means how good you think your life is. When "quality of life" is excellent, this means a patient is relatively untroubled by symptoms or pain. When it is poor, this means that pain or symptoms have interfered with a man's ability to function, to pursue his daily activities, and to enjoy his life.

R

Radiation "seeds": see **interstitial brachytherapy.**

Radiation therapy: see **external-beam radiation therapy** and **interstitial brachytherapy.**

Radical prostatectomy: the operation to remove the prostate, and the "gold standard" for curing localized prostate cancer.

Radioactive strontium 89: a highly effective radioactive substance, injected into the body, that is specially tailored for bone pain in cancer patients.

Radionuclide scintigraphy: see **bone scan.**

Randomize: Doctors use this verb when discussing medical studies in which some men are assigned one treatment or another at random.

Receptors: highly specific "locks" in cells that are opened, or activated, only by certain hormones or chemical signals, which act as "keys."

Regeneration: regrowth.

Resect *(verb):* to cut out, to remove surgically.

Resectoscope: an instrument used in the TURP procedure. Threaded through the penis, it shines a light that allows surgeons to view the prostate as they chip away at excess tissue.

Retreatment, reoperation: having to undergo a repeat procedure to treat the same initial problem.

Retrograde ejaculation: see **dry ejaculation.**

Retropubic *(adj.):* a surgical approach. In retropubic prostatectomy, the surgeon makes an incision in the lower abdomen, separates the abdominal muscles, and moves the bladder aside, unopened, to reach the prostate directly (as opposed to the suprapubic approach, in which the prostate is reached by cutting through the bladder).

RT-PCR: a technique (reverse transcriptase polymerase chain reaction) by which scientists examine cells from the blood to determine whether those cells can make PSA.

S

Salvage therapy: This is a medical term for Plan B. It means a patient is undergoing another form of treatment because Plan A, the first form of treatment the patient underwent, was not successful in curing the problem. Salvage therapy is often associated with a higher rate of complications.

Saturated fats: We should call these the "All American" fats, because the average American diet is full of them. These are the ones in red meats and in dairy fats. The Asian diet has hardly any saturated fat in it.

Selenium: a mineral in the soil, found in fruits and vegetables, meats, and fish, which may help prevent prostate cancer.

Semen: the fluid that transports sperm.

Seminal vesicles: glands that, like the prostate, are "sex accessory glands." Fluid secreted by these glands is critical in ensuring the consistency of semen.

Sex accessory tissues: glands such as the prostate, seminal vesicles, and Cowper's gland, which produce secretions that become part of the fluid in semen.

Sextant biopsy: an attempt to get a comprehensive picture of the prostate, by taking six tiny samples of cells from throughout the gland—one each from the top, middle, and bottom of the gland on the right and left sides.

Sinousoids: spongy chambers within the penis that become engorged with blood during an erection.

Small-cell carcinoma: a variety of prostate cancer. Cells in these tumors have a makeup similar to other small-cell cancers (of the lung, for example), and they respond to the same kinds of chemotherapy drugs used to treat these tumors.

Spinal anesthesia: a shot of local anesthetic in the small of the back through the dura, the membrane lining the spinal cord, and into the spinal fluid. Within minutes, the patient feels numb, relaxed, and heavy from the waist down.

Spinal cord compression: a very serious problem in men with metastatic prostate cancer. This happens when cancer eats away at the spine, causing part of the spinal column to collapse, trapping and sometimes crushing nearby nerves.

Spot radiation: localized external-beam radiation treatment, targeted at one or several painful bone metastases. It won't prevent new metastases from cropping up in bone, but it can ease pain dramatically in the sites it does treat.

Stage of prostate cancer: Determining the stage means finding out the extent of the disease—how big it is, and how far it has spread. The stage of prostate cancer has a major role in determining what treatment a man should receive. See also **clinical stage** and **pathologic stage.**

Staging pelvic lymphadenectomy: dissection of the pelvic lymph nodes to see whether they contain prostate cancer. This procedure is generally performed just before a radical prostatectomy.

Stents: tubes implanted and left in place to hold open a space that would otherwise collapse or be compressed.

Step-up hormonal therapy: a gradual approach to hormonal therapy. The idea here is to start modulating the male hormones with agents that have the fewest side effects, and then to escalate as needed if the disease progresses.

Stress incontinence: when urine leaks during certain activities, such as running or playing golf.

Stricture: a blockage caused by scar tissue.

Stromal cells: cells found in the prostate's smooth muscle tissue, which contract automatically to launch secretions into the urethra.

Subcapsular orchiectomy: a cosmetic approach to orchiectomy. In this operation, a surgeon opens the lining to the testicles and empties the contents of each testicle. The lining is closed again, and this empty shell is placed back inside the scrotum—so nothing looks different; in other words, no one can tell from outward appearance that there's nothing inside the testicles.

Suprapubic *(adj.):* an approach to the prostate.

Surgical margins: These are established when pathologists look at the edges of tissue that has been cut out during surgery. If no cancer appears on these edges and the margin is "clear," or "negative," then it's a pretty good bet that all the cancerous tissue was removed. If the margin is "positive," this means that the surgeon's ability to cut out all the cancer is not as certain.

Sutures: surgical stitches, used to close an incision.

T

Template: a highly sophisticated kind of "paint-by-numbers" map of the prostate that helps doctors know exactly where to insert radioactive seeds.

Testes, or testicles: Housed in the scrotum, these are a man's reproductive organs and the main source of the male hormone, testosterone, and of sperm.

Testosterone: the male hormone, or androgen, which is important to the prostate and is essential for sex drive and fertility. It is also responsible for such "manly" characteristics as postpuberty body hair and deepening of the voice. Lowering testosterone is a major goal of hormone therapy to treat prostate cancer.

Thermal therapy: using heat to destroy tissue.

Three-dimensional conformal radiation: In this approach to external-beam radiation, many X-ray beams, shaped to fit the target area, are focused on the prostate, delivering a homogenous, high dose of radiation.

Three-glass urine collection: an important test for prostatitis. When a man urinates, the first urine to come out contains fluid from the urethra: urine collected in midstream comes from the bladder. The last collection of urine is taken after a brief prostate massage, and this contains fluid from the prostate.

Total androgen blockade, or ablation: a form of hormone therapy to treat prostate cancer. The theory here is that even low levels of testosterone and DHT, engendered by the adrenal androgens, can stimulate cancer in the prostate, and they must be stopped. This can be accomplished by combining whatever achieves a castrate level of testosterone—surgical castration, estrogen, or an LHRH agonist—with an antiandrogen.

Transabdominal *(adj.):* through the abdomen.

Transition zone: the innermost ring of the prostate, tissue that surrounds the urethra. This is the sole site of BPH.

Transperineal *(adj.):* through the perineum.

Transrectal *(adj.):* through the rectum.

Treatment-planning CT scan: CT images to show the physical terrain of the targeted area, the prostate and surrounding organs, before radiation treatment.

Trilobar enlargement: a type of BPH involving three (two lateral and one middle) lobes, in which obstruction can occur in the bladder neck as well as the urethra.

TURP: transurethral resection of the prostate, the "gold standard" operation to treat symptoms of BPH. It does not require an incision; instead, prostate tissue is reached, chipped away, and removed in tiny fragments through the urethra.

U

Ultrasound: a painless, noninvasive way of imaging that creates a picture with high-frequency sound waves, like sonar on a submarine. It may be done either from outside, through the abdomen, or transrectally, via a wand inserted in the rectum. Transrectal ultrasound can determine the size of the prostate and direct the needle used for biopsies.

Ureters: muscular, one-way channels that work like toothpaste tubes, squeezing urine out from the kidneys and onward to the bladder.

Urethra: a tube that, like the prostate, is involved in both the urinary and reproductive systems. It serves as a conduit not only for urine, but for secretions from the ejaculatory ducts and the prostate.

Urethral sphincter: the muscle responsible for urinary control.

Urethral stricture: scar tissue that blocks the urethra.

Urethritis: inflammation of the urethra, often caused by an infection. If left untreated, this can result in a urethral stricture or a nasty infection that progresses back into the vas deferens and involves the epididymis.

Urge, or urgency, incontinence: when a man knows he has to go to the bathroom, but some urine leaks as he's trying to get there.

Urinalysis: microscopic and chemical examination of urine.

Urinary retention: when the bladder stays completely or partly full. Acute urinary retention means someone can no longer urinate. This is a very serious condition, and it requires immediate treatment.

Urodynamic studies: tests that measure urinary flow, pressures, and volumes to find out whether urinary trouble is caused by BPH or from a problem with the bladder.

Uroflowmetry: a test to measure the amount of urine a man passes, and the speed of his urinary stream.

Urologist: a physician who specializes in diagnosis and medical and surgical treatment of problems in the urinary and male reproductive systems.

UTI: urinary tract infection. The presence of bacteria in the urine, sometimes associated with fever.

V

Vacuum erection device: an apparatus that creates suction using an airtight tube, which is placed temporarily around the penis. An attached pump withdraws air, creating a reduced atmospheric pressure—a vacuum—around the penis, causing it to become engorged with blood. The penis becomes erect. Then a constricting ring, like a rubber band around the neck of a balloon, keeps the blood trapped in the penis so the erection can be sustained.

Vascular *(adj.):* involving blood vessels.

Vas deferens: There are actually two of these hard, muscular cords, but doctors often speak of the vas deferens as a single unit. The vas deferens winds its way from the epididymis to the base of the prostate, where it meets with the duct of the seminal vesicle to form the ejaculatory duct.

Vasectomy: a surgical procedure that is a form of male contraception. When the vas deferens is cut, sperm cannot exit the penis through ejaculation and instead are reabsorbed into the body.

Vasodilators: drugs that open up blood vessels, making a wider channel for blood to go through. In the penis, they also cause the smooth muscle tissue to relax and the veins to close; some vasodilators, injected in tiny amounts in the penis, are used to produce erections.

Venous *(adj.):* relating to the veins.

Venous leak: a common cause of erection problems. Even though the arteries fill the penis with blood, producing a partial erection, the veins don't clamp down to keep this blood trapped inside the penis, so a full erection can't be achieved.

Vitamin E: an antioxidant that may help prevent prostate cancer.

W

Watchful waiting: the most conservative treatment there is. It means following someone's symptoms closely but delaying treatment until these symptoms become severe enough to warrant it. Some doctors also call this "following expectantly."

Wide excision: During a radical prostatectomy, this means that a surgeon cuts out as much tissue as possible surrounding the prostate in an aggressive attempt to get every last bit of cancer.

X

X-ray therapy: see **external-beam radiation therapy.**

Z

Zones of the prostate: There are five distinct regions of the prostate. The two most commonly referred to are the transition zone and the peripheral zone.

Where to Get Help

The first thing you need to know is that you're not alone. There are many sources of good information available to help you. Here are a few of them:

American Cancer Society
1599 Clifton Rd., NE
Atlanta, GA 30329
(404) 320-3333
(808) ACS-2345
www.cancer.org

National, community-based organization that provides comprehensive information and resources, makes referrals to treatment centers, provides free publications, and sponsors a support group called Man to Man.

American Foundation for Urologic Diseases
1128 N. Charles St.
Baltimore, MD 21201
(410) 468-1800
(800) 242-2383
www.afud.org

Supports research and provides educational material on prostate cancer, erectile dysfunction, and other urological conditions. Also sponsors US TOO, a support group for prostate cancer survivors and their families. (See below.)

The Brady Urological Institute
The Johns Hopkins Hospital
Baltimore, MD 21287-2101
(410) 955-6707
www.prostate.urol.jhu.edu

This Web site has many news articles about the latest research in prostate cancer at Johns Hopkins, which we will update regularly.

Cancer Care, Inc.
1180 Avenue of the Americas
New York, NY 10036
(212) 302-2400
(800) 813-HOPE
www.cancercare.org

A nonprofit organization that provides free professional help to patients and families through counseling, education, information and referral, and direct financial assistance.

CaPCURE
1250 Fourth St., Suite 360
Santa Monica, CA 90401
(310) 458-2873
www.capcure.org

CaPCURE's mission is to identify and support prostate cancer research that will rapidly translate into treatments and cures; has information about clinical trials.

National Association for Continence
(formerly, Help for Incontinent People)
P.O. Box 8310
Spartanburg, SC 29305-8310
(864) 579-7900
(800) BLADDER (800-252-3337)
www.nafc.org

National Cancer Institute Cancer Information Service
Public Inquiries:
Building 31, Room 10A31
31 Center Drive, MSC 2580
Bethesda, MD 20892-2580
(301) 435-3848
(800) 4-CANCER
www.nci.nih.gov/hpage/cis.htm

National clearinghouse, with an extensive health information database and educational material. To learn about National Cancer Institute cancer trials, see this Web site: *www.cancertrials.nci.nih.gov*

National Hospice Organization
Suite 901
1901 North Moore St.
Arlington, VA 22209
(703) 243-5900
(800) 658-8898
www.nho.org

National Library of Medicine
www.nlm.nih.gov

This Web site helps you gain access to millions of scientific publications and abstracts.

Prostate Cancer Support Network (PCSN)
1218 North Charles St.
Baltimore, MD 21201
300 W. Pratt St., Suite 401
Baltimore, MD 21201
(800) 828-7866
www.ustoo.com

PCSN, affiliated with the American Foundation for Urologic Disease, provides services for several support groups, self-help organizations, and their members, including "Us Too."

Index